Bio-Inspired Algorithms and Devices for Treatment of Cognitive Diseases Using Future Technologies

Shweta Gupta
Jain University, Bengaluru, India

IGI Global
PUBLISHER of TIMELY KNOWLEDGE

A volume in the Advances in Medical Technologies and Clinical Practice (AMTCP) Book Series

Published in the United States of America by
IGI Global
Medical Information Science Reference (an imprint of IGI Global)
701 E. Chocolate Avenue
Hershey PA, USA 17033
Tel: 717-533-8845
Fax: 717-533-8661
E-mail: cust@igi-global.com
Web site: http://www.igi-global.com

Library of Congress Cataloging-in-Publication Data

Names: Gupta, Shweta, 1979- editor.
Title: Bio-inspired algorithms and devices for treatment of cognitive diseases using future technologies / Shweta Gupta, editor.
Description: Hershey, PA : Medical Information Science Reference, [2022] | Includes bibliographical references and index. | Summary: "This book will discuss new tools for early detection of Cognitive Brain Diseases like Depression , Epilepsy , Parkinson's Disease etc. using devices and algorithms whose basic concept is taken from nature in the absence of available proper medical tests, highlighting design , analysis and application of various bionics or bio-inspired based Algorithms or devices that would predict various Cognitive diseases or brain diseases, beforehand through medical tests"-- Provided by publisher.
Identifiers: LCCN 2021049855 (print) | LCCN 2021049856 (ebook) | ISBN 9781799895343 (hardcover) | ISBN 9781799895367 (ebook)
Subjects: MESH: Brain Diseases--diagnosis | Cognition Disorders--diagnosis | Algorithms
Classification: LCC RC386.6.N48 (print) | LCC RC386.6.N48 (ebook) | NLM WL 141 | DDC 616.8/0475--dc23/eng/20211015
LC record available at https://lccn.loc.gov/2021049855
LC ebook record available at https://lccn.loc.gov/2021049856

This book is published in the IGI Global book series Advances in Medical Technologies and Clinical Practice (AMTCP) (ISSN: 2327-9354; eISSN: 2327-9370)

British Cataloguing in Publication Data
A Cataloguing in Publication record for this book is available from the British Library.

For electronic access to this publication, please contact: eresources@igi-global.com.

Advances in Medical Technologies and Clinical Practice (AMTCP) Book Series

Srikanta Patnaik
SOA University, India
Priti Das
S.C.B. Medical College, India

ISSN:2327-9354
EISSN:2327-9370

Mission

Medical technological innovation continues to provide avenues of research for faster and safer diagnosis and treatments for patients. Practitioners must stay up to date with these latest advancements to provide the best care for nursing and clinical practices.

The **Advances in Medical Technologies and Clinical Practice (AMTCP) Book Series** brings together the most recent research on the latest technology used in areas of nursing informatics, clinical technology, biomedicine, diagnostic technologies, and more. Researchers, students, and practitioners in this field will benefit from this fundamental coverage on the use of technology in clinical practices.

Coverage

- Biomedical Applications
- Clinical Nutrition
- Medical Informatics
- Clinical Studies
- Telemedicine
- E-Health
- Biomechanics
- Diagnostic Technologies
- Biometrics
- Clinical Data Mining

IGI Global is currently accepting manuscripts for publication within this series. To submit a proposal for a volume in this series, please contact our Acquisition Editors at Acquisitions@igi-global.com or visit: http://www.igi-global.com/publish/.

The Advances in Medical Technologies and Clinical Practice (AMTCP) Book Series (ISSN 2327-9354) is published by IGI Global, 701 E. Chocolate Avenue, Hershey, PA 17033-1240, USA, www.igi-global.com. This series is composed of titles available for purchase individually; each title is edited to be contextually exclusive from any other title within the series. For pricing and ordering information please visit http://www.igi-global.com/book-series/advances-medical-technologies-clinical-practice/73682. Postmaster: Send all address changes to above address.

Titles in this Series

For a list of additional titles in this series, please visit: http://www.igi-global.com/book-series/advances-medical-technologies-clinical-practice/73682

Futuristic Design and Intelligent Computational Techniques in Neuroscience and Neuroegineering
Harjit Pal Singh (CT Institute of Engineering and Technology, Punjab, India) Anurag Sharma (GNA University, Punjab, India) and Vikas Khullar (CT Institute of Engineering and Technology, Punjab, India)
Medical Information Science Reference • © 2022 • 253pp • H/C (ISBN: 9781799874331) • US $295.00

Cases on Virtual Reality Modeling in Healthcare
Yuk Ming Tang (Hong Kong Polytechnic University, China) Ho Ho Lun (Hong Kong Polytechnic University, China) and Ka Yin Chau (City University of Macau, China)
Medical Information Science Reference • © 2022 • 287pp • H/C (ISBN: 9781799887904) • US $345.00

Emerging Advancements for Virtual and Augmented Reality in Healthcare
Luis Pinto Coelho (Polytechnic of Porto, Portugal) Ricardo Queirós (Polytechnic of Porto, Portugal) and Sara Seabra Reis (Polytechnic of Porto, Portugal)
Medical Information Science Reference • © 2022 • 308pp • H/C (ISBN: 9781799883715) • US $295.00

Assistive Technologies for Assessment and Recovery of Neurological Impairments
Fabrizio Stasolla (University Giustino Fortunato of Benevento, Italy)
Medical Information Science Reference • © 2022 • 396pp • H/C (ISBN: 9781799874300) • US $295.00

Ethical Implications of Reshaping Healthcare With Emerging Technologies
Thomas Heinrich Musiolik (Berlin University of the Arts, Germany) and Alexiei Dingli (University of Malta, Malta)
Medical Information Science Reference • © 2022 • 242pp • H/C (ISBN: 9781799878889) • US $295.00

Innovative Approaches for Nanobiotechnology in Healthcare Systems
Touseef Amna (Albaha University, Saudi Arabia) and M. Shamshi Hassan (Albaha University, Saudi Arabia)
Medical Information Science Reference • © 2022 • 424pp • H/C (ISBN: 9781799882510) • US $395.00

Machine Learning and Data Analytics for Predicting, Managing, and Monitoring Disease
Manikant Roy (Lovely Professional University, India) and Lovi Raj Gupta (Lovely Professional University, India)
Medical Information Science Reference • © 2021 • 241pp • H/C (ISBN: 9781799871880) • US $395.00

IGI Global
PUBLISHER of TIMELY KNOWLEDGE

701 East Chocolate Avenue, Hershey, PA 17033, USA
Tel: 717-533-8845 x100 • Fax: 717-533-8661
E-Mail: cust@igi-global.com • www.igi-global.com

Editorial Advisory Board

Table of Contents

Detailed Table of Contents

According to WHO, around 50 million people are affected with cognitive disorders with nearly 10 million new cases per year. It is a neuropsychiatric disorder that mainly affects the elderly, and it leads to deterioration in memory, thinking ability, behaviour, attention, executive dysfunction, perception, and activities of daily living. The etiology of cognitive disorders is multifactorial including structural damages to brain, genetic, nutritional, and environmental factors. Three major categories include delirium, mild neurocognitive disorders, and major neurocognitive disorders. Some common examples of these disorders are dementia, corticobasal degeneration, Alzheimer's disease, mild cognitive impairment, vascular dementia, etc. Therefore, the chapter will emphasize the different types of cognitive disorders along with their causes and symptoms.

The word "cognitive disorder" is assigned to behavioral and personality changes leading to a gradual decline of various cognitive realms which further disturbs the day-to-day social as well as professional activities. Acute disseminated encephalomyelitis (ADEM) and agenesis of the corpus callosum (ACC) are the irreversible and growing brain conditions destroying the memory and thinking ability causing dementia. Though there exists an exponential increase in both the patients, they are well demarcated clinically with various biomarkers. However, the limited efficiency of the available therapeutic agents for treating AD is a spotlight to develop novel drugs. Herein, the chapter deals with the basic information on symptoms, stages, causes, and even treatment methods for ADEM and ACC.

This chapter describes three types of cognitive diseases: depression, obsessive-compulsive disorder (OCD), and schizophrenia. Depression is a frequent kind of mental illness. More than 264 million individuals of all ages suffer from depression across the world. Women are more likely than males to suffer from depression. Suicide can be caused by depression. For mild and severe depression, there are effective psychological and pharmaceutical therapies. Obsessive-compulsive disorder (OCD) or obsessive-compulsive ailment is an anxiety disorder. It is divided into two parts: obsessions and compulsions. Obsessions are recurring thoughts, ideas, visions, or impulses that are unpleasant and distressing. Compulsions are behaviors, routines, or mental acts that you engage in to relieve the distress brought on by your obsessions. Schizophrenia is a severe mental illness in which patients have distorted perceptions of reality. Schizophrenia can include hallucinations, delusions, and severely disorganized thought and behavior, which can make it difficult to operate on a daily basis.

Parkinson's disease is a neurodegenerative disorder characterized by severe cognitive impairments. This is a condition of degeneration of substantia nigra of basal ganglia. Parkinsonism adversely influences the mental health of the person too. Parkinson's disease was first described in 1817 by James Parkinson. Parkinsonism patients may get severe complications like cognitive deficiency, which include loss of memory, attention difficulties, visual abnormalities, slow thinking, problems with word finding, and motor symptoms. Symptoms of this disease range from Parkinson's disease mild cognitive impairment (PD-MCI) to Parkinson's disease dementia (PDD). The primary motor symptoms are trembling in hands, arms, legs, jaw, and face; rigidity or stiffness of the limbs and trunk; slowness of movement; postural instability; and impaired balance and coordination. Studies on treatments of Parkinson's disease are progressing to prevent complications and sustain the normal functions of patients.

The chapter explores the research done so far on neuropsychological deficits in major depressive disorder (MDD). The most prominent deficits have been reported in executive function and the cognitive control networks. These deficits have also been shown to affect various cognitive aspects of a patient, such as metacognitions and emotional regulation. They are also predictors of socio-occupational functioning and of recovering and relapse in patients. This makes it pertinent that these newer treatments for MDD account for these deficits and work on ameliorating them for long-term gains.

ADHD is a neurodevelopmental disorder that affects children. ADHD can often persist in adulthood too. Children diagnosed with ADHD have significantly increased across the globe and range between 3-10% of the population. The cardinal features of ADHD are inattention, hyperactivity, and impulsivity. Clinically significant impairment affects bio-psychosocial functioning. Theoretical understanding reveals the central role of genetics, environmental factors, and cognition in ADHD symptoms. The gold standard for ADHD diagnosis relies on clinical history, mental status examination, and diagnostic tools. Pharmacological intervention is the first-line evidence-based treatment for ADHD. However, studies also report that children don't respond to or can't tolerate medications and suffered from adverse side effects. There are also evidence-based treatments such as neurofeedback training that uses technology to regulate brain activity through modifying brain waves. Hence, developing devices for assessment and intervention using technology that targets the cognitive deficits is the need of the hour.

Dementia is a neurological illness that causes diversion from a variety of important cognitive activities. Common examples include memory, reasoning, orientation, understanding, computation, verbal communication, and decision making. Alzheimer's disease (AD) is one of the most common dementias affecting the elderly. It was projected that more than 47 million people globally will be affected by dementia in 2015; these predictions were verified, and forecasts for 2050 are much more concerning, with 131 million people living with dementia. The basic objective of AI is to improve human decision-making and automate operations that are too time-consuming or resource-intensive for people to accomplish. AI can operate as a fast, accurate, and in the long run, cost-effective method to assist human experience and intuition through predictive analytics. AI is an effective technique for AD detection as these methods are employed as a computer-aided diagnosis (CAD) system in clinical practices and play a crucial role in identifying variations in the brain images to detect AD.

Chapter 10
The Influence of Artificial Intelligence on People With Autism Spectrum Disorder: A Methodical Literature Review 156
Shushma G. B., GITAM University, India
I. Jeena Jacob, GITAM University, India

This literature review examines the past and recent relevant research on autism disorder. As undergoing many changes in the whole world, especially after the deadly effect of the COVID-19 widespread in the year 2020, has led to drastic adoption of more intelligent devices for quicker detection of certain human diseases and delivering the results quicker via electronic media, the research will focus on the autism disorder intelligent device detection and feed these data to machine learning models to predict the issues without human intervention. Based on the outcome of the results, the diseases can be treated accordingly in an appropriate manner. The individual suffering from autism disorder can be detected early using AI or machine learning, and this domain can be integrated with the IoT sensors. Such sensors can be combined with the human body, and this sensor will extract the data and send it to the centralized healthcare system. Such data will be removed from the data storage and processed using the AI algorithm to get the desirable results to give an appropriate treatment at the correct stages.

Chapter 11
Artificial Intelligence, Machine Learning, and Internet of Drones in Medical Applications 180
Kavya J., ICAR Sugarcane Breeding Institute, Coimbatore, India
Prasad G., Dayananda Sagar University, Bangalore, India
Bharanidharan N., Dayananda Sagar University, Bangalore, India

Internet of drones (IOD) plays an important role in the delivery of emergency medicine to remote locations. Furthermore, it is employed for blood transfer, disaster assistance, missing persons, discovering lost hikers in the hill station, and a variety of other emergency services. The use of drones for emergency response services, particularly in medical circumstances, offers new avenues for life-saving interventions. Using drones to have "eyes" on a risky scenario or to transport medical supplies to stranded patients may increase the capacity of emergency response physicians to provide care in dangerous conditions. IOD provides several emergency response services that have an influence on daily life. The Federal Aviation Administration (FAA) conducts completely autonomous missions beyond visual range and flights above people to provide critical medical supplies. Artificial intelligence and machine learning are the future of the unmanned aerial vehicle in multiple applications.

Extracorporeal shock wave therapy in orthopaedics and traumatology is a relatively new treatment modality. The advancement of shock wave treatment has been quick in recent years. Shock waves have significantly altered therapy. Shock waves are now the treatment of choice for kidney and urethral stones. Urology has traditionally been the sole medical profession that uses shock waves. Meanwhile, shock waves have been utilised to treat insertion tendinitis, avascular necrosis of the head of the femur, and other necrotic bone changes in orthopaedics and traumatology. In veterinary medicine, another field of shock wave use is the therapy of tendons, ligaments, and bones. The basic theory and applications of shock waves, as well as their history in medicine, are discussed in this study. The goal of utilising shock wave treatment for orthopaedic disorders is to stimulate healing in the tendons, surrounding tissue, and bones. Shock waves have emerged as the preferred therapy for kidney and ureteral stones.

Traditional analytic strategies for investigating neuroimaging biomarkers for neuropsychiatric illnesses have relied on mass univariate statistics, assuming that various brain areas function separately. Machine learning (ML) methods that take into account intercorrelation across areas have recently become a popular and important part of computer-assisted analytical procedures and are now frequently used for the automated diagnosis and analysis of neuropsychiatric illnesses. The goal of this chapter is to provide a detailed overview of CNN and RNN applications in medical image comprehension. The overarching goal is to encourage medical image understanding experts to use CNNs extensively in their research and diagnosis. This chapter describes the development of various novel DL-based approaches and models as well as advancements in high-speed computing techniques, which provide a once-in-a-lifetime chance to anticipate and control Alzheimer's disease.

Epilepsy is long-term neurological seizures of various types, some of which are defined by involuntary repetitive convulsions and have a substantial impact on patients' everyday lives. Several approaches for diagnosing these types of seizures and observing the patient have been proposed in the literature; however, these approaches fall short in terms of ergonomics and proper integration with the health system. The precision measuring that this study looks into shows what an epileptic detection and monitoring tool should be able to do. This chapter describes specific epilepsy detection and monitoring platforms that specify the conditions. The information is gathered from the wearable part of the system.

The aim of the chapter is to provide the enormous profits of the IoT systems (or) devices vulnerable to highly capable intrusions of different attackers. The vital security necessities such as authorization and authentication do not satisfactorily meet the requirements, and prevailing events are not capable of securing the IoT innovative healthcare environment from data gaps of the system security. With the number of IoT application domains growing to incorporate smart homes, mobile healthcare, autonomous intelligent healthcare communication, and smart cities in day-to-day human life, the significance of an attack in the IoT intelligent healthcare networks will become serious. As there are many issues in applying present cryptographic principles to resource-constrained IoT sensor devices, the recommended new security features solutions come with a compromise between security, feasibility, and performance. These research topics focus on evolving lightweight cryptographic results that specifically implement the post-quantum McEliece cryptography algorithm to encrypt the IoT intelligent healthcare device data, which is integrated into the classical blockchain with hashing function SHA-512. The evolving quantum computing integration with AI is together a transformational technology. The AI requires quantum computing power to attain substantial advancement to analyze the enormous data set faster, specifically the mental medical images or patient data.

Foreword

The book is exemplary in its field and contributes to new medical techniques in the treatment of cognitive diseases like Parkinson, attention deficit hyperactivity disorder (ADHD), epilepsy, autism disorder, depression, etc. It focusses on the treatment using latest and upcoming future technologies like artificial intelligence, machine leaning, internet of things (IoT), internet of drones, etc. in which the software algorithms used are inspired by nature. It would lead to breakthrough in the field of medical science and would provide proper medical tests for cognitive diseases, thus preventing incorrect diagnosis of cognitive disease and wrong treatment.

As you would go through the book the first chapter speaks about bioinspired algorithms for treatment of cognitive diseases which is integral part of the theme of the book. Then the second chapter speaks about the different parts of brain which leads to understanding of the book contents to an individual who does not know or is not from cognitive or medical background. The third chapter speaks about different kinds of cognitive disorder to acquaint the reader about the cognitive diseases in very simple language without necessarily requiring him to any deep understanding of the brain diseases. So, the book is written in this way that it is easily comprehensible to reader of any background without him having any background knowledge of medical science or information technology. Chapter 4 and Chapter 5, Chapter 6, Chapter 7 and Chapter 8 talk about uncommon cognitive diseases like acute disseminated encephalomyelitis (ADEM), agenesis of the corpus callosum (ACC), depression, schizophrenia, obsessive compulsive disorder, and attention deficit cognitive disorder (ADHD). Chapter 8 and Chapter 9 speak about depression and Parkinson's Disease. Chapter 10 speaks about application of artificial intelligence for treatment of Alzheimer's Disease and artificial intelligence for Autism Disorder. Chapter 11 and Chapter 12 discuss new software technologies like internet of drones and aerodynamic shock wave for treatment of cognitive diseases and their medical applications. Chapter 13 speaks about neurocognitive prediction in Alzheimer Disease. Chapter 14 discusses about internet of things for epilepsy detection and control which in itself is a new venture and breakthrough in medical science. Chapter 15 discusses about Quantum AI and IoT about data security of cognitive diseases which are highly vulnerable intrusions of different attackers.

Thus, on the whole book is an asset in the field of medical science and easily comprehensible to any person who does not have basic knowledge of brain diseases or medical science. It would bring breakthrough in world of medical Science providing medical solutions for brain diseases.

Amit Kumar
Uttarakhand Technical University, Dehradun, India

Preface

It happens to be scientific research level book which brings out the technical content that happens to be boon to society and people suffering from cognitive diseases because as of now, no medical tests are available for the cognitive diseases and this book brings about the same. This book involves bio-inspired algorithms implies algorithms inspired from nature like algorithm based on how beetle changes color, algorithm based on camouflage of chameleon etc. for various Cognitive diseases like Epilepsy, Parkinson's Disease, Alzheimer's, depression etc. which is need of the day, since there are no proper medical tests available to predict the diseases at early stage. Various emerging future technologies like Industrial Internet of Things, Artificial Intelligence, Machine Learning, Data Sciences, Big Data and various communication protocols could be analysed and designed for application in prediction of various cognitive diseases which would be boon to society. Comparing present technologies or devices available for cognitive diseases to newly designed equipment using future technologies would be an asset of the book. Various parameters like power consumption, productivity, safety should be taken into account during the analysis, design and application of product. Machine learning algorithms, Artificial Intelligence and Cloud – based Industrial Internet of Things could be used be key parameters to achieve the desired objective. The book encompasses on the novel approaches to achieve the same.

OBJECTIVE

This book would be very useful to know new tools for early detection of Cognitive Brain Diseases like Depression, Epilepsy, Parkinson's Disease, etc. using devices and algorithms whose basic concept is taken from nature, since no proper medical tests are available, as though. This book would discuss design, analysis and application of various bionics or bio-inspired based algorithms or devices that would predict various Cognitive diseases or brain diseases, beforehand through medical tests. This book would be an exemplary in its context.
Various examples are:

1. We don't till date have tools or medical tests to differentiate between Depression and Schizophrenia or even initial tests to detect and confirm the same. As far as, Epilepsy or Parkinson's Disease are concerned which are dangerous diseases but still no proper medical tests are available. So, this book would be an asset for providing solution for early prediction of Cognitive Diseases.
2. Related specifically with Cognitive/Brain Diseases.

3. Novel and Proper design, analysis of cognitive or brain disease tests are described in the book which is breakthrough in medical science and society.
4. Book in itself is the discussion of invention and novel products.

TARGET AUDIENCE

This book would be utilized by

1.Various Medical Research Centers like:

a) John Hopkins Alzheimer's Research Center
b) Regional Medical Research Center
c) Alzheimer's Research Center

2. Engineering Institutions (UG, PG. Ph.D.) across the world.
3. Medical Colleges across the world.
4. Biomedical Research Centers.
5. Electronics and Communication Research Centers.
6. Medical Instrument Companies: Medtronic, PubMed.

Chapter 1 is "Bio-Inspired Algorithms/Devices for Diagnosis and Treatment of Parkinson's Disease" which describes Parkinson's disease (PD) which is a common neurodegenerative disorder with a high prevalence rate in geriatric population and more than 10 million people are afflicted with this disease worldwide. Striatal dopamine deficiency and intracellular inclusions containing aggregates of alpha-synuclein are the neuropathological signs caused by neuronal loss in the substantia nigra. PD causes motor and nonmotor symptoms. A diagnostic test or medical tool which is reliable for Parkinson disease is not yet available. Thus, the diagnosis of PD is primarily based on clinical symptoms. Optimized Bio-Inspired Algorithms are the novel and heuristic approach for diagnosis and treatment of Parkinson disease. In this chapter, various Bio-Inspired Algorithms are discussed such as Optimized Cuttlefish Algorithm, Optimized Grasshopper Algorithm, Wolf Search Algorithm, Crow Search Algorithm & Ant-lion Algorithm. Other useful approaches include Bionics Institute Rigidity Device, Sawtooth Waveform Inspired Pitch Estimator (SWIPE), Brain Stimulation Therapies and Bioinspired Nanomedicine.

Chapter 2 is "The Human Brain: Its Structure and Functions" which describes human brain that is a very complex entity with a distinctive organisation and function. There are three main structures in brain: the cerebrum, the cerebellum and brain stem. Further, these structures are subdivided into more parts depending on their position in the brain. The cerebrum is the major portion of brain with sulcus and gyrus of folded structure and deep structures too. Corpus callosum connects the right and left hemisphere of brain to communicate among them. Each hemisphere of brain is further classified into four regions: frontal, temporal, parietal, occipital lobes. Each lobe deals with different functions. Since, for understanding any disease or doing research or treatment, one should have depth knowledge of brain, its parts and functioning of different lobes and regions. Therefore, this chapter will deal with in depth knowledge brain parts, not only anatomically but also based on its functionality in detail.

Chapter 3 is "Introduction to Different Kinds of Cognitive Disorders" which describes according to WHO, around 50 million people are affected with Cognitive disorders and nearly 10 million new cases per year. It is a neuropsychiatric disorder that mainly affects elderly and it leads to deterioration in memory, thinking ability, behaviour, attention, executive dysfunction, perception and activities of daily living. The etiology of Cognitive Disorders is multifactorial including structural damages to brain, genetic, nutritional and environmental factors. Three major categories include: Delirium, Mild Neurocognitive Disorders and Major Neurocognitive Disorders. Some common examples of these disorders are: Dementia, Corticobasal degeneration, Alzheimer's disease, Mild Cognitive Impairment, Vascular dementia, etc. Therefore, the chapter will emphasize on the different types of cognitive disorders along with their cause and symptoms.

Chapter 4 is "Brief Discussion on Acute Disseminated Encephalomyelitis (ADEM) and Agenesis of the Corpus Callosum (ACC)" which describes a word cognitive disorder that is assigned to behavioral and personality changes leading to a gradual decline of various cognitive realms which further disturbs the day to day social as well as professional activities. Acute disseminated encephalomyelitis (ADEM) and Agenesis of the corpus callosum (ACC) are the irreversible and growing brain condition destroying the memory and thinking ability causing dementia. Though there exists an exponential increase in the both the patients, they are well demarcated clinically with various biomarkers. However, the limited efficiency of the available therapeutic agents for treating AD is a spotlight to develop novel drugs. Herein, the chapter deals with the basic information on symptoms, stages, causes and even treatment methods for ADEM and ACC.

Chapter 5 is "A Brief Discussion on Depression, Schizophrenia and Obsessive Compulsive Disorder" which describes three types of cognitive diseases that is Depression, Obsessive-compulsive disorder (OCD) and Schizophrenia. Depression is a frequent kind of mental illness. More than 264 million individuals of all ages suffer from depression across the world. Women are more likely than males to suffer from depression. Suicide can be caused by depression. For mild and severe depression, there are effective psychological and pharmaceutical therapies. Obsessive-compulsive disorder (OCD) or obsessive-compulsive ailment is an anxiety disorder. It is divided into two parts: obsessions and compulsions. Obsessions are recurring thoughts, ideas, visions, or impulses that are unpleasant and distressing. Compulsions are behaviors, routines, or mental acts that you engage in to relieve the distress brought on by your obsessions. Schizophrenia is a severe mental illness in which patients have distorted perceptions of reality. Schizophrenia can include hallucinations, delusions, and severely disorganized thought and behavior, which can make it difficult to operate on a daily basis.

Chapter 6 is "Parkinson's Disease: Neuro-Cognitive Perspective" which describes Parkinson's disease is a neurodegenerative disorder characterized by severe cognitive impairments. This is a condition of degeneration of Substantia Nigra of basal ganglia. Parkinsonism adversely influences the mental health of the person too. Parkinson's disease was first described in 1817 by James Parkinson. Parkinsonism patients may get severe complications like cognitive deficiency, which include, loss of memory, attention difficulties, visual abnormalities, slow thinking, problems with words finding and motor symptoms. Symptoms of this disease range from Parkinson's Disease Mild Cognitive Impairment (PD-MCI) to Parkinson's Disease Dementia (PDD). The primary motor symptoms are trembling in hands, arms, legs, jaw, and face; rigidity or stiffness of the limbs and trunk; or slowness of movement; and postural instability or impaired balance and coordination. Researches on treatments of Parkinson's disease are progressing to prevent complications and sustain normal functions of patients.

Chapter 7 is "Neuropsychological and Cognitive Control Deficits in Depression" which describes the research done so far on neuropsychological deficits in Major depressive disorder (MDD). The most prominent deficits have been reported in executive function and the cognitive control networks. These deficits have also been shown to effect various cognitive aspects of a patient, such as metacognitions and emotional regulation. They are also predictors of socio-occupational functioning and of recovering and relapse in patient. This makes it pertinent that these newer treatments for MDD account for these deficits and work on ameliorating them for long term gains.

Chapter 8 is "Characterising Attention Deficit Hyperactivity Disorder" which describes ADHD as a neurodevelopmental disorder that affects children. ADHD can often persist in adulthood too. Children diagnosed with ADHD have significantly increased across the globe that ranges between 3-10%. The cardinal features of ADHD are inattention, hyperactivity, and impulsivity. Clinically significant impairment affects bio-psychosocial functioning. Theoretical understanding reveals the central role of genetics, environmental factors, and cognition in ADHD symptoms. The gold standard for ADHD diagnosis relies on clinical history, mental status examination, and diagnostic tools. Pharmacological intervention is the first-line evidence-based treatment for ADHD. However, studies also report that children don't respond to or can't tolerate medications and suffered from adverse side effects. There are also evidence-based treatments such as Neurofeedback training that uses technology to regulate brain activity through modifying brain waves. Hence developing devices for assessment and intervention using technology that targets the cognitive deficits is the need of the hour.

Chapter 9 is "Artificial Intelligence in the Detection of Alzheimer's Disease" which describes dementia as a neurological illness that causes diversion from a variety of important cognitive activities. Common examples include memory, reasoning, orientation, understanding, computation, verbal communication and decision making. Alzheimer's disease (AD) is one of the most common dementias affecting the elderly. It was projected that more than 47 million people globally will be affected by dementia in 2015; these predictions were verified, & forecasts for 2050 are much more concerning, with 131 million people living with dementia. The basic objective of AI is to improve human decision-making and automate operations that are too time-consuming or resource-intensive for people to accomplish. AI can operate as a fast, accurate, and in the long run, cost-effective method to assist human experience and intuition through predictive analytics. AI is an effective technique for AD detection as these methods are employed as a computer-aided diagnosis (CAD) system in clinical practices and play a crucial role in identifying variations in the brain images to detect AD.

Chapter 10 is "The Influence of Artificial Intelligence on People with Autism Spectrum Disorder: A Methodical Literature Review" which describes the literature review that examines the past and recent relevant research on Autism disorder. As undergoing many changes in the whole world, especially after the deadly effect of the Covid19 widespread in the year 2020, has led to drastic adoption of more intelligent devices for quicker detection of certain human diseases and delivering the results quicker via electronic media. Our research will focus on the Autism disorder intelligent device detection and feed these data to machine learning models to predict the issues without human intervention. Based on the outcome of the results, the diseases can be treated accordingly in an appropriate manner. The individual suffering from the Autism disorder can be early detected using AI or machine learning as well as this domain can be integrated with the IoT sensors, and such sensors can be combined with the human body.

Chapter 11 is "Artificial Intelligence, Machine Learning, and Internet of Drones in Medical Applications" which describes Internet of Drones (IOD) that plays an important role in the delivery of emergency medicine to remote locations. Furthermore, it is employed for blood transfer, disaster assistance, missing persons discovering lost hikers in the hill station, and a variety of other emergency services. The use of drones for emergency response services, particularly in medical circumstances, offers up new avenues for life-saving interventions. Using drones to give "eyes" on a risky scenario or to transport medical supplies to stranded patients may increase the capacity of emergency response physicians to provide care in dangerous conditions. IOD provides several emergency response services that have an influence on daily life. The Federal Aviation Administration (FAA) conducts completely autonomous missions beyond visual range and flights above people to provide critical medical supplies.

Chapter 12 is "Application of Aerodynamic Shock Wave in Medical Treatment" which describes Extracorporeal shock wave therapy in orthopaedics and traumatology is a relatively new treatment modality. The advancement of shock wave treatment has been fast in recent years. Shock waves have significantly altered the therapy. Shock waves are now the treatment of choice for kidney and urethral stones. Urology has traditionally been the sole medical profession that uses shock waves. Meanwhile, shock waves have been utilised to treat insertion tendinitis, avascular necrosis of the head of the femur, and other necrotic bone changes in orthopaedics and traumatology. In veterinary medicine, another field of shock wave use is the therapy of tendons, ligaments, and bones. The basic theory and applications of shock waves, as well as their history in medicine, are discussed in this study. The goal of utilising shock wave treatment for orthopaedic disorders is to stimulate healing in the tendons, surrounding tissue, and bones. Shock waves have emerged as the preferred therapy for kidney and ureteral stones.

Chapter 13 is "Diagnostic Categorization and Neurocognitive Prediction Employing Neuroimaging Data Using Deep Learning in Alzheimer's Illness" which describes traditional analytic strategies for investigating neuroimaging biomarkers for neuropsychiatric illnesses have relied on mass univariate statistics, assuming that various brain areas function separately. Machine learning (ML) methods that take into account intercorrelation across areas have recently become a popular and important part of computer-assisted analytical procedures, and are now frequently used for the automated diagnosis and analysis of neuropsychiatric illnesses. The goal of this chapter is to provide a detailed overview of CNN and RNN applications in medical image comprehension. The overarching goal is to encourage medical image understanding experts to use CNNs extensively in their research and diagnosis. This article describes survey on the development of various novel DL-based approaches and models, as well as advancements in high-speed computing techniques, provide a once-in-a-lifetime chance to anticipate and control Alzheimer.

Chapter 14 is "An Industry Internet of Things Framework for Epilepsy Detection, Monitoring, and Control" which describes Epilepsy is a long-term neurological Seizures of various types, some of which are defined by involuntary repetitive convulsions and have a substantial impact on the patients' everyday lives. Several approaches for diagnosing these types of seizures and observing the patient have been proposed in the literature; however, these approaches fall short in terms of ergonomics and proper integration with the health system. The precision measuring that this study looks into what an epileptic detection and monitoring tool should be able to do. This article describes specific epilepsy detection and monitoring platform that specifies the conditions. The information will be gathered from the wearable part of the system.

Chapter 15 is "Quantum AI and IoT Cognitive Disease Data Security to Evade Quantum Computing Attacks" which aims at providing the larger profits of the IoT systems or devices that are vulnerable to highly vulnerable intrusions of different attackers when the vital security necessities such as authorization and authentication are not satisfactorily meet the requirements and prevailing events are not capable of securing the IoT smart health care environment from data gaps of the system security With the number of IoT application domains growing to include smart homes mobile health care autonomous intelligent health care communication and smart cities in day-to-day human life.

CONCLUSION

The book is the boon in field of medical science with literary contributions from various medical practitioners and world renowned engineers from India and abroad providing solutions to various brain diseases with algorithms inspired by Nature and implementing them in latest software technologies like Artificial Intelligence, Machine Learning, Internet of Things, Aerodynamic Shock Wave. The initial part of the book describes various bioinspired algorithms, description of novel brain diseases and then move onto implementation using latest software technologies like Extracorporeal shock wave therapy in orthopaedics and traumatology is a relatively new treatment modality. Since the book caters to description of development of newest algorithms for treatment of cognitive diseases it happens to bring breakthrough in the field of medical sciences.

Acknowledgment

First and foremost, I would like to acknowledge doctors from NIMHANS Hospital, bengaluru which happens to be best hospital for brain diseases across India, who not only gave their references for my book proposal but Dr. Meenakshi Baneerjee, Former Clinical phycologist in NIMHANS, now Assistant Professor in O.P. Jindal University, Sonepat and Dr. Mishab A. K., Former Clinical psychologist in NIMHANS, now Joint Director in Department of Psychology, University of Calicut, Kerela wrote chapters for my book. Then, eminent software technologies expert professors from Dayanand Sagar University, Bengaluru, Jain University, Bengaluru, Chitkara University, Chandigarh, Dayanand Sagar College of Engineering and Punjab University, Bengaluru wrote meticulously defining and applying all the aspects of newest software technologies pertaining to treatment of Brain diseases in the book. Besides that, a very young, diligent research scholar from Department of Neurology, Institute of Medical Sciences, Banaras Hindu University, India wrote for my Book. And last and not the least, three chapters of the book are contributed by abroad professors from University Of Technology and Applied Sciences, Oman, and College Of Business and Economics Management, Salale University, Ethopia, Catholic University in Erbil, Erbil, Kurdistan Region, Iraq.

Without the support of these authors from diverse backgrounds the crux of the book would not have been achieved. I thank all my authors and reviewers for their continued support in all the phases of the book.

Chapter 1
Bio-Inspired Algorithms:
Devices for Diagnosis and Treatment of Parkinson's Disease

Sumit Kumar
Panjab University, Chandigarh, India

Alka Bali
Panjab University, Chandigarh, India

Nishu Bali
Chitkara University, India

ABSTRACT

Parkinson's disease (PD) is a common neurodegenerative disorder with a high prevalence rate in the geriatric population, and more than 10 million people are afflicted with this disease worldwide. Striatal dopamine deficiency and intracellular inclusions containing aggregates of alpha-synuclein are the neuropathological signs caused by neuronal loss in the substantia nigra. PD causes motor and nonmotor symptoms. A diagnostic test or medical tool that is reliable for Parkinson's disease is not yet available. Thus, the diagnosis of PD is primarily based on clinical symptoms. Optimized bio-inspired algorithms are the novel and heuristic approach for diagnosis and treatment of Parkinson's disease. In this chapter, various bio-inspired algorithms are discussed such as optimized cuttlefish algorithm, optimized grasshopper algorithm, wolf search algorithm, crow search algorithm, and ant-lion algorithm. Other useful approaches include bionics institute rigidity device, sawtooth waveform-inspired pitch estimator (SWIPE), brain stimulation therapies, and bioinspired nanomedicine.

INTRODUCTION

Parkinson's disease is a common neurodegenerative disorder with prevalence to 4% of the population over 80 and with 160/100000 in western europe (davie, 2008). The driving sources of disability around the world are neurological disorders and the predominance of Parkinson's disease is expanding more

DOI: 10.4018/978-1-7998-9534-3.ch001

quickly than other neurological disorders (armstrong & okun, 2020). Parkinson's disease is associated with a loss of cells in the substantia nigra and James Parkinson was the first person to describe the cognitive syndrome- parkinson's disease in *an essay on the shaking palsy* in 1817 (jankovic, 2008). Carlsson and colleagues discovered dopamine as a putative neurotransmitter at lund, sweden in 1957 (jankovic, 2008). Deficiency of dopamine in the striatum (as a result of degeneration of dopaminergic neurons in the substantia nigra) and intracellular inclusions containing aggregates of alpha-synuclein called lewy bodies are the common neuropathological sign of pd (poewe, et al., 2017). The loss of dopaminergic terminals in the basal ganglia, is crucial for onset of motor symptoms (simon, tanner, & brundin, 2020).

Parkinson's disease manifests itself as a combination of motor as well as non-motor symptoms. Motor symptoms comprise of physical features such as tremors, ataxia, slowness, stiffness in limb movements and postural imbalance (dauer & przedborski, 2003). The non-motor symptoms are heterogeneous in nature, impacting several organ systems, such as gastrointestinal and genitourinary systems (armstrong & okun, 2020). Constipation, hyposmia, orthostatic hypotension and urogenital dysfunction are some of the non-motor symptoms which are the significant part of parkinson disease. Bradykinesia, hypokinesia, and akinesia are variety of symptoms including decreased voice volume, normal facial expression paucity, and drooling, decreased stride length during walking and decreased size and speed of handwriting (dauer & przedborski, 2003). Epidemiologic studies suggest that constipation is associated with an increased risk of parkinson disease and this often appears years prior to the appearance of significant motor symptoms (hopfner, et al., 2017). There are many disorders that can have at least some of these clinical symptoms and this clinical syndrome is known as *parkinsonism*. The disorders in which parkinsonism is a prominent part are called as *parkinsonian disorders* and the examples are parkinson's disease, progressive supranuclear palsy, multiple system atrophy, corticobasal degeneration and vascular parkinsonism (williams & litvan, 2013) (dickson, 2012).

There are two forms of parkinson disease, i.e., familial, which is hereditary in origin, and sporadic (idiopathic), which develops from gene-environment interactions. Familial form accounts for 10–15% of reported pd cases whereas, remaining 85-90% cases are sporadic ones. There are seven genes which have been identified for familial pd. These are; alpha-synuclein (snca), glucocerebrosidase (gba), parkin rbr e3 ubiquitin protein ligase (park2), leucine-rich repeat kinase 2 (lrrk2), parkinson protein 7 (park7), vacuolar protein sorting-associated protein 35 (vps35), phosphatase and tensing homolog-induced kinase 1 (pink1), these genes have been used to research for possible early detection methods for pd along with their specific metabolites and pd-associated biomarkers. Early diagnosis of pd is very crucial as almost 70% of neuronal death has occurred by the time actual symptoms of the disease are manifested. The genotypes of humans are unique and therefore, individuals exposed to same environmental factors are also affected varyingly, leading to diverse phenotypes of the disease. The combined impact of genetic and environmental factors leads to structural alterations in dna, which may affect the occurrence of human disease. Pesticides and heavy metals are known to increase pd by altering genes linked to familial pd (park1, lrrk2, pink1) causing oxidative stress, mitochondrial dysfunction and deterioration in protein degradation (ball et al., 2019). Drug induced parkinsonism is also a common etiology in many elderly patients. Nearly 40% of patients on drug therapy with conventional antipsychotics like chlorpromazine or haloperidol exhibit extrapyramidal side effects which include parkinsonism-like symptoms due to dopaminergic blockade in the nigrostriatal region (shin & chung, 2012).

The study of the bionic functions, biological structures, and organizational principles found in nature with modern technologies has led to the development of numerous mathematical and metaheuristic algorithms based upon the knowledge transferring process from life form to human technologies. Output of the bionic study includes not only physical products, but also various computation methods that can be applied in various areas. People have learnt from biological systems and structures to design and develop a number of different kinds of optimization algorithms, that have been widely used in theoretical studies as well as for practical application (zang, zhang, & hapeshi, 2010). Evolutionary algorithms are a part of ai which mainly focus on biological evolution. These algorithms are mainly genetic based algorithms and nature inspired. The concepts of mutation and survival of the fittest based on the calculation of a fitness function are used. Feature selection plays an important role in model construction in machine learning. There are several types of evolutionary algorithms, in which there are some genetic algorithms, estimation of distribution algorithms, evolutionary strategies and differential evolution (corne & lones, 2018). In recent years, artificial intelligence and bioinspired computing methodologies have risen rapidly and have been successfully applied to many fields. Bio-inspired techniques are founded on maxims, or models, of natural biological systems. Several bio-inspired methods have been successfully used to solve diverse problems linked to computer networks. Bio inspired network systems are fields of biology and computer science, having a good relation to the bio inspired computing and bio inspired systems. These have the self-organizing and self-healing characteristics that help them in achieving complex tasks with much ease in network environment (chiang, sangaiah, chen, & liu, 2020). Bio inspired algorithms have been found to be useful as clinical decision support system for reliable diagnosis and prediction of various diseases, e.g., heart disease (bethel & sandhya, 2020), cancer (venkatesh & bojja, 2020), covid-19 (singh, kumar, mahmud, kaiser, & kishore, 2021) (martínez-álvarez, et al., 2020), bionic based dust sized wireless sensor which is battery less, placed in cortex region of brain to sense the tremors of epilepsy (gupta, sundaram, khanna, hassanien, & de albuquerque, 2018) etc. This chapter is intended to review various algorithms used for prediction of parkinson's disease, a complex neurological disorder afflicting a sizeable part of human population.

BACKGROUND

Parkinson's disease (PD) is a progressive neurodegenerative disorder affecting a significant part of the population aged over 60 years, all over the world (ball, teo, chandra, & chapman, 2019). The incidence of parkinson's disease increases in sixth to ninth decade of life up to 5 to 10 folds (poewe, et al., 2017). A diagnostic test or medical tool which is reliable for pd is not yet available. Thus, in epidemiological studies, the diagnosis of pd is primarily based on clinical symptoms. The diagnosis of parkinson's disease in current criteria requires the presence of at least two of the following symptoms - postural imbalance, resting tremors, bradykinesia or rigidity. Single-photon-emission ct or pet may be more helpful to diagnose pd with modern imaging in particular settings. However, despite the fact that these techniques have gotten to be more broadly accessible and easier to use, their usefulness for population-based epidemiological research is still constrained (de lau & breteler, 2006).

In model construction in machine learning, feature selection plays an important role (gupta & ahlawat, usability feature selection via mbbat: a novel approach, 2017). Feature selection is defined as the process of choosing an optimal subset of features representing the whole dataset, also known as variable selection and the part of dimensional reduction (eesa, orman, & brifcani, a novel feature-selection approach based on the cuttlefish optimization algorithm for intrusion detection systems, 2015), (gupta & ahlawat, usability feature selection via mbbat: a novel approach, 2017). In feature selection, a relevant features subset is chosen from a set of features in such a way that the precision of the original model (preceding feature selection) is comparable to the model after feature selection. The computation cost of the model as well as complexity of the dataset is reduced by feature selection. It could also be used to make the model less prone to over-fitting. Feature selection can be categorized in wrapper, filter and embedded methods (gupta & ahlawat, usability feature selection via mbbat: a novel approach, 2017). Fs has been used in many fields, such as data mining, classification, object recognition etc. It is very effective in removing redundant and irrelevant features from the dataset (eesa, orman, & brifcani, a novel feature-selection approach based on the cuttlefish optimization algorithm for intrusion detection systems, 2015).

Optimization is a process in which searching an optimal solution to solve a particular problem is carried out. Optimization algorithms can be classified into: a. Deterministic algorithm, in which identical solutions are produced if initial values are same when solving the same problem. B. Stochastic algorithms, which are generally gradient free algorithms, where random steps are taken to reach the optimum) (brownlee, 2011). Stochastic algorithms are further divided into two types, i.e., heuristic and metaheuristic (yang, gandomi, talatahari, & alavi, 2012).

Several algorithms have been successfully explored and applied for accurate diagnosis of various diseases like cancers, heart diseases, covid-19, etc. Accurate timely diagnosis of parkinson's disease is crucial for arresting the progression of this disease through various therapeutic interventions because considerable neuronal degeneration has already occurred in patients by the time, they manifest recognizable clinical symptoms of the disease. Several algorithms have been utilized successfully in this regard which are compiled in the succeeding sections.

OPTIMISED CUTTLEFISH ALGORITHM

Optimized cuttlefish algorithm is a metaheuristic procedure which is a very recent solution to a wide range of optimization tasks (kowalski, łukasik, charytanowicz, & kulczycki, 2018). It is inspired from the color changing characteristics of cuttlefish effecting change in visibility, reflectivity of light rays (eesa, brifcani, & orman, a new tool for global optimization problems-cuttlefish algorithm, 2014). Cuttlefish is a type of cephalopod which is a very famous for its abilities to change its colour so that it can apparently disappear into its surroundings or it can produce stunning colour displays (eesa, brifcani, & orman, cuttlefish algorithm-a novel bio-inspired optimization algorithm, 2013). This ability obtained by a combination of chromatophores, leucophores and iridophores. Chromatophores comprise of a group of cells which include an elastic saccule carrying a pigment along with about 15-25 muscles attached to this saccule. When the muscles contract, this saccule gets stretched and consequently, the pigment inside covers a larger surface area. Conversely, the saccule shrinks and hides the pigment when the muscles relax. Leucophores are responsible for the white spots occurring on certain species of cuttlefish. These are branched, flattened cells that scatter and reflect incoming light. So, the predominant wavelength of light is reflected by the colour of the leucophore in the environment, *viz,* white in white light, or blue in blue light. Iridophores are found in the next layer under the chromatophores, and these work by reflecting light. They are generally used to conceal organs and can additionally, assist in communication (eesa, brifcani, & orman, a new tool for global optimization problems-cuttlefish algorithm, 2014). Various cells are interacting with each other and combining with the reflecting light to output different colors (gupta, et al., 2018). Cuttlefish algorithm mimics the light reflection process through a combination of three cell layers. To match its background, cuttlefish uses matching pattern process (eesa, brifcani, & orman, a new tool for global optimization problems-cuttlefish algorithm, 2014). The aim of the algorithm is to do efficient feature selection and get ideal solution features from the given set of the features without compromising on accuracy (eesa, brifcani, & orman, cuttlefish algorithm-a novel bio-inspired optimization algorithm, 2013). Optimized cuttlefish algorithm was developed by adel sabry eesa, zeynep orman and adnan mohsin abdulazeez brifcani in 2013 (mäthger, denton, marshall, & hanlon, 2009) (gupta, et al., 2018). This algorithm considers two main processes: reflection and visibility. The process of reflection is used to simulate the light reflection mechanism and to output different colours and patterns, whereas, the visibility of matching patterns and optimization of output patterns according to its environment is simulated by visibility process. The combination of reflection and visibility process gives rise to six different cases giving new possible solutions (gupta, et al., 2018). These processes are used as a key to find the optimal solution figure 1.

Figure 1. Six different cases giving new possible solution

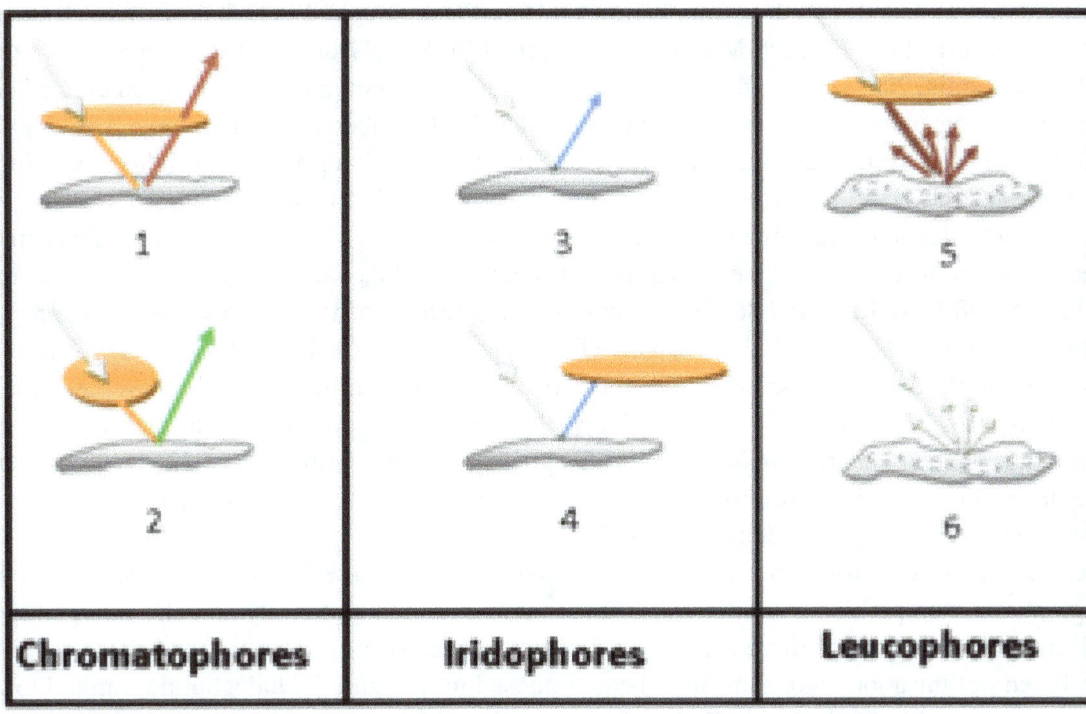

The optimized Cuttlefish Algorithm is actualized using python and its libraries. It has been applied to diagnose the occurrence of PD at earlier stages and also on the Parkinson's Datasets to optimize the issue using feature selection (Gupta, et al., 2018).

Several changes have been proposed in the optimized cuttlefish algorithm over the traditional cuttlefish algorithm. These include implementation on multiple features in the optimized cuttlefish algorithm compared to the traditional version which was designed to be implemented on a singular feature. Further, two-dimensional structures of cells are used in original algorithm, whereas 3D structure is taken to incorporate all the features in the optimized algorithm.

Feature selection is done based on weights. Weights act as a measure and control the importance of each attribute. Data is normalized to a range from 0 to 1. The dataset is also fitted to other models such as KNN and decision trees and the accuracy is compared (Eesa, Brifcani, & Orman, A new tool for global optimization problems-cuttlefish algorithm, 2014).

MACHINE LEARNING MODELS

There are two most popular and classic machine learning classifier models which are used to compare results. First is a supervised learning algorithm, KNN which is working on the principle of nearest neighbors and distance between the records in a Euclidean space. The second ML model is Decision Tree which is also a supervised algorithm. It fits the data into a tree where every node splits the data based on an inference rule developed by the algorithm (Gupta, et al., 2018). Various datasets for speech with many types of sound recordings and Parkinson HandPD are applied in OCFA such as, Speech PD Dataset, Voice PD Dataset, HandPD Meander Dataset, HandPD Spiral Datasets (Little, McSharry, Hunter, Spielman, & Ramig, 2008). These datasets are tested in terms of accuracy. It has been calculated using computational time and (True Positive + True Negative / Total number of testing samples) by KNN and Decision tree and the results are compared (Gupta, et al., 2018). In first stage, the weights are optimized as per the algorithm and the corresponding weight function. In 2nd stage the accuracy is determined without feature selection, and in the next stage, features are based on the values of their weights and the accuracy is determined by fitting the model to the test data (Gupta, et al., 2018). The average accuracy of 92.19%, 83.48%, 87.12%, and 88.46% is achieved in detection of Parkinson's disease by proposed algorithm on datasets- Speech PD dataset, Voice PD Dataset, Parkinson Hand PD Meander Dataset and Parkinson Hand PD Spiral Dataset, with an estimated computational time of 2.59 seconds, 1.84 seconds, 1.28 seconds and 1.31 seconds respectively (Gupta, et al., 2018). The optimized cuttlefish algorithm can be used in foreseeing the Parkinson's disease with a precision of approximately 94% thus, providing the proof that this bio-inspired algorithm is very reliable in prediction of PD, thus, enabling treatment of the disease at an early stage (Gupta, et al., 2018).

There are many swarm-based algorithms proposed in the literature for solving complex and challenging optimization problems in different area search due to their simplicity and efficiency in global optimization. The number of these algorithms has a steep increase over the last decade. A variety of swarm-based optimization algorithms have been proposed in literature include, but not limited to PSO (Eberhart & Kennedy, 1995), Flower Pollination Algorithm (FPA) (Yang, Karamanoglu, & He, Flower pollination algorithm: a novel approach for multiobjective optimization, 2014), Bat Algorithm (BA) (Cai, Gao, & Xue, 2016), Ant Colony Optimization (ACO) (Dorigo, Maniezzo, & Colorni, 1996), Ant Lion Optimization (ALO) (Mirjalili, The ant lion optimizer, 2015), Grey Wolf Optimization (GWO) (Mirjalili, Mirjalili, & Lewis, Grey wolf optimizer, 2014), Dragonfly Algorithm (DA) (Mirjalili & Lewis, The whale optimization algorithm, 2016), Moth-Flame Optimization (MFO) (Mirjalili, Moth-flame optimization algorithm: A novel nature-inspired heuristic paradigm, 2015), and Whale Optimization Algorithm (WOA) (Mirjalili & Lewis, The whale optimization algorithm, 2016). Almost all of these approaches are originally proposed for continuous optimization problems and after that, these were binarized to be used for the binary optimization problems such as feature selection in data classification where they show superior performance (Hichem, Elkamel, Rafik, Mesaaoud, & Ouahiba, 2019).

Figure 2. General principle of Cuttlefish algorithm

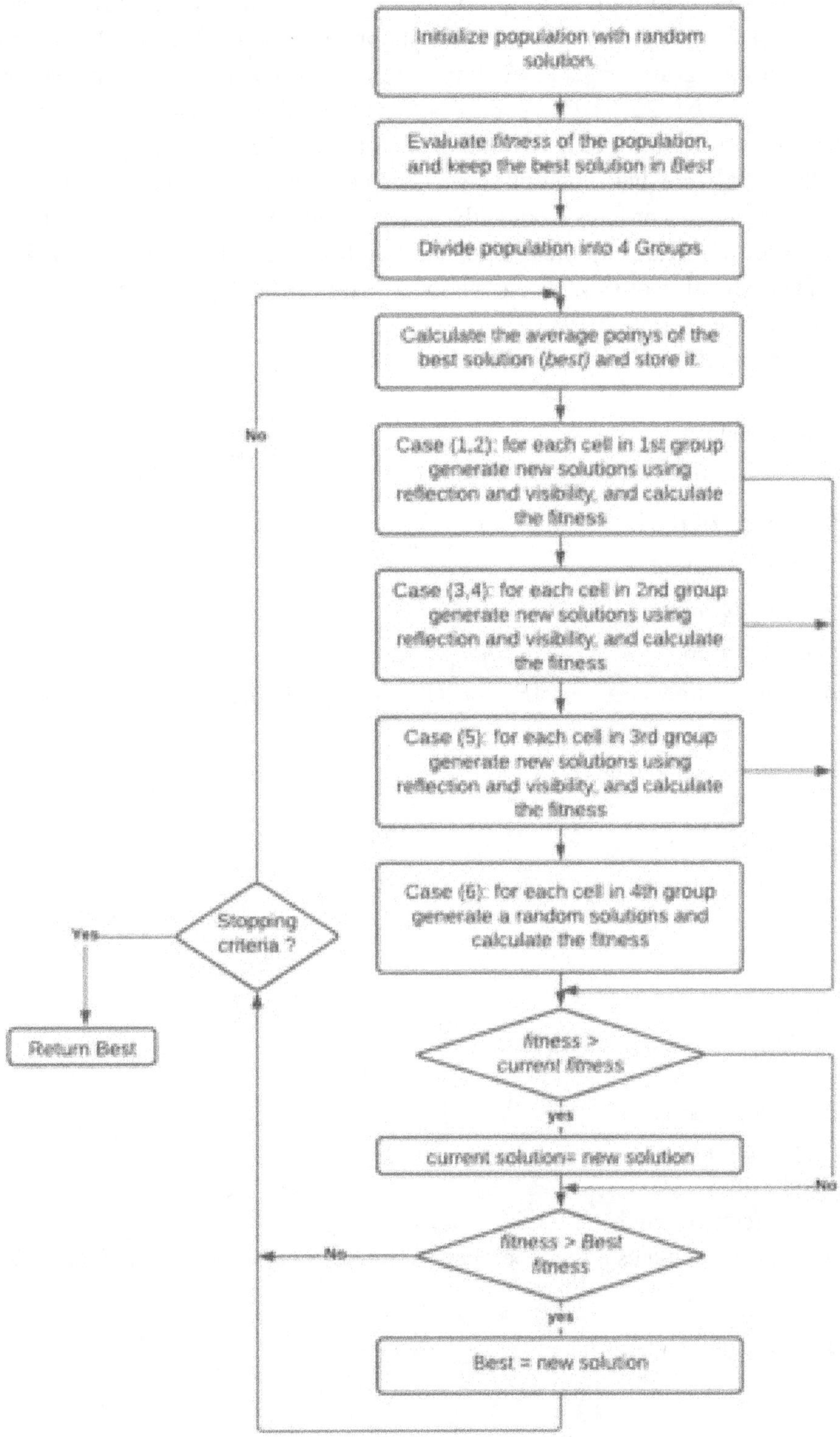

GRASSHOPPER OPTIMIZATION ALGORITHM

Grasshopper Optimization Algorithm GOA, proposed in 2016 (Aljarah, et al., 2018), is a metaheuristic optimization algorithm inspired from the lives of grasshoppers (Ibrahim, Mazher, Ucan, & Bayat, 2019). The swarming behavior of grasshoppers in nature is mimicked by this algorithm (Hichem, Elkamel, Rafik, Mesaaoud, & Ouahiba, 2019). GOA mimics the behavior of grasshopper swarms in nature for solving optimization problems (Ewees, Abd Elaziz, & Houssein, 2018). Egg, nymph and adulthood are the three parts of their life cycle. In the nymph stage, the swarm progresses slowly with short paces but in the adulthood stage, the swarm progresses quickly and with long paces. So, this optimization algorithm is applied in two phases which are exploration and exploitation (Hichem, Elkamel, Rafik, Mesaaoud, & Ouahiba, 2019). The utilization of GOA is encouraged by rapid convergence and extensive exploration (Ibrahim, Mazher, Ucan, & Bayat, 2019).
To simulate above, the model is designed as;

$X_i = S_i + G_i + A_i$ (equation 1)

where, X_i is the location of the i_{th} insect,
S_i is the social communications,
G_i is the gravity strength on i_{th} insect,
and A_i is the wind advection.
Note that Eq. (1) can be written as $X_i = r1S_i + r2G_i + r3A_i$, where r1, r2, r3 are random values inside [0,1].
The components of Eq. (1) can be attained as:

$\text{si} = \sum_{j=1, j\neq 0}^{N} \text{s (dij) d\^{} ij, dij} = |\text{xj - xi}|, \text{ d\^{} ij}$

= (xj – xi)/ dij
Gi = -ge^g
A i = -ue^w (equation 2)
where, d_{ij} is the distance of two grasshoppers,
$d\hat{}_{ij}$ is a unit vector,
g denotes the gravitational constant,
eˆg is the unity vector of gravity,
u denotes a constant drift,
and eˆw is the unity vector of wind.
The s function in Eq. (2) calculates either social attraction or repulsion forces and can be attained by:

$s(r) = fe^{-\frac{r}{l}} - e^{-r}$ (equation 3)

Where the amplitude of attraction is represented by f and the length scale by l (Heidari, Faris, Aljarah, & Mirjalili, 2019).

However, equation 1 cannot be applied to find the solution of the optimization problem, it was reformulated (Saremi, Mirjalili, & Lewis, 2017) as follows:

$$xi = \mathrm{c}(\sum_{\mathrm{j=1,\ i\neq j}}^{N} \left(\mathrm{c}\,\frac{\mathrm{u}-\mathrm{l}}{2} s\left(\left|xj - xi\right|\right) \mathrm{x}\, \frac{xj - xi}{dij} \right) + \mathrm{T\^{}\ d\ (equation\ 4)}$$

Where, 'u' represents the upper bound and 'i' represents the lower bound of the search space, T^d represents the value of the best solution found.

However, in equation 3, gravity is not considered, and the direction of wind is always considered to be towards T^d.

c is a decreasing coefficient to shrink the comfort zone, and attraction zone as follows:

$$c = \mathrm{cmax} - \mathrm{t}\frac{\mathrm{cmax} - \mathrm{cmin}}{\mathrm{tmax}}\mathrm{(equation\_5)}$$

where, c^{max} represents the maximum value (i.e., 1), cmin represents the minimum value (equal to 0.00001) of c; 't' refers to the current iteration, and tmax is the maximum number of iterations.

Finally, the pseudo code of the GOA is given as:

1. 1: Initialize the value of the parameters including population size (N), Initialize cmin, cmax and maximum number of iteration tmax
2. 2: Generate a random population (X)
3. 3: Set the current iteration to t = 1
4. 4: while (t < tmax) do
5. 5: Update $c1$ and $c2$
6. 6: **for** i D 1 to *N* (all *N* grasshoppers in the population) **do**
7. 7: Normalize the distance between grasshoppers in the range [1,4]
8. 8: Update the position of the current grasshopper
9. 9: Bring the current grasshopper back if it goes outside the boundaries
10. 10: **end for**
11. 11: Update *T* if there is a better solution
12. 12: *t* D *t* C 1
13. 13: **end while**
14. 14: Return the best solution *T* (Meraihi, Gabis, Mirjalili, & Ramdane-Cherif, 2021).

where the GOA starts by generating a population X (which is random) of size N. Then, calculate the fitness function for each solution x_i, i = 1…., N, and the best solution, T^ d, is then selected according to the best fitness function. Thereafter, for each xi, the following two steps are performed:

1. normalize the distance between the solutions in X to [1,4]

2. Update the current solution xi.

The next step is to update the current iteration and repeat the previous steps until the stopping conditions are achieved (Ewees, Abd Elaziz, & Houssein, 2018).

Figure 3. Flowchart of Grasshopper optimization algorithm

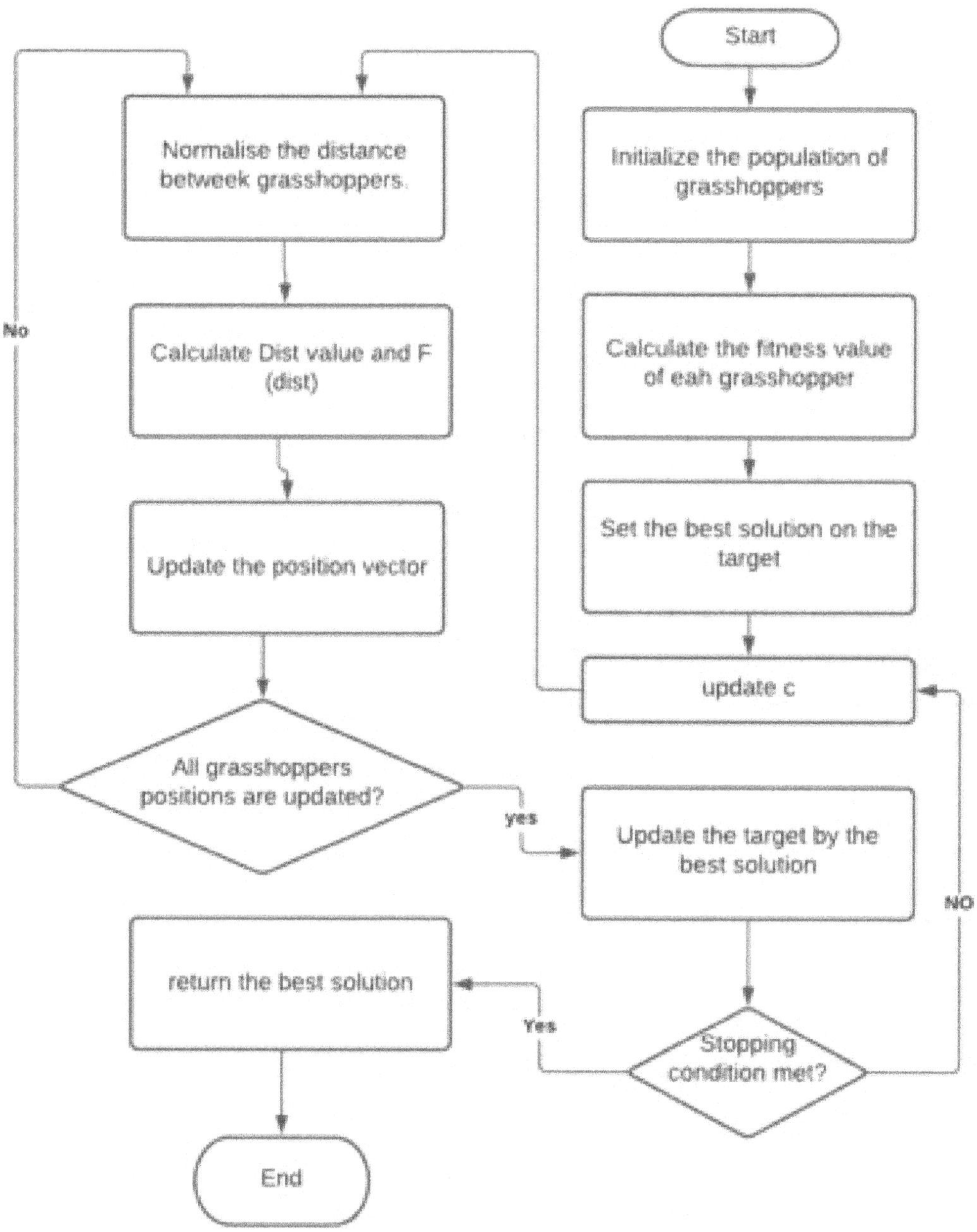

MODIFIED GRASSHOPPER OPTIMIZATION ALGORITHM

Traditional algorithm may be enhanced through the application of fitness function and sigmoid function resulting in the Modified Optimized Grasshopper Algorithm (MGOA). MGOA algorithm has been actualized by employing Python programming language for feature selection. Details of the implemented functions are as follows:

1. Init function

It initializes Grasshopper's position in space. Grasshoppers [each] position is set to 1.

2. Fitness function

This involves calculation of each agent's fitness by using following equation and the fitness value of each grasshopper is returned as:

fitness_GOA = imp + bf × (1 − (selected_features / total_features)) (Gupta & Ahlawat, Usability feature selection via MBBAT: a novel approach, 2017).

In this equation, *imp* is the sum of each selected feature's importance (Feature's importance is a characteristic of Random Forest Classifier from sclera library which possesses a value ranging from 0 to 1 for every feature according to their importance in prediction of target. Sum of all feature's importance is always equal to 1). The term 'bf' represents the balancing factor, which when implemented on all forms of Parkinson's disease, generates a balance between the feature importance, "imp" and selected features count.

selected_feature is the count of features which are shortlisted and total_feature is the count of all features present in dataset.

Machine Learning Models

Random forest, k-Nearest Neighbour (k-NN) and decision tree (Sehgal et al., 2018) are the three popular machine learning models used in MGOA for classification and regression. These are utilized for the visualization of target (Sehgal et al., 2019).

Datasets

Various datasets are compiled including the HandPD dataset, Speech PD dataset, Voice PD dataset, etc and are applied on GOA algorithm. On applying the MGWO classifiers to datasets; Accuracy (AR) shows how often the classifier correctly recognizes diseased as well as normal individuals. It is given as:

AR = No. of Correctly recognized cases / Total number of cases in the test set * 100

Detection rate (DR) shows how many times the classifier model identifies a Parkinson patient correctly, and is given as:

DR = No. of correctly recognized patient / Total no. of Parkinson patient in the test set ∗ 100

False alarm rate (FAR) shows the number of times, a normal individual is falsely identified as a Parkinson patient, out of an 'all normal individual' test set.

FAR = No. of normal individuals falsely recognized as Parkinson patients / Total no. of normal individual in the test set * 100

When FAR values are on lower side and AR, DR values are on higher side, the Classifier performance is considered good.

The MGOA processes feature work as input and give output as the reduced feature set which upgrades the performance of model. This bio-inspired algorithm is satisfactorily relentless and can identify the optimal feature set. The outcome reveals that the Modified Grasshopper Optimization Algorithm helps in improving the accuracy and in reducing the selected features. MGOA can be used for several optimization problems including Parkinson disease for getting improved and better results. Study results show that AR and DR (100%) are highest, FAR is least for classifier MGOA using Random Forest. (Sehgal, Agarwal, Gupta, Sundaram, & Bashambu, 2020).

WOLF SEARCH ALGORITHM

There are many other versions of heuristic algorithms for feature selection. Binary Particle Swarm Optimization (BPSO) was created by Kennedy and Russel, and Russel extended the BPSO research for feature selection. This led to a change in the traditional feature selection pattern towards processing a binary optimization problem. Tang proposed the Wolf Search Algorithm WSA (Li, Fong, Wong, Millham, & Wong, 2017). Wolves belong to the Canidae family and are considered as apex predators, which implies that they are placed at the top of the food chain. Wolves mostly prefer to live in a pack and the average group size ranges from 5-12. Their particular interest is that they maintain a strict social dominant hierarchy (Mirjalili, Mirjalili, & Lewis, Grey wolf optimizer, 2014). Wolves typically commute in a nuclear family. Wolves remain silent and use stealth when they are hunting for prey together. WSA forgoes a kind of communication, which reduces the run time of the search. WSA is based on the social behavior of the wolves in their nuclear families for hunting and avoiding enemies. Wolves move in a group in a loosely coupled formation but tend to take down prey individually (Ahmadebrahimpour, 2019).

In WSA method, multiple wolves move to find the best solution in multiple directions, without a single leader to scout for prey. In the WSA, each wolf moves independently of others in order to get a better position according to its characteristics. WSA does not engage in communication such as in ant colony optimization which decreases searching run time of the WSA. The feature of wolves of trying to hide while approaching the prey suggests hunters to continually change their position to find better positions which are less vulnerable. Wolves generally track their prey with their excellent sense of smell, thus, in WSA, each wolf creates a sensing radius having a visual range.
The basic rules of the WSA algorithm are summarized as follows:

1. Each wolf can see wolves only in his visual range. The Minkowski distance, which is estimated in the hyper plane domination by multiple features, is the fixed visual range in WSA with radius (r).
2. Wolf continually works to move to the better positions. That includes a companion. The wolf changes position randomly, if no options better than the current location of the wolf are available.
3. If the wolf finds an enemy, it tries to avoid it by escaping to a random location which is beyond the visual range of the enemy.

Pseudo code of Wolf Search Algorithm:

```
Initialize the population of wolves xi (i=1, 2..., W)
Define and initialize parameters: (r: radius of the visual range, s: step size by which a wolf moves
at a time, α: velocity factor of wolf, pa = a user defined threshold [0...1])
while t <generations && stopping criteria do
for i= 1 to W do
initiative_prey ()
generate_location ()
if (dist(xi,xj) < r && xj
xi moves towards xj
else if
xi = initiative_prey ()
end if
generate_location ()
if rand () > pa
xi = xi + rand () + v
end if
end for
end while (Parlar, 2021).
```

Classification dataset is collected from the voice records and applied on random forest (RF) support vector machines (SVM), logistic regression (LR), and artificial neural network (ANN) to classify the PD dataset and evaluate the classification performance by using the micro-average of F-score with five-fold cross validations. In Random Forest, low correlation is important to produce collective predictions because de-correlation models protect from individual errors (Hastie, Tibshirani, & Friedman, 2009). The most accurate performance classification results are obtained with reliefF method among all the other methods. After running the classifiers, ANN shows the most accurate results of all classifiers for the PD dataset. The only disadvantage of ANN method is that this method needs greater computation times compared to other methods (Parlar, 2021).

ANT-LION ALGORITHM

Ant-Lion Algorithm ALA is a recently proposed algorithm which can be implemented for the diagnosis of Parkinson's disease. It mimics the hunting pattern of ant lion (doodle bergs). ALA is used to find the minimum number of features which ultimately results in higher accuracy in diagnosis using machine learning classifiers. The optimal features for the two different Parkinson's datasets are extracted by the proposed modified version of ALA with improved accuracy and computational time. The maximum accuracy achieved by the classifier after feature selection is 95.91% (optimal) (Sharma, Jain, Sharma, & Gupta, 2019).

CROW SEARCH ALGORITHM

The Crow Search Algorithm CSO is based on the intelligent behaviors of the crows (Askarzadeh, 2016). The performance accuracy of the Optimized Crow Search Algorithm is 100% and it can be used in predicting the PD. This ultimately helps an individual to get a proper treatment and early stage of disease. The performance has been measured for 20 benchmarks of datasets and the results have been compared with original chaotic Crow Search Algorithm. Most experimental results show that the CSO, nature inspired algorithm gets an optimal subset of features which maximize the accuracy and minimize a number of features selected hence, is more stable (Gupta, Sundaram, Khanna, Hassanien, & De Albuquerque, 2018).

MORE AVENUES FOR DIAGNOSIS AND TREATMENT

Dopamine Transporter Single-Photon Emission Computed Tomography

A very sensitive method for detecting pre-synaptic dopamine neural dysfunction is Dopamine transporters (DAT) imaging, which is a sign of Parkinsonism which is neurodegenerative. Dopamine transporter single-photon emission computed tomography (DaT SPECT) (Kägi, Bhatia, & Tolosa, 2010) determines the presynaptic dopamine neuronal dysfunction present in PD. It demonstrates the reduced uptake of a radioactive tracer which binds to dopamine transporters in the basal ganglia. It is 98%-100% sensitive and specific in identifying nigrostriatal cells in Parkinson's disease (Mirjalili & Lewis, The whale optimization algorithm, 2016). DAT-SPECT is helpful in diagnosis of psychogenic, drug induced and vascular Parkinsonism by underlying true nigrostriatal dysfunctions. According to a study (Bega et al., 2015), Over a two years period 83 DAT-SPECT scans were ordered. Scans were ordered to differentiate PD from Essentials Tremors (ET) 21.7%, or from drug induced Parkinsonism 21.7%, A change in clinical diagnosis or medication regimen occurred in 59% of cases within one visit after the scan. Further, 72% had a change in diagnosis, management and both which is a strong impact that was seen for ET vs. PD indication (Bega et al., 2015).

Bionics Institute Rigidity Device

Bionics Institute Rigidity Device (BiRD) is a palm-worn instrument designed to measure the force required to flex the third digit of the hand. The digit is flexed and extends by a miniature on-board electric motor. The digit required greater force for flex to increase rigidity, so this device aims to monitor the clinical rating scale albeit limited to the metacarpophalangeal joint (Perera, et al., 2019). This device has sensors to accurately measure tremors, stiffness, and slowness of movement. It takes less than 2 minutes for assessment and gives precise information about rigidity, tremors, movement.

Sawtooth Waveform Inspired Pitch Estimator (SWIPE)

To detect PD, different kinds of methods have been proposed with measurements including force tracking data, speech data, gait patterns, smell identification data and spontaneous cardiovascular oscillations. Sawtooth waveform inspired pitch estimator (SWIPE) scheme is used to determine speech disorders (caused by PD) recorded via Smartphone (Wang, Lee, Harrou, & Sun, 2020).

BRAIN STIMULATION THERAPIES

The Wireless Log-based Closed-loop Deep Brain Stimulation (CDBS) with two-way wireless telemetry emerged as the new research (Gupta, Singh, & others, Bionics Based Solar Powered Clothing for Treating Parkinson's Disease and Epilepsy, 2015). Thus, bionics based embedded solar photovoltaic cell-based fabric which converts solar energy into electrical energy to charge the polymer embedded electronic circuit came up. Silicon based polymer is used to make Solar Powered Clothing. The electronic circuit can sense the tremors of Parkinson's disease and to prevent the tremors, it can pass the medicine to specific regions of the brain (Gupta S., Repetitive Transcranial Magnetic Stimulation (RTMS) for the Treatment of Depression, Migraine and Parkinson's Disease). Brain stimulation therapies involve activating the brain with electricity, magnets, or implants for treatment of cognitive disorders. Repetitive transcranial magnetic stimulation [rTMS] involves targeting specific areas of brain that are affected by mood disorders (depression, etc). It modulates activity in small areas of the brain. This technique can particularly use in the condition of depression associated with Parkinsonism. TMS uses an electromagnet placed on the scalp that imparts magnetic field pulses which stimulate a small area of the brain (Gupta S., Repetitive Transcranial Magnetic Stimulation (RTMS) for the Treatment of Depression, Migraine and Parkinson's Disease, 2014).

BIOINSPIRED NANOMEDICINE

The approach of bioinspired nanomedicine to brain diseases is more reliable and inert with no autoimmune reactions. The Blood Brain Barrier BBB is more amenable to biomimetic nanomedicine than exogenic one. Only about 2% of the drugs can pass through the BBB (Mitragotri, 2013). Despite the fact that nanotechnology is at starting stages to cure brain diseases, their natural analogy to the cell architecture makes them more appropriate for biomedicine. In near future, it may get access to clinical practices. Only few available drugs can pass through the BBB, and amongst these, very few drugs are effective in the treatment of various brain disorders, including Parkinson's disease (PD) (Rehman, 2020).

DEEP LEARNING-BASED TECHNIQUES

Deep learning-based techniques have gained extraordinary consideration in PD diagnosis due to their capacity to handle huge data and accomplishing high accuracy with free assumption on data distribution (Das, 2010). Random Forest (RF), or support vector machine (SVM), Neural Network and machine learning algorithms, are used to detect PD based on acoustic analysis of speech. Performance of four classifier- DMneural, Decision Trees, Regression, and Neural network (NN) has been compared, and high accuracy (92.9%) is obtained employing the NN algorithm (Wang, Lee, Harrou, & Sun, 2020). The occurrence of Parkinson's disease can also be predicted by the signals of Electroencephalogram (EEG). Support Vector Machine (SVM) is used in this case that converts EEG into single signal from multiple channels and improve signal- to- noise- ratio (SNR) (Gupta S., Smartphone based Early Detection of Epileptic Seizures Using Machine Learning, 2020).

These above techniques offer reasonably good capacity for handling of data, achievement of high accuracy and free assumption on data distribution (Gunduz, 2019; Ashour, El-Attar, Dey, Abd El-Kader, & Abd El-Naby, 2020).

Table 1. Comparison between algorithms

Algorithms	Basics	Test data or Data sets	Accuracy of prediction	Classifiers and Machine learning techniques
OCFA	Inspired from the colour changing characteristics of cuttlefish effecting change in visibility, reflectivity of light rays.	Speech PD Dataset, Voice PD Dataset, HandPD Meander Dataset, HandPD Spiral Datasets	**94%**	
GOA	Mimics the behaviour of grasshopper swarms in nature for solving optimization problems.	Speech PD Dataset, Voice PD Dataset, HandPD Meander Dataset, HandPD Spiral Datasets	**100%**	Random forest, k-Nearest Neighbour (k-NN) and decision tree
WSA	It is based on the social behaviour of the wolves in their nuclear families for hunting and avoiding enemies.	Speech PD Dataset, Voice PD Dataset, HandPD Meander Dataset, HandPD Spiral Datasets		Random forest (RF), support vector machines (SVM), logistic regression (LR), and artificial neural network (ANN)
ALA	Mimics the hunting pattern of ant lion (doodle bergs).		**96%**	
CSA	It is based on the intelligent behaviours of the crows.		**100%**	

Figure 4. Accuracy comparison between GOA, WSA, CFA

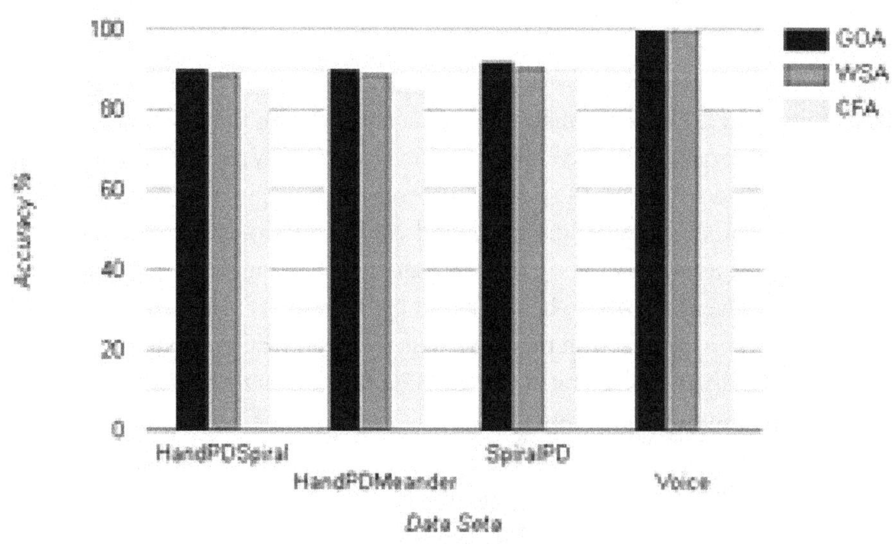

Among Modified Grasshopper Optimization Algorithm, Crow Search Algorithm and Wolf Search Algorithm, MGOA is most accurate and has smallest count of features which are shortlisted. The main reason of achieving low run time by the MGOA is its quick convergence ability, even in search space is unknown. It facilitates fast convergence by specifying the number of main iterations. MGOA possess better accuracy percentage, least false alarm rate and best detection rate.

FUTURE RESEARCH DIRECTIONS

The bio-inspired algorithms are being widely implemented for diagnosis for various diseases including the Parkinson's disease. More work can be done to combine traditional machine learning algorithms with the evolutionary algorithms. These algorithms can be applied to resolve other classification problems to predict the results with better accuracy & fewer computations than the other machine learning algorithms. These algorithms can also be applied to image datasets for classification and to compare with other algorithms present to do the same (Eesa, Brifcani, & Orman, Cuttlefish algorithm-a novel bio-inspired optimization algorithm, 2013). To solve the problem of convergence, these bio-inspired algorithms could hybridize with other methods and approaches such as chaotic theory and quantum computing to enhance their performance in future (Darwish, 2018). Further, application of these algorithms for prediction of drug-related Parkinsonian-like adverse effects can also be tried, thus, helping in recognizing individuals more likely to suffer from such extra-pyramidal symptoms.

CONCLUSION

Early diagnosis of Parkinson's disease is crucial for its timely treatment because, the disease has progressed significantly by the time its symptoms are noticed in afflicted patients. Several bio-inspired algorithms have been utilized in this regard. Optimized Cuttlefish Algorithm is a modified bio-inspired algorithm which is inspired from the colour changing characteristics of cuttlefish effecting reflectivity of light rays and change in visibility. This is obtained by a combination of chromatophores, leucophores and iridophores cells which are interacting with each other and are combined with the reflecting light to output different colours. The optimized Cuttlefish Algorithm (OCFA) has been successfully applied on the Parkinson's Datasets to optimize feature selection and this algorithm can be used in foreseeing the disease with a precision of approximately 94%. Grasshopper Optimization Algorithm is another heuristic optimization swarm intelligence algorithm based on movement of grasshoppers in search for food. Algorithms like k-Nearest Neighbour classifier, Random Forest and Decision Tree are utilized in determination of selected features. This GOA algorithm is highly effective in identification of Parkinson's disease, enabling the treatment of the disease at early stages with less complications and higher survival rates. Modified grasshopper optimization algorithm (MGOA) has been actualized using Python programming language for feature selection with the ultimate goal to minimize the value of fitness function to find the solution for Parkinson's disease detection. MGOA helps in improving the accuracy of prediction and in reduction of the selected features. The wolf search algorithm (WSA) is an algorithm inspired from the hierarchy and hunting behaviour of wolves, which has been applied for PD detection. Several other algorithms can also be used in early detection of Parkinson's disease such as; Ant lion algorithm, Crow search algorithm, etc. Dopamine Transporter Single-Photon Emission Computed Tomography determines the presynaptic dopamine neuronal dysfunction present in Parkinson's disease. Bionics Institute Rigidity Device accurately measure tremors, stiffness, and slowness of movement, Sawtooth Waveform Inspired Pitch Estimator (SWIPE) is used to determine speech disorders. Brain Stimulation Therapies stimulate a small area of the brain and treat the cognitive disorders. Bioinspired nanomedicines are less effective & Deep learning-based techniques such as Random Forest, support vector machine, DMneural, Decision Trees, Regression, and Neural network have been used for diagnosis of Parkinson's disease.

REFERENCES

Ahmadebrahimpour, E. (2019). Optimal operation of reservoir systems using the Wolf Search Algorithm (WSA). *Water Supply*, *19*(5), 1396–1404. doi:10.2166/ws.2019.005

Aljarah, I., Al-Zoubi, A. M., Faris, H., Hassonah, M. A., Mirjalili, S., & Saadeh, H. (2018). Simultaneous feature selection and support vector machine optimization using the grasshopper optimization algorithm. *Cognitive Computation*, *10*(3), 478–495. doi:10.100712559-017-9542-9

Armstrong, M. J., & Okun, M. S. (2020). Diagnosis and treatment of Parkinson disease: A review. *Journal of the American Medical Association*, *323*(6), 548–560. doi:10.1001/jama.2019.22360 PMID:32044947

Ashour, A. S., El-Attar, A., Dey, N., Abd El-Kader, H., & Abd El-Naby, M. M. (2020). Long short term memory based patient-dependent model for FOG detection in Parkinson's disease. *Pattern Recognition Letters*, *131*, 23–29. doi:10.1016/j.patrec.2019.11.036

Askarzadeh, A. (2016). A novel metaheuristic method for solving constrained engineering optimization problems: Crow search algorithm. *Computers & Structures*, *169*, 1–12. doi:10.1016/j.compstruc.2016.03.001

Ball, N., Teo, W.-P., Chandra, S., & Chapman, J. (2019). Parkinson's disease and the environment. *Frontiers in Neurology*, *10*, 218. doi:10.3389/fneur.2019.00218 PMID:30941085

Bega, D., Gonzalez-Latapi, P., Zadikoff, C., Spies, W., & Simuni, T. (2015). Is there a role for DAT-SPECT imaging in a specialty movement disorders practice? *Neurodegenerative Diseases*, *15*(2), 81–86. doi:10.1159/000370116 PMID:25592727

Brownlee, J. (2011). *Clever algorithms: Nature-inspired programming recipes*. Jason Brownlee.

Cai, X., Gao, X., & Xue, Y. (2016). Improved bat algorithm with optimal forage strategy and random disturbance strategy. *International Journal of Bio-inspired Computation*, *8*(4), 205–214. doi:10.1504/IJBIC.2016.078666

Chiang, H.-S., Sangaiah, A. K., Chen, M.-Y., & Liu, J.-Y. (2020). A novel artificial bee colony optimization algorithm with SVM for bio-inspired software-defined networking. *International Journal of Parallel Programming*, *48*(2), 310–328. doi:10.100710766-018-0594-6

Corne, D. W., & Lones, M. A. (2018). *Evolutionary algorithms*. arXiv preprint arXiv:1805.11014.

Darwish, A. (2018). Bio-inspired computing: Algorithms review, deep analysis, and the scope of applications. *Future Computing and Informatics Journal*, *3*(2), 231–246. doi:10.1016/j.fcij.2018.06.001

Das, R. (2010). A comparison of multiple classification methods for diagnosis of Parkinson disease. *Expert Systems with Applications, 37*(2), 1568–1572. doi:10.1016/j.eswa.2009.06.040

Dauer, W., & Przedborski, S. (2003). Parkinson's disease: Mechanisms and models. *Neuron, 39*(6), 889–909. doi:10.1016/S0896-6273(03)00568-3 PMID:12971891

Davie, C. A. (2008). A review of Parkinson's disease. *British Medical Bulletin, 86*(1), 109–127. doi:10.1093/bmb/ldn013 PMID:18398010

De Lau, L. M., & Breteler, M. M. (2006). Epidemiology of Parkinson's disease. *Lancet Neurology, 5*(6), 525–535. doi:10.1016/S1474-4422(06)70471-9 PMID:16713924

Dickson, D. W. (2012). Parkinson's disease and parkinsonism: Neuropathology. *Cold Spring Harbor Perspectives in Medicine, 2*(8), a009258. doi:10.1101/cshperspect.a009258 PMID:22908195

Dorigo, M., Maniezzo, V., & Colorni, A. (1996). Ant system: Optimization by a colony of cooperating agents. *IEEE Transactions on Systems, Man, and Cybernetics. Part B, Cybernetics, 26*(1), 29–41. doi:10.1109/3477.484436 PMID:18263004

Eberhart, R., & Kennedy, J. (1995). A new optimizer using particle swarm theory. *MHS'95. Proceedings of the Sixth International Symposium on Micro Machine and Human Science*, 39–43. 10.1109/MHS.1995.494215

Eesa, A. S., Brifcani, A. M., & Orman, Z. (2013). Cuttlefish algorithm-a novel bio-inspired optimization algorithm. *International Journal of Scientific and Engineering Research, 4*, 1978–1986.

Eesa, A. S., Brifcani, A. M., & Orman, Z. (2014). A new tool for global optimization problems-cuttlefish algorithm. *International Journal of Mathematical, Computational. Natural and Physical Engineering, 8*, 1208–1211.

Eesa, A. S., Orman, Z., & Brifcani, A. M. (2015). A novel feature-selection approach based on the cuttlefish optimization algorithm for intrusion detection systems. *Expert Systems with Applications, 42*(5), 2670–2679. doi:10.1016/j.eswa.2014.11.009

Ewees, A. A., Abd Elaziz, M., & Houssein, E. H. (2018). Improved grasshopper optimization algorithm using opposition-based learning. *Expert Systems with Applications, 112*, 156–172. doi:10.1016/j.eswa.2018.06.023

Gunduz, H. (2019). Deep learning-based Parkinson's disease classification using vocal feature sets. *IEEE Access: Practical Innovations, Open Solutions, 7*, 115540–115551. doi:10.1109/ACCESS.2019.2936564

Gupta, D., & Ahlawat, A. K. (2017). Usability feature selection via MBBAT: A novel approach. *Journal of Computational Science, 23*, 195–203. doi:10.1016/j.jocs.2017.06.005

Gupta, D., Julka, A., Jain, S., Aggarwal, T., Khanna, A., Arunkumar, N., & de Albuquerque, V. H. (2018). Optimized cuttlefish algorithm for diagnosis of Parkinson's disease. *Cognitive Systems Research, 52*, 36–48. doi:10.1016/j.cogsys.2018.06.006

Gupta, D., Sundaram, S., Khanna, A., Hassanien, A. E., & De Albuquerque, V. H. (2018). Improved diagnosis of Parkinson's disease using optimized crow search algorithm. *Computers & Electrical Engineering, 68*, 412–424. doi:10.1016/j.compeleceng.2018.04.014

Gupta, S. (2020). Smartphone based Early Detection of Epileptic Seizures Using Machine Learning. *Proceedings of the 2020 12th International Conference on Bioinformatics and Biomedical Technology*, 38–42. 10.1145/3405758.3405763

Gupta, S. (2014). *Repetitive Transcranial Magnetic Stimulation (RTMS) for the Treatment of Depression*. Migraine and Parkinson's Disease.

Gupta, S., HariPrasad, S. A., & Kumar, A. (2018). Bionics Based Emergency Contact for Treatment of Epilepsy. *Proceedings of the 2018 10th International Conference on Bioinformatics and Biomedical Technology*, 46–50. 10.1145/3232059.3232064

Gupta, S., Singh, V. K., & ... (2015). Bionics Based Solar Powered Clothing for Treating Parkinson's Disease and Epilepsy. *International Journal of Life Sciences Biotechnology and Pharma Research, 4*, 132.

Hastie, T., Tibshirani, R., & Friedman, J. H. (2009). Statistics The Elements of Statistical Learning. *The Mathematical Intelligencer, 27*, 83–85.

Heidari, A. A., Faris, H., Aljarah, I., & Mirjalili, S. (2019). An efficient hybrid multilayer perceptron neural network with grasshopper optimization. *Soft Computing, 23*(17), 7941–7958. doi:10.100700500-018-3424-2

Hichem, H., Elkamel, M., Rafik, M., Mesaaoud, M. T., & Ouahiba, C. (2019). A new binary grasshopper optimization algorithm for feature selection problem. *Journal of King Saud University-Computer and Information Sciences*.

Hopfner, F., Künstner, A., Müller, S. H., Künzel, S., Zeuner, K. E., Margraf, N. G., Deuschl, G., Baines, J. F., & Kuhlenbäumer, G. (2017). Gut microbiota in Parkinson disease in a northern German cohort. *Brain Research, 1667*, 41–45. doi:10.1016/j.brainres.2017.04.019 PMID:28506555

Ibrahim, H. T., Mazher, W. J., Ucan, O. N., & Bayat, O. (2019). A grasshopper optimizer approach for feature selection and optimizing SVM parameters utilizing real biomedical data sets. *Neural Computing & Applications, 31*(10), 5965–5974. doi:10.100700521-018-3414-4

Jankovic, J. (2008). Parkinson's disease: Clinical features and diagnosis. *Journal of Neurology, Neurosurgery, and Psychiatry, 79*(4), 368–376. doi:10.1136/jnnp.2007.131045 PMID:18344392

Kägi, G., Bhatia, K. P., & Tolosa, E. (2010). The role of DAT-SPECT in movement disorders. *Journal of Neurology, Neurosurgery, and Psychiatry, 81*(1), 5–12. doi:10.1136/jnnp.2008.157370 PMID:20019219

Kowalski, P. A., Łukasik, S., Charytanowicz, M., & Kulczycki, P. (2018). Optimizing clustering with cuttlefish algorithm. *Conference on Information Technology, Systems Research and Computational Physics*, 34–43.

Li, J., Fong, S., Wong, R. K., Millham, R., & Wong, K. K. (2017). Elitist binary wolf search algorithm for heuristic feature selection in high-dimensional bioinformatics datasets. *Scientific Reports, 7*(1), 1–14. doi:10.103841598-017-04037-5 PMID:28659577

Little, M., McSharry, P., Hunter, E., Spielman, J., & Ramig, L. (2008). Suitability of dysphonia measurements for telemonitoring of Parkinson's disease. *Nature Proceedings*, 1–1. doi:10.1038/npre.2008.2298.1

Martínez-Álvarez, F., Asencio-Cortés, G., Torres, J. F., Gutiérrez-Avilés, D., Melgar-García, L., Pérez-Chacón, R., Rubio-Escudero, C., Riquelme, J. C., & Troncoso, A. (2020). Coronavirus optimization algorithm: A bioinspired metaheuristic based on the COVID-19 propagation model. *Big Data*, *8*(4), 308–322. doi:10.1089/big.2020.0051 PMID:32716641

Mäthger, L. M., Denton, E. J., Marshall, N. J., & Hanlon, R. T. (2009). Mechanisms and behavioural functions of structural coloration in cephalopods. *Journal of the Royal Society, Interface*, *6*(suppl_2), S149–S163. doi:10.1098/rsif.2008.0366.focus PMID:19091688

Meraihi, Y., Gabis, A. B., Mirjalili, S., & Ramdane-Cherif, A. (2021). Grasshopper optimization algorithm: Theory, variants, and applications. *IEEE Access: Practical Innovations, Open Solutions*, *9*, 50001–50024. doi:10.1109/ACCESS.2021.3067597

Mirjalili, S. (2015). Moth-flame optimization algorithm: A novel nature-inspired heuristic paradigm. *Knowledge-Based Systems*, *89*, 228–249. doi:10.1016/j.knosys.2015.07.006

Mirjalili, S. (2015). The ant lion optimizer. *Advances in Engineering Software*, *83*, 80–98. doi:10.1016/j.advengsoft.2015.01.010

Mirjalili, S. (2016). Dragonfly algorithm: A new meta-heuristic optimization technique for solving single-objective, discrete, and multi-objective problems. *Neural Computing & Applications*, *27*(4), 1053–1073. doi:10.100700521-015-1920-1

Mirjalili, S., & Lewis, A. (2016). The whale optimization algorithm. *Advances in Engineering Software*, *95*, 51–67. doi:10.1016/j.advengsoft.2016.01.008

Mirjalili, S., Mirjalili, S. M., & Lewis, A. (2014). Grey wolf optimizer. *Advances in Engineering Software*, *69*, 46–61. doi:10.1016/j.advengsoft.2013.12.007

Mitragotri, S. (2013). Devices for overcoming biological barriers: The use of physical forces to disrupt the barriers. *Advanced Drug Delivery Reviews*, *65*(1), 100–103. doi:10.1016/j.addr.2012.07.016 PMID:22960787

Parlar, T. (2021). A heuristic approach with artificial neural network for Parkinson's disease. *International Journal of Applied Mathematics Electronics and Computers*, *9*(1), 1–6. doi:10.18100/ijamec.802599

Perera, T., Lee, W.-L., Jones, M., Tan, J. L., Proud, E. L., Begg, A., Sinclair, N. C., Peppard, R., & McDermott, H. J. (2019). A palm-worn device to quantify rigidity in Parkinson's disease. *Journal of Neuroscience Methods*, *317*, 113–120. doi:10.1016/j.jneumeth.2019.02.006 PMID:30776378

Poewe, W., Seppi, K., Tanner, C. M., Halliday, G. M., Brundin, P., Volkmann, J., Schrag, A.-E., & Lang, A. E. (2017). Parkinson disease. *Nature Reviews. Disease Primers*, *3*(1), 1–21. doi:10.1038/nrdp.2017.13 PMID:28332488

Rehman, F. U. (2020). Impact of bioinspired nanotechnology on brain diseases amelioration. *Biometrical Letters*, *6*, 17–22.

Saremi, S., Mirjalili, S., & Lewis, A. (2017). Grasshopper optimisation algorithm: Theory and application. *Advances in Engineering Software, 105*, 30–47. doi:10.1016/j.advengsoft.2017.01.004

Sehgal, S., Agarwal, M., Gupta, D., Sundaram, S., & Bashambu, A. (2020). Optimized grass hopper algorithm for diagnosis of Parkinson's disease. *SN Applied Sciences*, *2*(6), 1–18. doi:10.100742452-020-2826-9

Sharma, P., Jain, R., Sharma, M., & Gupta, D. (2019). Parkinson's diagnosis using ant-lion optimisation algorithm. *International Journal of Innovative Computing and Applications*, *10*(3/4), 138–146. doi:10.1504/IJICA.2019.103370

Shin, H.-W., & Chung, S. J. (2012). Drug-induced parkinsonism. *Journal of Clinical Neurology (Seoul, Korea)*, *8*(1), 15–21. doi:10.3988/jcn.2012.8.1.15 PMID:22523509

Simon, D. K., Tanner, C. M., & Brundin, P. (2020). Parkinson disease epidemiology, pathology, genetics, and pathophysiology. *Clinics in Geriatric Medicine*, *36*(1), 1–12. doi:10.1016/j.cger.2019.08.002 PMID:31733690

Singh, A. K., Kumar, A., Mahmud, M., Kaiser, M. S., & Kishore, A. (2021). COVID-19 Infection detection from chest X-ray images using hybrid social group optimization and support vector classifier. *Cognitive Computation*, 1–13. doi:10.100712559-021-09848-3 PMID:33688379

Venkatesh, C., & Bojja, P. (2020). Lung cancer detection using bio-inspired algorithm in CT scans and secure data transmission through IoT cloud. *International Journal of Advanced Computer Science and Applications*, *11*(11), 2020. doi:10.14569/IJACSA.2020.0111148

Wang, W., Lee, J., Harrou, F., & Sun, Y. (2020). Early detection of Parkinson's disease using deep learning and machine learning. *IEEE Access: Practical Innovations, Open Solutions*, *8*, 147635–147646. doi:10.1109/ACCESS.2020.3016062

Williams, D. R., & Litvan, I. (2013). Parkinsonian syndromes. *Continuum: Lifelong Learning in Neurology, 19*, 1189.

Yang, X.-S., Gandomi, A. H., Talatahari, S., & Alavi, A. H. (2012). *Metaheuristics in water, geotechnical and transport engineering*. Newnes.

Yang, X.-S., Karamanoglu, M., & He, X. (2014). Flower pollination algorithm: A novel approach for multiobjective optimization. *Engineering Optimization*, *46*(9), 1222–1237. doi:10.1080/0305215X.2013.832237

Zang, H., Zhang, S., & Hapeshi, K. (2010). A review of nature-inspired algorithms. *Journal of Bionics Engineering*, *7*(S4), S232–S237. doi:10.1016/S1672-6529(09)60240-7

Chapter 2
The Human Brain:
Its Structure and Functions

Priya Dev
Institute of Medical Sciences, Banaras Hindu University, India

ABSTRACT

The human brain is a very complex entity with a distinctive organisation and function. There are three main structures in brain: the cerebrum, the cerebellum, and brain stem. Further, these structures are subdivided into more parts depending on their position in the brain. The cerebrum is the major portion of brain with sulcus and gyrus of folded structure and deep structures too. Corpus callosum connects the right and left hemisphere of brain to communicate. Each hemisphere of the brain is further classified into four regions: frontal, temporal, parietal, occipital lobes. Each lobe deals with different functions. For understanding any disease or doing research or treatment, one should have a depth of knowledge of the brain, its parts, and the functioning of different lobes and regions. Therefore, this chapter will deal with in-depth knowledge of the brain parts, not only anatomically but also their functionality.

INTRODUCTION

The Human Brain

The brain is the most volatile body part in the anthropological body. It creates all our considerations, activity, memory, sensation and involvement of the world. This organ like mass of tissue, slanting the scales at around 1.4 kilograms, contains one hundred billion nerve cells, or neurons.

The complexity of the accessibility between these cells is stunning. Each neuron can associate with thousands or even colossal quantity of others, through little developments called synapses. Model and strength of the affiliations is consistently changing and no two brain organs are comparable. It is in these changing affiliations that memories are taken care of, inclinations learned and characters shaped, by developing explicit instances of brain activity, and bringing up the rear others.

The brain consists of three main structures called cerebrum, cerebellum and brain stem. (Fig.1: Different parts of brain and their function) The brain is divided in to two parts left and right hemisphere

DOI: 10.4018/978-1-7998-9534-3.ch002

which is connected by a group of neural fibres called the corpus callosum. The corpus callosum allows the communication between two hemispheres thereby coordination between the two sides of the body. The word split brain syndrome indicates the neurological condition caused by severing or lesioning of corpus callosum. It causes the disruption in the white matter connection between two parts of the brain. The condition may lead to the incoordination between the both sides of the body. Among the major three parts the cerebrum occupies the greatest surface area of the human brain which has grooves and folds, Known as sulci and gyri respectively. The second largest area of the brain cerebellum is situated at the back of the head. it is responsible for the constant streams of information between brain and body. Third part of the brain named brain stem or hind brain is situated in the bottom of the brain and is the top part of the spinal cord. It controls the autonomic functions which are not under conscious control. Based on the position the brain can be divided as frontal, temporal, parietal and occipital lobes. As the name suggest the frontal lobe (left and right) is situated in the front part of the brain. The temporal lobes are located ventral to the Sylvian fissure and the parietal lobes. The smallest region called occipital lobes is located back of the brain.

Figure 1. Different parts of brain and their function

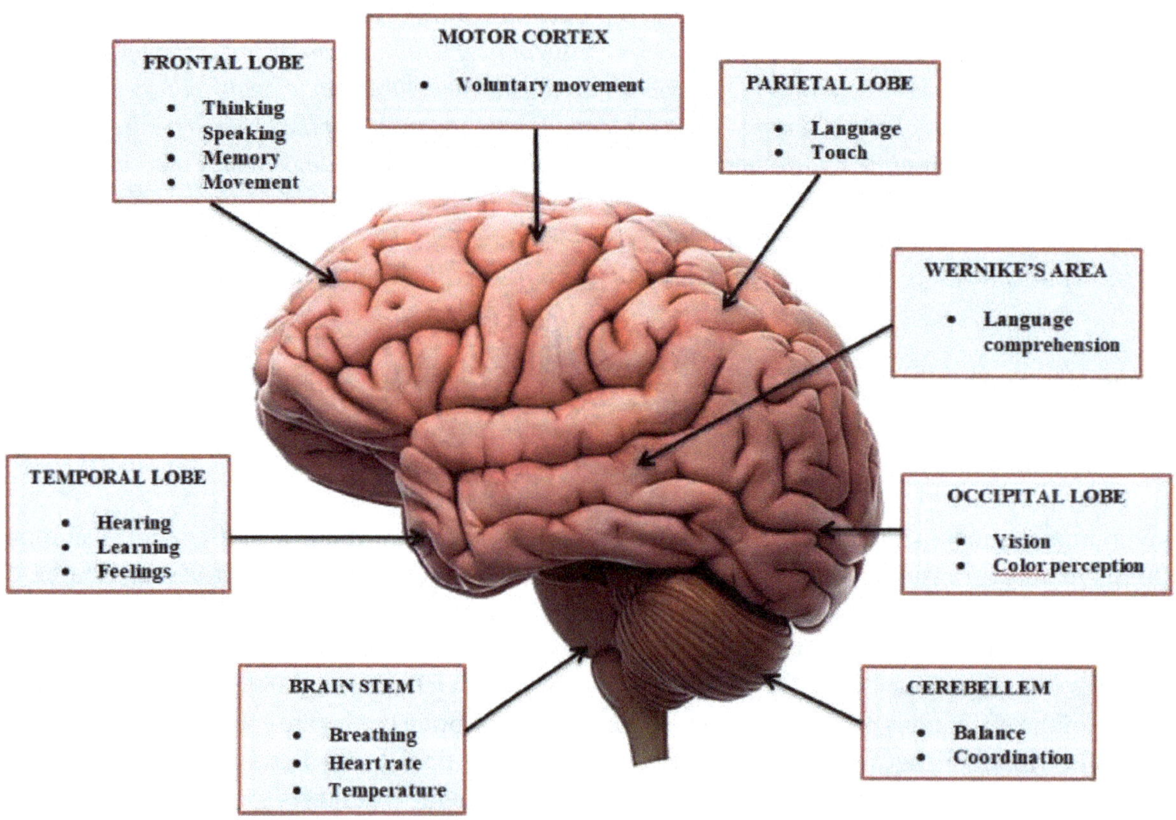

Grey Matter

Despite the fact people oftentimes talk about their "faint matter", the brain similarly contains grey matter. The faint matter is the telephone gatherings of the neurons, while the white matter is the growing organization of string like rings – called dendrites and axons – that spread out from the telephone bodies to connect with various neurons.

Notwithstanding, "the brain similarly has another, substantially more different kind of cell, called glial cells. These bantam neurons on different occasions over. At the point when thought to be support cells, they are presently known to improve neural signs and to be practically pretty much as huge as neurons in mental calculations. There are a wide scope of kinds of neuron, only one of which is novel to individuals and the other uncommon gorillas, the supposed shaft cells."

Brain structure is formed part of the way by qualities, yet generally by experience. Just generally as of late it was found that new brain cells are being brought into the world for the duration of our lives – an interaction called neurogenesis. The brain has eruptions of development and afterward times of combination, when overabundance associations are pruned. The most prominent blasts are in the initial a few years of life, during pubescence, and furthermore a last barged in youthful adulthood.

Anatomy of Brain

The brain is the point of convergence of the tangible framework in all vertebrate. The scientists say that, "It is arranged in the head, ordinarily close to the fundamental substantial organs for such resources as vision, hearing, harmony, taste, and smell. The brain of a vertebrate is the most baffling organ in its body. In a typical human the cerebral cortex (the greatest part) is evaluated to contain about 15–33 billion neurons (Pelvig et al., 2008), each related by synapses to a couple thousand distinct neurons. These neurons talk with one another through long protoplasmic strands called axons, which pass on trains of sign pulses called action prospects to distant bits of the brain or body zeroing in on unequivocal recipient cells. As per an evolutionary-biological point of view, the limit of the brain is to apply bound together control over various organs of the body. The brain circles back to the rest of the body either by making instances of muscle development or by driving discharge of engineered materials called synthetic substances. This joined control allows fast and worked with responses to changes in the environment. Some crucial kinds of responsiveness, for instance, reflexes can be interceded by the spinal line or periphery ganglia, yet current purposeful control of direct ward on complex material data requires the information-integrating capacities of a consolidated brain. According to a philosophical perspective, what makes the brain exceptional in contrast with different organs is that it frames the actual construction that produces the psyche. As Hippocrates put it: ″Men should realize that from nothing else except for the brain come delights, enjoyments, giggling and sports, distresses, pain's, dejection, and groans Hippocrates (400 BCE)." In the early piece of brain research, the psyche was believed to be independent from the brain. Nonetheless, after early researchers led tests it was resolved that the psyche was a segment of a working brain that communicated certain practices dependent on the outside climate and the improvement of the organism. (Rosenberger et al., 2011) The components by which brain movement leads to cognizance and thought have been exceptionally difficult to comprehend: notwithstanding fast logical advancement, much about how the brain works stays a secret. The tasks of individual brain cells are presently perceived in significant detail, however the manner in which they participate in gatherings of millions has been extremely challenging to translate. The most encouraging methodologies treat the brain as an organic

PC, totally different in instrument from electronic PCs, yet comparative as in it obtains data from the encompassing scene, stores it, and cycles it in an assortment of ways.
The main vertebrate brain parts are:

- The medulla, alongside the spinal string, contains numerous little cores associated with a wide assortment of tangible and engine capacities.
- The pons mendacities in the brainstem straight over the medulla. In addition to other things, it contains cores that control rest, breath, gulping, bladder work, balance, eye development, looks, and stance (Seigel, 2010).
- The operational hub is a little district at the establishment of the prosencephalon, whose complexity and position distorts its size. It is made out of different little centres, each with undeniable affiliations and neurochemistry. The operational hub oversees rest and wake cycles, eating and consumption, synthetic conveyance, and various other essential inherent limits (Swaab et al., 2003). The thalamus is another assortment of cores with different capacities. Some are associated with transferring data to and from the cerebral sides of the equator. Others are engaged with inspiration. The subthalamic region appears to contain action-generating frameworks for a few sorts of ″consummatory″ practices, including eating, drinking, crap, and sex (Yen CT et al., 1985).
- The cerebellum tweaks the yields of other brain frameworks to make them exact. Expulsion of the cerebellum doesn't keep a creature from doing anything specifically, yet it makes activities reluctant and cumbersome. This exactness isn't built-in, however scholarly by experimentation.
- The optic tectum permits activities to be coordinated toward focuses in space, most regularly in light of visual information. In warm blooded animals it is normally alluded to as the unrivaled work is to coordinate eye developments. It likewise coordinates arriving at developments and other object-directed activities (Saitoh et al., 2007).
- The pallium is a deposit of dim matter that lies on the outside of the prosencephalon. In reptiles and warm-blooded animals, it is known as the cerebral cortex. Different capacities include the pallium, together with olfaction and spatial retention. In warm blooded creatures, where it turns out to be so huge as to overwhelm the brain, it assumes control over capacities from numerous other brain regions. In numerous warm-blooded creatures, the cerebral cortex comprises of collapsed swells considered gyri that make profound wrinkles or crevices termed sulci. The folds increment the exterior space of the cortex and thusly increment the measure of dark matter and the measure of data that can be prepared (Puelles, 2001).
- The hippocampus, rigorously talking, is discovered distinctly in vertebrates. Notwithstanding, the region it gets from, the average pallium, has partners in all vertebrates (Salas et al. 2003). The basal ganglia tends to be a gathering of interconnected constructions in the forebrain. The essential capacity of the basal ganglia seems, by all accounts, to be activity choice: they convey inhibitory messages to all pieces of the organ that can create engine practices, and in the right conditions can deliver the restraint, so the frameworks can execute their activities. Prize and discipline apply their most significant neural impacts by changing associations inside the basal ganglia (Grillner et al., 2005)

Physiology

Also the author develops that, "The elements of the brain rely upon the capacity of neurons to communicate electrochemical signs to different cells, and their capacity to react suitably to electrochemical signs got from different cells. The power-driven properties of neurons are constrained by a wide assortment of biochemical and metabolic cycles, most prominently the cooperation among synapses and receptors that happen at neurotransmitters. Synapses are synthetics that are delivered at neurotransmitters when an activity potential initiates them—synapses connect themselves to receptor particles on the film of the synapse's target cell, and along these lines adjust the electrical or compound properties of the receptor atoms. With few special cases, every neuron in the brain delivers a similar compound synapse, or mix of synapses, at all the synaptic associations it makes with different neurons." In this manner, a neuron can be described by the synapses that it discharges.

Functions of Brain

According to an evolutionary-biological point of view, the capacity of the brain is to give lucid authority over the activities. A brought together brain permits gatherings of muscles to be co-activated in complex examples; it additionally permits boosts impinging on one piece of the body to summon reactions in different parts, and it can keep various pieces of the body from acting at cross-purposes to one another (Sutton MA and Carew, 2000). To create intentional and brought together activity, the brain initially brings data from receptors together at a focal area. It then, at that point measures this crude information to remove data about the design of the climate. Next it consolidates the prepared tactile data with data about the current requirements and with memory of past conditions.

Knowledge - One of the fundamental components of a brain is to eliminate organically material information from substantial wellsprings of data. The human brain is outfitted with information about light, sound, the compound design of the air, temperature, head bearing, member position, the substance course of action of the dissemination framework, and that is only the start. By one way or another, these material modalities are from the start perceived by explicit sensors that adventure signals into the brain.

Motor control: Motor systems are spaces of the brain that are clearly or by suggestion drew in with making body improvements, that is, in starting muscles. Except for the muscles that control the eye, which are driven by centres in the midbrain, all of the deliberate muscles in the body are directly innervated by motor neurons in the spinal string and hindbrain. Spinal motor neurons are controlled both by neural circuits trademark for the spinal rope, and by inputs that slip from the brain. The natural spinal circuits execute various reflex responses, and contain plan generators for melodic improvements like walking or swimming.

The diving relationship from the brain thinks about more present day control. The brain contains a couple of motor districts that project clearly to the spinal string. At the most diminished level is motor locales in the medulla and pons, which control summed up advancements like walking, breathing, or swallowing. At a more raised level are districts in the midbrain, similar to the red centre, which is liable for arranging advancements of the arms and legs. At a more huge level yet is the fundamental motor cortex, a segment of tissue arranged at the back edge of the forward looking projection. The fundamental motor cortex sends projections to the subcortical motor locales, yet moreover sends an immense projection directly to the spinal rope, through the pyramidal part. This direct corticospinal projection considers careful intentional control of the fine nuances of improvements. Other motor-related brain locales apply assistant effects by projecting to the fundamental motor districts. Among the fundamental discretionary locales are the premotor cortex, basal ganglia, and cerebellum. The human brain controls the central tangible framework, by means of the cranial nerves and spinal line, the periphery tactile framework and directs for all intents and purposes all human action. Compulsory, or "lower," activities, for example, pulse, breath, and absorption, are unknowingly administered by the brain, explicitly through the autonomic sensory system. Complex, or "higher," mental action, like idea, reason, and reflection, is intentionally controlled. Anatomically, the brain can be isolated into three sections: the forebrain, midbrain, and hindbrain; the forebrain incorporates the few flaps of the cerebral cortex that control higher capacities, while the mid and hindbrain are more engaged with oblivious, autonomic capacities. During encephalization, human brain mass expanded past that of different species comparative with weight. This interaction was particularly articulated in the neocortex, a segment of the brain engaged with language and cognizance.

The neocortex represents about 76% of the mass of the human brain; with a neocortex a lot bigger than different creatures, people appreciate novel intellectual abilities notwithstanding having a neuroarchitecture like that of more crude species. Essential frameworks that ready people to boosts, sense occasions in the climate, and keep up with homeostasis are like those of fundamental vertebrates. Human awareness is established upon the all-encompassing limit of the cutting edge neocortex, just as the significantly evolved constructions of the brain stem. A cerebral half of the globe (hemispherium cerebrale) is characterized as one of the two districts of the brain that are outlined by the body's middle plane. The brain would thus be able to be depicted as being partitioned into left and right cerebral halves of the globe. Every one of these halves of the globe has an external layer of dark matter considered the cerebral cortex that is upheld by an internal layer of white matter. The sides of the equator are connected by the corpus callosum, an extremely huge heap of nerve strands, and furthermore by other more modest commissures, including the foremost commissure, back commissure, and hippocampal commissure. These commissures move data between the two halves of the globe to arrange confined capacities.

The engineering, sorts of cells, kinds of synapses and receptor subtypes are completely conveyed among the two sides of the equator in a particularly hilter kilter design. Practically around 20 years prior neuro-scientist recommended that the hardware of the cerebellum looks like the learning machine known as the "perceptron." A perceptron figures out how to relegate a proper yield to each contribution by submitting to the ideas of its "instructor". The instructor gives support when the perceptron is fruitful and demoralization in any case. Marr and Albus recommended that the climbing filaments in the cerebellum assume the part of the instructor, and the overgrown strands assume the part of the contribution to which the perceptron should allocate yield.

Perceptions are at this point not stylish. Nonetheless, the overall perspective on the cerebellum as a learning machine has gotten a lot of exploratory help. Vestibulo-ocular reflex — the reflex which keeps the look of the eye at a fixed point, paying little mind to head development depends on an exceptionally itemized program, yet it is additionally situation-dependent in specific regards; and it is currently evident that the cerebellum can change the increase of the vestibulo-ocular reflex in a versatile manner. The cerebellum, in itself, isn't fit for organizing complex developments. In any case, Fabre and Buser (1980) have recommended that comparative learning happens in the engine cortex — the piece of the cortex that is straightforwardly associated with the cerebellum. To get familiar with a perplexing development, one should accomplish something beyond change a couple of mathematical qualities in a past movement for example the addition of a reflex circular segment, the speed of a muscle development and so forth (Fabre and Buser, 1980)

Psychological Functions of Human Brain

Discernment is consistent; believing is our specialty. The investigation of discernment has huge consequences for a general comprehension of how you perform on an everyday premise. The investigation of comprehension likewise loans bits of knowledge past brain science. Neuroscience endeavours to indicate the connection among psyche and brain. Psychological neuroscience includes relating intellectual cycles to their neural substrates that is the thing that the brain is doing when the psyche is thinking. There is a great deal that science doesn't comprehend about the learning interaction. Each individual conceived can learn at some level. The brain is considered as the "equipment" of the human PC framework and the various psychological cycle as the "product"; taking part in various mental activities which is closely resembling running distinctive programming bundles.

"The human brain is the focal organ of the human material system and with the spinal line makes up the focal substantial structure. The arrangement of brain incorporates the frontal cortex, the brainstem and the cerebellum. It controls a large portion of the exercises of the body, preparing, intertwining, and organizing the data it gets from the receptors, and settling on choices concerning the headings moved off the remainder of the body. The brain is contained in, and got by, the skull bones of the head. The frontal cortex is the best piece of the human brain. It is segregated into two cerebral sides of the equator. The cerebral cortex is an external layer of weak matter, covering the point of convergence of white matter. The cortex is isolated into the neocortex and the fundamentally more modest allocortex. The neocortex is included six neuronal layers, while the allocortex has three or four. Each side of the equator is generally allocated into four overlays the forward looking, transient, parietal, and occipital projections. The forward looking fold is associated with pioneer limits including limitation, arranging, thinking, and determined idea, while the occipital projection is focused on vision. Inside each crease, cortical areas are associated with express restricts, like the undeniable, engine and union districts. However the left and right sides of the equator are totally close to fit and, several cutoff points are associated with one side, like language in the left and visual-spatial cutoff pushed. The sides of the equator are connected by commissural nerve divides, most noteworthy being the corpus callosum. The frontal cortex is connected by the brainstem to the spinal rope. The brainstem includes the midbrain, the pons, and the medulla oblongata. The cerebellum is connected with the brainstem by sets of packs. Inside the frontal cortex is the ventricular framework, remembering four interconnected ventricles for which cerebrospinal liquid is passed on and streamed. Under the cerebral cortex several basic turns of events, including the thalamus, the epithalamus, the pineal organ, the functional center, the pituitary organ, and the subthalamus; the limbic plans, including the amygdala and the hippocampus; the claustrum, the different focuses of the basal ganglia; the basal forebrain structures, and the three circumventricular organs. The cells of the brain unite neurons and predictable glial cells. There are in excess of 86 billion neurons in the brain, and an essentially equivalent number of different cells. Brain movement is made conceivable by the interconnections of neurons and their appearance of synapses because of nerve motivations. Neurons structure elaborate neural organizations of neural pathways and circuits. The entire gear is driven by the example of neurotransmission. The brain is gotten by the skull, suspended in cerebrospinal liquid, and limited from the circulatory structure by the blood–brain obstacle. Edge the brain is presented to harm, infection, and debasement."

Laterisation of Brain Function

Laterality implies the plan and limit of coordinated with organs or of two in like manner arranged spaces of non-paired organs, passed on the right and left sides. It deduces that particular limits are differentially tended to in the various sides of the brain. While the contemplations of brain lateralization and hemispheric transcendence are smart since long the picture is at this point not agreeable past a general clarification that there are different sides of the equator which shift in specialization and there is hemispheric lop-sidedness. Verification, kind of procedure, extent of sense modalities, and the work of various organismic and setting focused variables is yet not palatable. Laterality is essential comparably utilitarian. Essentially, the cortex is isolated anatomically into equal parts of the globe, the right and the left. The different sides of the equator are for the most part adjusted clearly, anyway not in plan and limits. For instance, while the left 50% of the globe (LH) is found to have longer sylvian fissure, decently more dim matter, greater planum temporale, and more broad occipital projection, the right half of the equator (RH) is recorded to be heavier, having greater Herschel's gyrus and a broader forward looking fold.

This fundamental irregularity prompts reasonable lop-sidedness. While the LH invests huge energy in taking care of information that is dominatingly logical, straight, consecutive, and transient, the RH addresses impressive expert in planning information that is made, configurational, coordinated, and exhaustive in nature. Accurate evidence recommends that in a bigger piece of the human people, however the RH is superior to the LH for visuo-spatial limits. In any case, in a liberal minority of the general population, hemispheric lop-sidedness doesn't follow this model. The minority with odd hemispheric awkwardness may show a pivoted heading of hemispheric lop-sidedness or various degrees of bilateralization of language and visuo-spatial limits. Solitary assortments in hemispheric unevenness have been credited to countless factors, similar to heredity, cytoplasmic left-right point, foetal testosterone levels, loss of epic axons, and birth pressure (Krupski et al, 1971). A longitudinal hole secludes the human brain into two specific cerebral parts of the globe, related by the corpus callosum. The sides seem as though each other and each hemisphere's structure is generally reflected by the contrary side. Anyway despite the strong anatomical likenesses, the components of each cortical portion of the globe are directed in an unforeseen manner. For example, the level sulcus all around is longer in the left half of the equator than in the right 50% of the globe.

Expansive speculations are frequently made in famous brain science around one side or the other having trademark marks, for example, ″logical″ or ″creative″. These marks should be dealt with cautiously; albeit a sidelong predominance is quantifiable, these qualities are truth be told existent in the two sides (Westen et al. 2006) and test proof offers little help for corresponding the underlying contrasts between the sides with useful contrasts. The degree of any measured quality, or specialization of brain work by region, stays being scrutinized. On the off chance that a particular locale of the brain or even a whole half of the globe is either harmed or annihilated, its capacities can now and then be expected by an adjoining district, even in the contrary side of the equator, contingent on the space harmed and the patient′s age. At the point when injury meddles with pathways starting with one region then onto the next, elective (aberrant) associations may come to exist to discuss data with disengaged regions, regardless of the failures. While capacities are lateralized, these are just a propensity. The pattern across numerous people may likewise shift essentially with respect to how a particular capacity is executed.

The spaces of examination of this causal or helpful difference of a particular brain work join its gross anatomy, dendritic development, and neural connection appointment. The essential and compound change of a particular brain work, between the different sides of the equator of one brain or between comparative portions of the globe of two unmistakable brains, is at this point being thought of. Brain work lateralization is evident in the wonders of right- or left-handedness and of right or left ear tendency, anyway a person's supported hand is authentically not a conspicuous indication of the space of brain work. "Though 95% of right-handed people have left-hemisphere strength for language, only 18.8% of left-handed people have right-hemisphere transcendence for language work. Besides, 19.8% of the left-handed have separate language limits. (Taylor, 1990) Even inside various language limits (e.g., semantics, phonetic design, prosody), degree (and surprisingly 50% of the globe) of solidarity may shift. Handedness is the clearest kind of scholarly and lead disparity declared in individuals. It insinuates the tendency to play out a couple of tasks with one hand rather than the other. Moreover, the brain part covered up handedness is so much that handedness is contra at the edge related to the two parts of the globe, passed nearby to and right hand to the LH. There is evidence that left- and right handers contrast when investigated on a grouping of social measures. This undoubtedly lean toward the right hand for manual activities, to be more capable and stunning with the right-hand, and to have language lateralized to the contra sidelong left cerebral portion of the globe. Appropriately, in right- handers the neural circumstance that add to these practices are lateralized dominatingly to the LH, and the hand used to create is contralateral to the side of the equator intervening language limits. Alternately, in numerous lefthanders language is ipsilateral to the supported hand. LH dominating for language. Additionally, left handers will undoubtedly be isolated on extents of hand tendency, capacity and strength than right-handers. In various social orders including the Indian culture, the right hand is the supported hand and the left hand is avoided and serious approvals about its use are taken note. Past research has exhibited that in various non-western social orders the transcendence of right handedness is more important than that found in the Western social orders. (Scharoun and Bryden, 2014)

Handedness has ideas for task execution and raises stresses for making distinctive methodology game plans at the work place. This is huge considering the way that the environment and various gadgets and instruments are routinely organized for right-handed people. Handedness, regardless, has been moved nearer as per the perspective of tendency similarly as execution. While execution measures are social and fair-minded, the tendency measures incorporate self-reports and are essentially established on memory. Considering these and related differences a couple of subject matter experts battle that hand tendency and disproportionate endeavor execution incorporate commonly different wonders. This is in light of the fact that, first, the associations between's hand tendency and hand execution irregular characteristics are of simply subtle size. Second, the scores on tendency and execution gauges yield indisputable people spreads.

While the general population scattering of hand tendency scores is portrayed by a bimodal J-shaped apportionment, the flow of hand execution scores is portrayed by a normal spread with a mean shift towards prevalent execution of the right hand and lower execution of the mixed/ambiguous- handers underneath the middle zone. The author has exhibited that the J-shaped dissemination of tendency can be superimposed on the regular transport of execution disparity when the scatterings are exactly tended to. Contrary to the above see, a couple of assessments have shown that consistent hand tendency is connected with capable motor execution. They suggest that more lateralized people would be fewer factors in hemispheric specialization and, thusly, would show more expressed utilitarian deviations than the clashing individuals.

Unsurprising equal tendency is needed to incite worked with advancement plans showing fine motor control. The test verification on this issue is various. During the early years, right handers are found to differ from mixed-handers anyway not from lefthanders by strolling execution (Gabbard, 1989). Tremendous right and left hand differentiation has been represented on tasks like tapping and pegboard. The author has found that right-handers are more unequivocally lateralized than their left-hander sisters. Moreover, the preference-performance score associations are basically sure. In young adults, hand tendency is on a very basic level related to execution. Peters (1995) battled that tendency actuates lop-sidedness in a given capacity in view of extended use of the supported hand. Regardless, it has also been entrapped. Thusly, quick finger tapping has shown right hand advantage which is credited to that for the organization and control of successive turn of events.

Direct vs. All-Encompassing Measure

The left half of the brain measures data in a straight way. It measures from portion to entirety. It takes fragments, shapes them up, and orchestrates them in an intelligent request; then, at that point it makes determinations. The right intellect nonetheless, measures from entire to parts, comprehensively.

Consecutive vs. Irregular Processing

As well as suspecting in a direct way, the left-brain measures in succession. The left brained individual is a rundown producer. In case somebody is left brained, he will appreciate making ace timetables and every day arranging. The left brain is additionally grinding away in the straight and successive handling of math and in after ways. By contrasts, the methodologies of the right- brained individuals are irregular.

Representative vs. Substantial Processing

The left brain experiences no difficulty preparing images. Numerous scholarly pursuits manage symbols-such as letters, words, and numerical documentations. The left brained individual will in general be alright with phonetic and numerical undertakings. Left-brained individual will likely remember jargon confrontations or math recipes. The right brain, then again, needs things to be concrete. The right brain individual needs to see, sense, or contact the genuine item.

Coherent vs. Natural Processing

The left-brain measures in a direct, successive, coherent way. At the point when you measure on the left lateral, you use data portion by portion to tackle a numerical question or work out a science test. At the point when you peruse and tune in, you search for the pieces so you can make legitimate inferences. In the event that you interaction essentially on the right half of the brain, you use nature.

Verbal vs. Nonverbal Measure

Left brain individuals experience little difficulty putting themselves out there in words. Right brain people may know what they mean, yet regularly experience difficulty tracking down the right words. These are only a portion of the distinctions that exist between the left and right halves of the globe, yet one can see an example. Since left brain techniques are the ones utilized regularly in the study hall, right brain understudies now and then feel lacking. In any case, one can be adaptable and adjust material to the right half of brain. Similarly, the individuals who are dominatingly left brain realize that it is astute to utilize the two sides of the brain and utilize some right brain techniques.

Knowledge

"Information is an especially expansive intellectual ability that, notwithstanding different things, incorporates the ability to reason, plan, tackle issues, think powerfully, appreciate complex considerations, take in quickly and acquire in actuality" (Gottfredson et al.,1993). While information is maybe the most talked about subjects inside brain science, there is no standard significance of what definitely contains 'understanding.' Some researchers have suggested that information is a single, general limit, while other acknowledges that knowledge consolidates an extent of aptitudes, capacities and gifts. As demonstrated by L. Gottfredson et al., 1993, "Knowledge is an uncommonly wide mental capacity that, notwithstanding different things, incorporates the ability to reason, plan, deal with issues, think extraordinarily, comprehend complex musings, take in quickly and acquire for a reality." "Information is a property of brain that consolidates many related intellectual abilities, similar to the capacities to reason, plan, deal with issues, think reasonably, understand contemplations and language, and learn." "Understanding is everything except a single, unitary limit, however rather a composite of a couple of limits. The term connotes that mix of limits required for perseverance and progress inside a particular culture." (Anastasi, 1992). Thorndike E.L., 1927 has parceled clever activity into three sorts for instance (1) Social understanding, or ability to grasp and oversee individuals; (2) Concrete information, or ability to fathom and oversee things as in capable trades and intelligent devices, (3) Abstract knowledge, or ability to appreciate and oversee verbal and mathematical pictures. To the layman, the IQ isn't identified with a particular kind of score on a particular test, yet is routinely a shorthand task for information. One social event of definitions puts the emphasis upon change or change of the individual to his supreme environment, or to limited piece of it. According to implications of this sort, understanding is general mental flexibility to new issues and conditions of life or with everything taken into account, it is the capacity to reorganize one's very own lead standard to act even more suitably and every one of the more appropriately in smart conditions. "Understanding is everything except a singular, unitary limit, yet rather a composite of a couple of limits. The term shows that mix of limits required for perseverance and progress inside a particular culture." "Knowledge is the ability to handle issues, or to make things, that are regarded inside something like one group environments." (Gardner, 1993). "Information is assimilation to the extent that it joins all of the given data of association inside its design. There can be no doubt either, that mental life is in like manner comfort to the environment. Assimilation can never be unadulterated because by melding new parts into its earlier schemata the information constantly adjusts the last to transform them to new segments." There are a few investigations where speed of handling has been straightforwardly connected to focal sensory system working and to insight (Vernon, P.A, and Mori, M. (1992). Insight, Reaction times and fringe nerve conduction speed as referred to in Bee, H. (2000). The creating youngster (ninth ed.). Boston: Allyn and Bacon). Exploration shows that the speed with which individuals can recover data is identified with insight. Overall individuals with higher IQ scores respond rapidly on the data preparing and perceptual assignment. Studies have shown that during perceptual undertakings, right half of the globe is more enacted so astute individuals may have more particular right side of the equator (Barlow, 2001). Knowledge is certifiably not a steady develop from the birth till the passing. There are various elements, which add to the conflicting idea of IQ.

Theories of Intelligence

Spearman's Theory: According to Spearman, intelligence is the faculty to understand the complicated relationships between different things and ideas. The more intelligent the person, the greater will be the number of relations he sees in them. He will be able to understand those relationships which others can not understand easily. According to Spearman, a person has two kinds of faculties- 'G' factor or general factor and 'S' factor or specific factor. Spearman stated that every individual possesses general factor up to some extent. The greater the amount of general factors in a person, the higher the intelligence he possesses. According to Spearman's theory, besides general factor a person has also some specific factors. It is possible that a person without much general factor may acquire higher skill in some specific sphere, but had he received the same amount of support from his general factor, he would have done much better in that specific sphere too.

Thorndike's Theory: According to theory proposed by Thorndike, intelligence is of three kinds: mechanical, abstract and social. This Thorndike also finds lack of general element in nature of intelligence. As per this particular theory, attention, retention power, memory, recognition, organisation, induction, deduction and the faculty to learn and acquire knowledge are the necessary parts of intelligence. Thurstone's Theory According to Thurstone, intelligence consists of nine primary mental abilities i.e. visual or spatial ability, perceptual ability, numerical ability, logical or verbal relation ability, fluency in dealing with words, memory, inductive ability, deductive ability, and ability to restrict the solution of a problem. Thurstone propounded that a person uses in a combined manner all these abilities according to his/her needs.

Guilford's Theory: Guilford is of the view that each intellectual ability has its own uniqueness and some kind of intellectual ability in necessary for executing some task. Therefore, Guilford contends that that each intellectual ability should be measured separately.
Guilford places intelligence into three broad categories:

1. Process or operation:
   a. Cognition
   b. Memory
   c. Divergent thinking
   d. Convergent thinking
   e. Evaluation
2. Material and Content:
   a. Figure content
   b. Symbolic content
   c. Semantic content
   d. (iv) Behavioural content
3. Product
   a. Units: To grasp sensory perceptions into their uniqueness.
   b. Classes- The ability to categorise ideas.
   c. Relations: The ability to understand the relation existing between things.
   d. Systems: The ability to group ideas or problems into space or the ability to structure problems for solutions.

e. Transformations: The ability to give suggestions for the necessary transformation or the ability to predict the future shape of a certain object or situation under a certain circumstance.
f. Implications: The ability to understand the implied meaning.

Role of Homotopic Connections

We examined that piece of the unexplained change could reflect issues with the appraisal of SC from DWI, which can be expected taking into account limitations in current fiber following estimations and the issue of crossing point strands. We know for instance that various fibers going through the corpus callosum are inadequately evaluated in scattering imaging, explicitly those partner more equal bits of the cerebral cortex. Be that as it may, the corpus callosum is the essential of the vertebrate brain. It intentionally relates homologous spaces of the cerebral cortex across the two parts of the globe in a back slant, through a plan of myelinated homotopic strands or 'homotopic affiliations'. The hypothesis of an impact of SC appraisal issues on FC unexplained change was maintained by the insight that, in our results, affiliations yielded on typical significantly higher farsighted power than interhemispheric affiliations.

To extra test the work of white matter relationship in driving FC, we erroneously set all homotopic relationship with a consistent SC regard for the ordinary subject and reran all diversions. In this way, the perceptive power vehemently extended for all models, going from. Likewise, the distinction unexplained was diminished to 63%. Likewise, insightful power for intra and interhemispheric affiliations became same. Inquisitively, adding homotopic affiliations similarly provoked a huge extension in perceptive power for deviant affiliations, that is, sets of regions for which SC is zero (growing). The relationship on growing farsighted power was significantly express to homotopic affiliations. While applying the SAR model to the SC network with added homotopic affiliations and discretionarily permuting the 80 relating interhemispheric affiliations (one region in one portion of the globe was related with one and only one area in the opposite side of the equator), the perceptive power decidedly reduced, even stood out from results with the main SC. In addition, we further reviewed the expressness of this result by methodically controlling SC. In three unmistakable entertainments, we self-assertively dispensed with, added, and permuted basic affiliations. In all cases, the perceptive power lessened as a segment of the degree of affiliations controlled. Likewise, changes instigated by these controls remained close to nothing, far under the movements that we had the alternative to incite by adding homotopic affiliations. With everything considered, these results suggest that homotopic affiliations expect an indispensable part in shaping the organization components, in an unpredictable and non-immaterial way.

CONCLUSION

How the human brain functions is as yet an inquiry, just like its suggestion with brain design: the non-insignificant construction work relationship. The fundamental theory is that the anatomic design conditions, however doesn't decide, the neural organization dynamic. The useful network can't be clarified just thinking about the anatomical substrate. This includes mind boggling and dubious parts of the neuroscience field and that the techniques and approaches to acquire underlying and useful network are not in every case thoroughly applied. The current novel frameworks and neuroimaging methods with high resolutive physio-primary limit have achieved the improvement of a vital system of various underlying and morphometric apparatuses, for example, picture handling, computational displaying and chart hypothesis.

Examining the connection between brain design and capacity is a focal undertaking for neuroscience research. However, the systems forming this relationship to a great extent still need to be clarified and are profoundly discussed. Specifically, the presence and relative commitments of anatomical imperatives and dynamical physiological systems of various sorts still need to be set up. We resolved this issue by efficiently looking at utilitarian network (FC) from resting-state practical attractive reverberation imaging information with reproductions from progressively complex computational models, and by controlling anatomical availability acquired from fiber tractography dependent on dispersion weighted imaging.
Funding: NIL

REFERENCES

Anastasi, A. (1992). What counselors should know about the use and interpretation of psychological tests. *Journal of Counseling and Development, 70*(5), 610–615. doi:10.1002/j.1556-6676.1992.tb01670.x

Barlow, H. (2001). Redundancy reduction revisited. *Network (Bristol, England), 12*(3), 241–253. doi:10.1080/net.12.3.241.253 PMID:11563528

Bee, H. (2000). The developing child (9th ed.). Academic Press.

Fabre, M., & Buser, P. (1980). Structures involved in acquisition and performance of visually guided movements in the cat. *Acta Neurobiologiae Experimentalis, 40*, 95–116. PMID:7424596

Gabbard, C. (1989). Foot lateralization and psychomotor control in four-year-olds. *Perceptual and Motor Skills, 68*(2), 675–678. doi:10.2466/pms.1989.68.2.675 PMID:2717370

Gardner, H. (1993). *Multiple intelligences: The theory in practice*. Basic Books.

Gottfredson, G. D., Jones, E. M., & Holland, J. L. (1993). Personality and vocational interests: The relation of Holland's six interest dimensions to five robust dimensions of personality. *Journal of Counseling Psychology, 40*(4), 518–524. doi:10.1037/0022-0167.40.4.518

Grillner, S., Markram, H., De Schutter, E., Silberberg, G., & LeBeau, F. E. (2005). Microcircuits in action–from CPGs to neocortex. *Trends in Neurosciences, 28*(10), 525–533. doi:10.1016/j.tins.2005.08.003 PMID:16118022

Krupski, A., Raskin, D. C., & Bakan, P. (1971). Physiological and personality correlates of commission errors in an auditory vigilance task. *Psychophysiology, 8*(3), 304–311. doi:10.1111/j.1469-8986.1971.tb00460.x PMID:5093973

Pelvig, D. P., Pakkenberg, H., Stark, A. K., & Pakkenberg, B. (2008). Neocortical glial cell numbers in human brains. *Neurobiology of Aging, 29*(11), 1754–1762. doi:10.1016/j.neurobiolaging.2007.04.013 PMID:17544173

Puelles, L. (2001). Thoughts on the development, structure and evolution of the mammalian and avian telencephalic pallium. *Philosophical Transactions of the Royal Society of London. Series B, Biological Sciences, 356*(1414), 1583–1598. doi:10.1098/rstb.2001.0973 PMID:11604125

Rosenberger, A. L., Halenar, L., & Cooke, S. B. (2011). The making of platyrrhine semifolivores: Models for the evolution of folivory in primates. *Anatomical Record (Hoboken, N.J.)*, *294*(12), 2112–2130. doi:10.1002/ar.21510 PMID:22042497

Saitoh, K., Ménard, A., & Grillner, S. (2007). Tectal control of locomotion, steering, and eye movements in lamprey. *Journal of Neurophysiology*, *97*(4), 3093–3108. doi:10.1152/jn.00639.2006 PMID:17303814

Salas, C., Broglio, C., & Rodríguez, F. (2003). Evolution of forebrain and spatial cognition in vertebrates: Conservation across diversity. *Brain, Behavior and Evolution*, *62*(2), 72–82. doi:10.1159/000072438 PMID:12937346

Scharoun, S. M., & Bryden, P. J. (2014). Hand preference, performance abilities, and hand selection in children. *Frontiers in Psychology*, *5*, 82. doi:10.3389/fpsyg.2014.00082 PMID:24600414

Siegel, D. J. (2010). *The Mindful Therapist: A Clinician's Guide to Mindsight and Neural Integration (Norton Series on Interpersonal Neurobiology)*. WW Norton & Company.

Sutton, M. A., & Carew, T. J. (2000). Parallel molecular pathways mediate expression of distinct forms of intermediate-term facilitation at tail sensory–motor synapses in Aplysia. *Neuron*, *26*(1), 219–231. doi:10.1016/S0896-6273(00)81152-6 PMID:10798406

Swaab, D. F., Chung, W. C., Kruijver, F. P., Hofman, M. A., & Hestiantoro, A. (2003). Sex differences in the hypothalamus in the different stages of human life. *Neurobiology of Aging*, *24*, S1–S16. doi:10.1016/S0197-4580(03)00059-9 PMID:12829102

Taylor, R. (1990). Interpretation of the correlation coefficient: A basic review. *Journal of Diagnostic Medical Sonography: JDMS*, *6*(1), 35–39. doi:10.1177/875647939000600106

Thorndike, E. L. (1927). The refractory period in associative processes. *Psychological Review*, *34*(3), 234–236. doi:10.1037/h0072072

Vernon, P. A., & Mori, M. (1992). Intelligence, reaction times, and peripheral nerve conduction velocity. *Intelligence*, *16*(3-4), 273–288. doi:10.1016/0160-2896(92)90010-O

Westen, D., Blagov, P. S., Harenski, K., Kilts, C., & Hamann, S. (2006). Neural bases of motivated reasoning: An fMRI study of emotional constraints on partisan political judgment in the 2004 US presidential election. *Journal of Cognitive Neuroscience*, *18*(11), 1947–1958. doi:10.1162/jocn.2006.18.11.1947 PMID:17069484

Yen, C. T., Conley, M., & Jones, E. G. (1985). Morphological and functional types of neurons in cat ventral posterior thalamic nucleus. *The Journal of Neuroscience: The Official Journal of the Society for Neuroscience*, *5*(5), 1316–1338. doi:10.1523/JNEUROSCI.05-05-01316.1985 PMID:2987437

KEY TERMS AND DEFINITIONS

Cerebellum: Situated at the back of the head. it is responsible for the constant streams of information between brain and body.

Cerebrum: Occupies the greatest surface area of the human brain which has grooves and folds.

Corpus Callosum: Neural fibres that connects two hemispheres of the brain.

Grey Matter: Also called as faint matter. It is the gathering of neurons.

Human Brain: The most complex organ in the body. contains one hundred billion nerve cells, or neurons.

Intelligence: It is the faculty to understand the complicated relationships between different things and ideas.

Knowledge: Is an uncommonly wide mental capacity that, notwithstanding different things, incorporates the ability to reason, plan, deal with issues, think extraordinarily, comprehend complex musings, take in quickly and acquire for a reality.

Medulla: Alongside the spinal string, contains numerous little cores associated with a wide assortment of tangible and engine capacities.

White Matter: The growing organization of string like rings – called dendrites and axons.

Chapter 3
Introduction to Different Kinds of Cognitive Disorders

Priya Dev
Institute of Medical Sciences, Banaras Hindu University, India

ABSTRACT

According to WHO, around 50 million people are affected with cognitive disorders with nearly 10 million new cases per year. It is a neuropsychiatric disorder that mainly affects the elderly, and it leads to deterioration in memory, thinking ability, behaviour, attention, executive dysfunction, perception, and activities of daily living. The etiology of cognitive disorders is multifactorial including structural damages to brain, genetic, nutritional, and environmental factors. Three major categories include delirium, mild neurocognitive disorders, and major neurocognitive disorders. Some common examples of these disorders are dementia, corticobasal degeneration, Alzheimer's disease, mild cognitive impairment, vascular dementia, etc. Therefore, the chapter will emphasize the different types of cognitive disorders along with their causes and symptoms.

INTRODUCTION

Cognitive disorder and dementia influence the day by day life of individuals (and their family members) in a critical way. Instruments to help early finding may work with activities that may influence the advancement and effect of various intercessions. Since age is the principle hazard factor for the improvement of cognitive debilitation and dementia, discovery of dependable and legitimate approaches to help the finding and its suggestions for regular daily existence in the old people. Cognitive impedance or dementia can, nonetheless, influence more youthful individuals of working age, which requires important evaluation instruments. Dementia is the biggest reason for incapacity in more seasoned individuals and the reliance on others that regularly follows has been found to have a critical adverse impact on individuals' health related personal satisfaction (HRQoL). This theory means to give more proof in this field; in the accompanying presentation a portion of the current information in the field is introduced and a few ideas are clarified.

DOI: 10.4018/978-1-7998-9534-3.ch003

Cognitive capacity Cognition is about the cycles behind human reasoning and encounters. Comprehension alludes to "a cycle of distinguishing, choosing, deciphering, putting away, and utilizing data to figure out and collaborate with the physical and social world, to direct one's ordinary exercises, and to design and institute the course of one's word related life". In the writing on cognitive capacity, writers frequently allude to various cognitive areas like insight, consideration, memory, language, leader work (starting, arranging, coordinating, controlling and assessment of reasoning and acting) and psychomotor speed (Costafreda et al., 2011). A portion of those cognitive capacities decline inside ordinary maturing; for instance, transient memory and the manner in which we acquire new abilities, mental speed, intelligent reasoning and spatial critical thinking. In any case, the vast majority of our language measures are flawless all through maturing (Shafto and Tyler, 2014). Today, we realize that there are some danger factors for the advancement of cognitive debilitation; among these, age is the most serious danger factor. In any case, there are additionally a few good factors for keeping perception unblemished for longer like actual work, social investment and commitment, instruction and scholarly movement. Diet is likewise referenced as a significant factor (Costafreda et al., 2011).

MAJOR COGNITIVE DISORDER

A few illnesses can cause cognitive weakness in the old like despondency, long haul liquor misuse, absence of nutrient B12 and folic corrosive, diabetes, cardiovascular sicknesses, stress-related infections, or a blend of various illnesses (multimorbidity). Neurodegenerative sicknesses like Alzheimer infection (AD), frontotemporal dementia, Parkinson illness, and multiple sclerosis can likewise cause cognitive weakness. Early identification of cognitive decrease could prompt auxiliary counteraction since this data could be utilized to foster systems that control hazard factors. A significant speed increase of cognitive decay seems quite a long while before an analysis of dementia.

MILD COGNITIVE DISORDER

Gentle cognitive disorder is once in a while viewed as an antecedent of dementia or as the limit between typical maturing and dementia (Petersen et al., 2014). In an agreement meeting, the accompanying rules for not set in stone: (I) the individual is neither ordinary nor insane, (ii) there is proof of cognitive crumbling displayed by either unbiasedly estimated decrease over the long run or potentially an abstract report of decay without anyone else as well as witness related to target cognitive shortages; and (iii) exercises of day by day living are safeguarded and complex instrumental capacities are either unblemished or insignificantly weakened (Winblad et al., 2004). The predominance of MCI is assessed to be somewhere in the range of 10% and 20% among individuals more than 65 years old yet various figures have been referenced (Fig 1). About half of those with MCI progress to dementia inside 5 years of period (Rockwood et al., 1999).

Figure 1. Structural MRI of control, Mild cognitive impairment (MCI) and Vascular Dementia (VD) individual showing mild (MCI) and significant (VD) atrophy in the hippocampus cortex (shown by arrow) and significant ventricular enlargement (shown by asterisk)

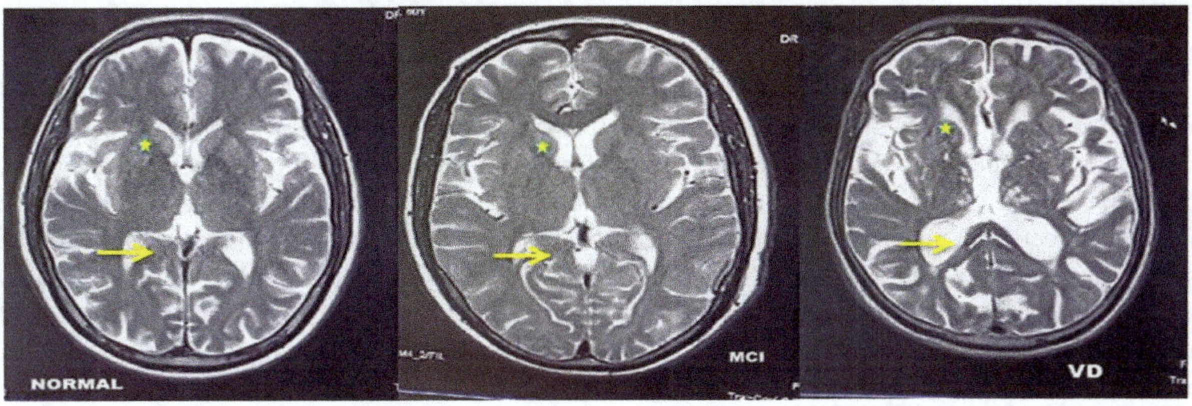

DEMENTIA

Dementia can be characterized as an aggravation in scholarly capacities and it is normal joined by changes in the individual's conduct and character. Dementia is a disorder as opposed to a determination and there are distinctive analytic rules just as various dementia analyze. The most widely recognized type of dementia is AD (around 50–60% surprisingly with dementia). Vascular dementia (VaD) is the second most normal infection (10–half surprisingly with dementia). Blended dementia alludes to a mix of AD and VaD and is especially normal among more established individuals. Different types of dementia incorporate Lewy body dementia and frontotemporal dementia. The quantity of individuals with dementia in Sweden has been assessed and it is expanding. Dementia is the most widely recognized and the most extreme reason for cognitive weakness and inability. Around the world, the pervasiveness of dementia is assessed to be in excess. As future increments around the world, so does the predominance of dementia. In 2050, those figures may have multiplied. The complete expense for dementia care in Sweden is determined to be 63 billion SEK. The expenses for local area care are the most elevated, about 78% of the complete expenses on society. Other than the high cultural expenses, dementia causes massive languishing over the people and their families. Dementia is the biggest reason for handicap on the planet among more seasoned individuals and the reliance on others for performing exercises of day by day living (ADL) is the principle factor that influences HRQoL contrarily (Andersen et al., 2004).

Dementia Examination

Examine dementia at a beginning phase to recognize any reparable conditions, convey the right clinical treatment and offer suitable help and help to patients and family members. Today, no single blood test or test can analyze a dementia illness. In Sweden, The Welfare has characterized the necessities that should be remembered for a dementia examination. A basal examination ought to be founded on appraisal of discernment utilizing cognitive tests and an organized evaluation of capacity and movement limit. Both have main goal. The basal examination ought to be done in essential medical services (PHC). The rules additionally suggest a multi-professional group based methodology. People with a dementia disease ought to have somewhere around a yearly development. This follow-up ought to incorporate evaluation of medicine, insight, and practical limit, general condition of wellbeing, conduct changes and the help that has been concurred on.

These rules have significantly better the work on focusing on individuals with dementia. In any case, in 2014 an assessment of the consideration of individuals with dementia expressed that PHC actually needs to work on their examinations and the multi-professional collaboration. The tests that are suggested in the rules are the Mini Mental State Examination (MMSE) along with the Clock Drawing Test (CDT) for cognitive screening. No instrument is suggested for organized appraisal of capacity and movement. The MMSE is the most regularly utilized test worldwide for evaluating cognitive capacity. The MMSE evaluates direction in time and location, consideration, memory, language and visual development. The MMSE has a limit of 30 focuses and higher scores show better comprehension. It requires around 10 minutes to regulate. MMSE has been censured for having roof impacts for high premorbid capacities and instruction, and not considering the impacts old enough and tactile disability. In clinical use, assess what subtests bombed as opposed to utilizing the absolute aggregate. The MMSE has been believed to be more helpful in precluding dementia in essential consideration and should be enhanced with different tests for best use. The CDT is a short test and requires 5 minutes to control. The CDT measures visuospatial and chief capacities. A shortcoming is that various forms and scoring strategies exist. There are other cognitive screening tests accessible yet these are not assessed as much as the MMSE and the CDT. A test that is for the most part directed by word related specialists in Sweden is Cognistat (some time ago known as the Neurobehavioral Status Examination) (Kiernan et al., 1987). As opposed to the MMSE and CDT, the test outcomes are not introduced as a general total. The outcomes are introduced graphically and contain data about the degree of disability (typical/normal, gentle, moderate, and serious debilitation). Cognistat has age-revised standards and requires around 20 minutes to oversee. It incorporates 10 subtests: direction, consideration, language (understanding, redundancy, and naming), constructional capacity, memory, computation, and thinking (similitudes and decisions). It is additionally incorporates a more subjective evaluation of word familiarity.

Word related advisors can add to the multi-professional group with their exceptional spotlight on word related execution and what cognitive impedances mean for regular day to day existence. While assessing cognitive disability and its results in regular daily existence, various techniques and approaches are frequently required (Hartman-Maeir et al., 2009): meetings or self-revealed evaluations with the individual and others (for example family members, parental figures), perception based evaluations, cognitive screening or more explicit cognitive tests. The cognitive assessment frequently begins with a meeting about the individual's own encounters of cognitive issues in regular daily existence along with a word related history and screening estimations (Hartman-Maeir et al., 2009). The job and the strategies rely upon the setting where the word related advisor works.

EXERCISES OF EVERYDAY LIVING

There is no broad meaning of the idea of ADL in spite of the fact that it is regularly utilized in the writing. ADL is regularly separated into individual or fundamental ADL (which incorporates exercises like individual cleanliness, dress, taking care of and toileting) and instrumental exercises of day by day living (IADL), which are normally alluded to as autonomous living capacities. Exercises remembered for this idea are family exercises, taking care of cash, shopping and transportation. These exercises have a more appeal for cognitive capacities than essential ADL and are significant for carrying on with a free life in the public arena. As a rule, exercises like pastimes or relaxation exercises or work are not engaged with the idea of IADL. A third ADL idea is portrayed by certain creators as cutting edge exercises of everyday living (AADL) or complex exercises of day by day living (CADL) (Tabert et al., 2002), both alluding to exercises like work, relaxation and social exercises. These three degrees of ADL ought to be assessed to cover all exercises in day by day life. In the word related treatment writing, the capacity to play out these three degrees of ADL are covered under word related execution spaces of self-care, play/relaxation and work. Occupations allude to "the ordinary exercises that individuals do as people, in families and with networks to possess time and rejuvenate importance and reason. Occupations incorporate things individuals need to, need to and are required to do" (WFOT, 2010). The Swedish Association of Occupational Therapists characterizes movement as "execution of an undertaking or activity by a person".

COGNIZANCE COMPARABLE TO ADL

In the dementia and geriatric writing, the capacity to perform ADL is frequently alluded to as utilitarian capacity and as an estimation of incapacity. Dementia influences individuals' capacity to perform exercises of day by day life, at first in complex exercises yet advancing to more fundamental exercises like the capacity to adapt to dressing and toileting later in the sickness course. More youthful individuals some of the time experience the principal changes at work. Past research shows that exercises that are influenced by cognitive decrease incorporate utilization of phones and public transportation and the executives of meds and accounts. Issues with these exercises along with cognitive deficiencies can be seen even before people foster dementia (Barberger-Gateau et al., 1999). MCI contrarily impacts a person's capacity to perform complex ADL and expands the danger for dementia (Palmer et al., 2003). The capacity to perform essential ADL is saved when the principal manifestations of cognitive crumbling happen, while the capacity to perform complex ADL is bound to diminish when memory, consideration, and leader capacities decay. Performing errands at a more slow speed may be an early marker of practical change in MCI. Cognitive decrease influences execution in IADL, though ADL is influenced when a specific level of cognitive brokenness is reached (Aguero-Torres et al., 2002). Hence, early identification of cognitive brokenness is vital in PHC. Moreover, appraisal of regular day to day existence exercises ought to be acted to realize when and how to intercede. The connection between cognitive brokenness and the capacity to perform regular daily existence exercises is a significant issue in clinical practice. Cognitive capacities like chief capacities, memory and consideration have been displayed to associate with disabled useful status. Evaluate cognitive capacities as well as the capacity to perform complex ADL in dementia examinations (Perneczky et al., 2006).

MILD COGNITIVE IMPAIRMENT

Over the top Cognitive Disorder is a charming and handicapping ailment portrayed by the presence of fixations (undesirable contemplations, pictures or driving forces) and additionally impulses (tedious conduct) (Khanna, 1990). Fig.1 Structural MRI of control, Mild cognitive impairment (MCI) and Vascular Dementia (VD) individual showing mild (MCI) and significant (VD) atrophy in the hippocampus cortex (shown by arrow) and significant ventricular enlargement (shown by asterisk). As of late as during the 1980s, Obsessive Compulsive Disorder was viewed as an uncommon disorder that was not really receptive to treatment. A significant part of the advancement in understanding the Obsessive Compulsive Disorder has happened following the finding of the National Epidemiological Catchment Area (ECA) study (0) that Obsessive Compulsive Disorder is the fourth most normal mental disorder. A significant extra stimulus to the expanded interest in diagnosing Obsessive Compulsive Disorder is the accessibility of compelling medicines. Notwithstanding, in spite of the great predominance just a minority of the victims looks for proficient assistance due to the mysterious idea of the ailment. The individuals who experience the ill effects of Obsessive Compulsive Disorder regularly think that it's humiliating to discuss their undesirable musings bringing about impressive postponement in looking for treatment. When clinical assistance is looked for, some long stretches of disease would have slipped by. Even in the wake of beginning with pharmacotherapy they neglect to hold fast to treatment because of absence of information about disorder. Henceforth with the assistance of Cognitive Behavior Therapy they comprehend the sickness, the course and anticipation and the significance of therapy continuation. This prompts better result. The fundamental component of over the top impulsive disorder (Obsessive Compulsive Disorder) is the indication of intermittent fixations or impulses adequately serious to make stamped trouble the individual. The fixations or impulses are tedious and meddle essentially with the individual's typical everyday practice, word related working, normal social exercises, or connections. A patient with Obsessive Compulsive Disorder might have a fixation or an impulse or both. A fixation is a repetitive and meddling idea, believing, thought or sensation. Rather than a fixation, which is a psychological occasion, an impulse is a conduct. In particular, an impulse is a cognizant, normalized, repetitive conduct, like tallying, checking or keeping away from. A patient with Obsessive Compulsive Disorder understands the madness of the fixation and encounters both the fixation and the impulse as personality dystonic (for example undesirable conduct). Albeit the urgent demonstration might be done trying to decrease the nervousness related with the fixation, it doesn't generally prevail with regards to doing as such. The consummation of the urgent demonstration may not influence the tension, and it might even expand the nervousness. Tension is additionally expanded when an individual opposes completing an impulse. Verifiable foundation and current nosography shows that Obsessive contemplations and urgent desires or activities are important for regular daily existence. We get back to watch that we locked an entryway and turned off the light. We can't quit contemplating the unpleasant occasion booked for the following week. We will not eat with the spoon that dropped on the floor, regardless of whether we know the opportunity of defilement is far off. These occasions are important for the ordinary criticism and control circle between our musings and our activities, and they have hereditary natural endurance esteem. It is just when over the top contemplations become incessant or exceptional, or unavoidable, or when these impulsive ceremonies become so unmistakable that they meddle with a person's working, that the finding of Obsessive Compulsive Disorder is made.

THE STUDY OF DISEASE TRANSMISSION

The lifetime pervasiveness of Obsessive Compulsive Disorder in everybody is assessed at 2 to 3 percent. A few analysts have assessed that the disorder is found in upwards of 10% of outpatients in mental facilities. These figures make Obsessive Compulsive Disorder the fourth most normal mental determination after fears, substance-related disorders, and significant burdensome disorder. Epidemiological examinations in various other countries have affirmed these rates across social limits. Among grown-ups, people are similarly liable to be influenced, however among teenagers; young men are more normally influenced than young ladies. The mean period of beginning is about 20years, in spite of the fact that men have a somewhat prior time of beginning (mean around 19 years) than ladies (mean around 22 years). By and large, the side effects of around 66% of influenced people have a beginning before age 25, and the indications of less than 15% have a beginning get-together 35. The beginning of the disorder can happen in pre-adulthood or youth, now and again as ahead of schedule as 2 years old. Single people are more as often as possible influenced with Obsessive Compulsive Disorder than are hitched people, albeit this finding likely mirrors the trouble that people with the disorder have keeping a relationship. Fanatical Compulsive Disorder happens less regularly among blacks than among whites, in spite of the fact that admittance to medical services as opposed to contrasts in pervasiveness might clarify the variety.

Comorbidity

Individual with Obsessive Compulsive Disorder is ordinarily influenced by other mental disorders. The lifetime predominance for significant burdensome disorder in people with Obsessive Compulsive Disorder is around 67% and for social fear, around 25%. Other normal co dreary mental judgments in patients with Obsessive Compulsive Disorder incorporate liquor use disorders, summed up uneasiness disorder, explicit fear, alarm disorder, dietary problems, and behavioral conditions. The rate of Tourette's disorder in patients with Obsessive Compulsive Disorder is 5 to 7 percent, and 20 to 30 percent of Obsessive Compulsive Disorder patients have a background marked by spasms.

Etiology

1. Serotonergic System

The numerous clinical medication preliminaries that have been directed help the theory that dysregulation of serotonin is engaged with the manifestation development of fixations and impulses in the disorder. Information shows that serotonergic drugs are more powerful than drugs that influence other synapse frameworks, yet regardless of whether serotonin is engaged with the reason for Obsessive Compulsive Disorder isn't clear. Clinical examinations have tested cerebrospinal liquid (CSF) convergences of serotonin metabolites (e.g., 5-hydroxyindoleacetic corrosive {5-HIAA}) and affinities and quantities of platelet-restricting destinations of tritiated imipramine (Tofranil), which ties to serotonin reuptake locales, and have detailed variable discoveries of these actions in patients with Obsessive Compulsive Disorder. In one investigation, the CSF convergence of 5-HIAA diminished get-togethers with clomipramine (Anafranil), zeroing in consideration on the serotonergic framework.

2. Noradrenergic System

Presently, less proof exists for brokenness in the noradrenergic framework in Obsessive Compulsive Disorder. Episodic reports show some improvement in Obsessive Compulsive Disorder indications with utilization of oral clonidine (Catapres), a medication that brings down the measure of norepinephrine delivered from the presynaptic nerve terminals.

3. Neuroimmunology

There has been some interest in a positive connection between streptococcal disease and Obsessive Compulsive Disorder. Gathering A hemolytic streptococcal disease can cause rheumatic fever, and roughly 10 to 30 percent of the patients foster Sydenham's chorea and show fanatical urgent indications.

4. Brain-Imaging Studies

Neuroimaging in Obsessive Compulsive Disorder patients has created merging information ensnaring modified capacity in the neurocircuitry between orbitofrontal cortex, caudate, and thalamus. Different practical brain-imaging reads – for instance, positron emanation tomography (PET) – have shown expanded movement (e.g., digestion and blood stream) in the front facing flaps, the basal ganglia (particularly the caudate), and the cingulum of patients with Obsessive Compulsive Disorder. The inclusion of these spaces in the pathology of Obsessive Compulsive Disorder shows up more connected with corticostriatal pathways than with the amygdale pathways that are the ebb and flow focal point of much tension disorder research. Pharmacological and conduct medicines supposedly switch these anomalies. Information from utilitarian brain-imaging contemplates are predictable with information from primary brain-imaging considers. Both figured tomographic (CT) and attractive reverberation imaging (MRI) examines have discovered respectively more modest caudate in patients with Obsessive Compulsive Disorder. Both utilitarian and underlying brain-imaging study results are additionally viable with the perception that neurological systems including the cingulum are at times successful in the treatment of Obsessive Compulsive Disorder patients. One late MRI study announced expanded T1 unwinding times in the cerebrum, a finding predictable with the area of irregularities found in PET examinations.

Psychosocial Factors

1. Personality Factors

Fanatical Compulsive Disorder contrasts from over the top impulsive behavioral condition. Most people with Obsessive Compulsive Disorder don't have premorbid urgent indications, and such character characteristics are neither essential nor adequate for the advancement of Obsessive Compulsive Disorder. Simply around 15 to 35 percent of Obsessive Compulsive Disorder patients have had premorbid obsessional qualities.

2. Psychodynamic Factors

Sigmund Freud initially conceptualized the condition we currently call Obsessive Compulsive Disorder as obsessional anxiety. He accepted there was a cautious retreat associated with the essence of uneasiness inciting Oedipal wishes. He hypothesized that the patient with an over the top enthusiastic depression relapsed to the butt-centric period of psychosexual turn of events. Freud's hypotheses are talked about underneath. Psychodynamic knowledge might be of extraordinary assistance in understanding issues with treatment consistence, relational challenges, and character issues going with the Axis I disorder. Numerous patients with Obsessive Compulsive Disorder might decline to help out powerful medicines, for example, specific serotonin reuptake inhibitors and conduct treatment. Despite the fact that the side effects of Obsessive Compulsive Disorder might be organically determined, psychodynamic implications might be joined to them. Patients might become put resources into keeping up with the symptomatology as a result of optional increases. For instance, a male patient, whose mother remains at home to deal with him, may unwittingly wish to hold tight to his Obsessive Compulsive Disorder side effects since they keep the consideration of his mom. Another commitment of psychodynamic understanding includes the relational measurements. Studies have shown that family members will oblige the patient through dynamic investment in customs or huge changes of their everyday schedules. This type of family convenience is connected with pressure in the family, dismissing perspectives toward the patient, and helpless family working. Frequently the relatives are engaged with a work to decrease the patient's nervousness or to control the patient's demeanors of outrage. This example of relatedness might become disguised and be reproduced when the patient enters a treatment setting. By taking a gander at repeating examples of relational connections according to a psychodynamic point of view, patients might figure out what their ailment means for other people. At long last, one other commitment of psychodynamic believing is acknowledgment of the precipitants that start or worsen manifestations. Regularly, relational challenges increment the patient's nervousness and in this manner increment the patients' symptomatology too. Examination recommends that Obsessive Compulsive Disorder might be accelerated by various natural stressors, particularly those including pregnancy, labor, or parental consideration of youngsters. A comprehension of the stressors might help the clinician in a general treatment plan that decreases the upsetting occasions themselves or their importance to the patient.

Clinical Features

Patients with Obsessive Compulsive Disorder frequently take their grievances to doctors other than therapists. Most patients with Obsessive Compulsive Disorder have the two fixations and impulse - upto 75% in some reviews. A few analysts and clinicians accept that the number might be a lot more like 100% in case patients are painstakingly evaluated for the presence of mental impulses notwithstanding conduct impulses. For instance, a fixation on harming a kid might be trailed by a psychological impulse to rehash a particular supplication a particular number of times. Different specialists and clinicians, nonetheless, accept that a few patients do have just over the top considerations without impulses. Such patients are probably going to have redundant contemplations of a sexual or forceful demonstration that is unforgivable to them. For lucidity, it is ideal to conceptualize fixations as contemplations and impulses as conduct. Fixations and impulses share certain highlights for all intents and purpose: A thought or a drive interrupts itself stubbornly and tirelessly into an individual's cognizant mindfulness. A sensation of restless fear goes with the focal sign and habitually drives the individual to take counter measures against the underlying thought or motivation. The fixation or the impulse is conscience outsider; that is, it is capable as unfamiliar to the individual's experience of oneself as a mental being. Regardless of how striking and convincing the fixation or impulse, the individual generally remembers it as crazy and unreasonable. The individual experiencing fixations and impulses normally feels a powerful urge to oppose them. In any case, about portion of all patients offer little protection from impulses, albeit around 80% of all patients accept that the impulse is silly. Once in a while patients exaggerate fixations and impulses – for instance, they might demand that habitual tidiness is ethically right, despite the fact that they have lost their positions on the grounds that for time spent cleaning.

COGNITIVE DISORDER SYMPTOM PATTERNS

The introduction of fixations and impulses is heterogeneous in grown-ups and in kids and teenagers. The indications of an individual patient might cover and change with time; however Obsessive Compulsive Disorder has four significant side effect designs.

1. Tainting

The most well-known example is a fixation of defilement, trailed by washing or joined by habitual evasion of the apparently sullied object. The dreaded item is regularly difficult to stay away from (e.g., excrement, pee, residue, or germs). Patients may in a real sense take the skin off their mind by exorbitant hand washing or might not be able to leave their homes due to dread of germs. Despite the fact that uneasiness is the most well-known enthusiastic reaction to the dreaded article, over the top disgrace and nausea are additionally normal. Patients with tainting fixations normally accept that the pollution is spread from one item to another or individual to individual by the smallest contact.

2. Fears

Perhaps the most pervasive fixations are a dread of tainting, which represents roughly a fourth of all fanatical topics in the US and is the most well-known Obsessive Compulsive Disorder concern around the world. Commonly the pollution stress depends on a dread of a type of sickness or disease (normally passing, yet at times different concerns, for example, a dread of visual impairment or strict concerns are a factor). For instance, one may fear creating malignancy or illness thus stress over harmful materials to a limit, for example, x-beams, asbestos, or numerous other various cancer-causing agents happening either normally or in regular items.

Plainly something, for example, asbestos is hazardous, in actuality (it is presently not utilized generally as it is unlawful, however a great deal of more seasoned homes fabricating still have things made out of asbestos or different perils, for example, lead paint), yet an individual with defilement Obsessive Compulsive Disorder would take the dread to the limit. When strolling past a home with asbestos siding, the Obsessive Compulsive Disorder victim may begin to envision that downpour water had washed the asbestos particles onto the side walk, and since it was dry that they may really be stepping on asbestos particles which were then surging into the air and connecting onto their garments. Or then again even that the asbestos siding had crumbled (regardless of whether it was plainly all around typified) such a lot of that it was noticeable all around and connecting to their garments and for sure contaminating everything in vicinity. Though a customary individual would understand that while destructive, the asbestos would truly possibly be hazardous if they somehow managed to split it up and begin sniffing in the residue, and that while there are a great deal of perils regular day to day existence, that in case everything was so perilous we would all be wiped out and dead effectively (for this situation by means of malignancy). Contingent upon where the tainting fixation dwells in an Obsessive Compulsive Disorder victims' chain of importance or the seriousness of the Obsessive Compulsive Disorder, decides the limits to which these fixations can show. Regularly an individual with defilement fears will quit wasting time where basically everything aside from a little protected region is sullied, since the tainting has spread. Since the fixation is concerning infection or disease one with Obsessive Compulsive Disorder regularly feels an awareness of certain expectations to shield others from the foreign substances. This is frequently where pressure is made or stress is brought about by those near an Obsessive Compulsive Disorder victim as they will demand companions and friends and family staying away from toxins inspired by a paranoid fear of them being defiled or spreading the germs to their protected zones. While dread of sickness or illness is the foundation of most pollution fixations, it isn't generally the situation. A genuine model is individuals that are annoyed by tacky or oily substances. In cases, for example, these frequently the justification being irritated by the substance can't be explained with the exception of a distress. Those with Obsessive Compulsive Disorder regularly experience the ill effects of an increased feeling of balance so maybe getting something tacky on one's hand prompts inconvenience.

PROGNOSIS

The greater part of patients with Obsessive Compulsive Disorder has an unexpected beginning of manifestations. The beginning of indications for around 50 to 70 percent of patients happens after an upsetting occasion, like a pregnancy, a sexual issue, or the passing of a family member. Since numerous people figure out how to stay quiet, there is regularly a deferral of 5 to 10 years before patients come to mental consideration, albeit the postponement is most likely shortening with expanded attention to the disorder. The course is typically long however factor; a few patients experience a fluctuating course, and others experience a steady one.

Around 20 to 30 percent of patients have critical improvement in their manifestations, and 40 to 50 percent have moderate improvement. The excess 20 to 40 percent of patients either stay sick or their manifestations decline. Around 33% of patients with Obsessive Compulsive Disorder have significant burdensome disorder, and self destruction is a danger for all patients with Obsessive Compulsive Disorder. A helpless anticipation is demonstrated by respecting (as opposed to opposing) impulses, youth beginning, peculiar impulses, the requirement for hospitalization, a coinciding significant burdensome disorder, whimsical convictions, the presence of exaggerated thoughts (i.e., some acknowledgment of fixations and impulses), and the presence of a behavioral condition (particularly schizotypal behavioral condition). A decent anticipation is demonstrated by acceptable social and word related change, the presence of an encouraging occasion, and a wordy nature of the indications, the obsessional substance doesn't appear to be identified with the forecast.

TREATMENT

With mounting proof that Obsessive Compulsive Disorder is to a great extent controlled by natural variables, exemplary psychoanalytic hypothesis has become undesirable. Also, in light of the fact that Obsessive Compulsive Disorder indications seem, by all accounts, to be generally unmanageable to psychodynamic psychotherapy and therapy, pharmacological and social medicines have gotten normal. Yet, psychodynamic components might be of extensive advantage in getting what encourages intensifications of the disorder and in getting different types of opposition therapy, like resistance with medicine. Numerous patients with Obsessive Compulsive Disorder determinedly oppose treatment endeavors. They might decline to take prescription and may oppose doing helpful schoolwork tasks and different exercises recommended by conduct advisors. The obsessive-compulsive manifestations themselves, regardless of how organically based, may have significant mental implications that make patients hesitant to surrender them. Psychodynamic investigation of a patient's protection from treatment might further develop consistence.

All around controlled examinations have discovered that pharmacotherapy, conduct treatment, or a blend of both is viable in altogether decreasing the side effects of patients with Obsessive Compulsive Disorder. The choice about which treatment to utilize depends on the clinician's judgment and experience and the patient's acknowledgment of the different modalities. Without satisfactory investigations of knowledge situated psychotherapy for Obsessive Compulsive Disorder, any substantial speculations about its adequacy are difficult to make, despite the fact that there are episodic reports of accomplishments. Singular examiners have seen striking and enduring improvements in patients with over the top habitual behavioral condition, particularly when they can grapple with the forceful motivations lying behind their person qualities. Similarly, examiners and progressively arranged specialists have noticed checked suggestive improvement in patients with Obsessive Compulsive Disorder over the span of investigation or delayed knowledge psychotherapy. Strong psychotherapy without a doubt has its place, particularly for those Obsessive Compulsive Disorder patients who, notwithstanding manifestations of differing levels of seriousness, can work and make social changes. With ceaseless and customary contact with an intrigued, thoughtful, and empowering proficient individual, patients might have the option to work by excellence of this assistance, without which their side effects would weaken them. Sometimes when obsessional customs and nervousness arrive at a heinous power, it is important to hospitalize patients until the sanctuary of an establishment and the expulsion from outer ecological anxieties lessen manifestations to an average level. A patient's relatives are regularly headed to the skirt of hopelessness by the patient's conduct. Any Psychotherapeutic undertakings should incorporate regard for the relatives through arrangement of enthusiastic help, consolation, clarification, and guidance on the best way to oversee and react to the patient.

1. Pharmacotherapy

The adequacy of pharmacotherapy in Obsessive Compulsive Disorder has been demonstrated in numerous clinical preliminaries and is upgraded by the perception that the examinations discover a fake treatment reaction pace of just around 5%. The medications, some of which are utilized to treat burdensome disorders or other mental disorders, can be given in their standard measurements ranges. Introductory impacts are for the most part seen following 4 to about a month and a half of treatment, albeit 8 to about four months are typically expected to get maximal remedial advantage. Treatment with upper medications is as yet dubious, and huge extents of patients with Obsessive Compulsive Disorder who react to treatment with stimulant medications appear to backslide if the medication treatment is ended. The standard methodology is to begin treatment with a SSRI or clomipramine and afterward move to other pharmacological procedures if the serotonin-explicit medications are not powerful. The serotonergic drugs have expanded the level of patients with Obsessive Compulsive Disorder who are probably going to react to treatment to the scope of 50 to 70 percent.

2. Stereo Therapy

Albeit barely any straight on examinations have been made, conduct treatment is just about as successful as pharmacotherapies in Obsessive Compulsive Disorder, and a few information show that the useful impacts are longer enduring with conduct treatment. Along these lines, numerous clinicians consider conduct treatment the treatment of decision for Obsessive Compulsive Disorder. Conduct treatment can be led in both outpatient and inpatient settings. The important conduct approaches in Obsessive Compulsive Disorder are openness and reaction counteraction. Desensitization, thought halting, flooding, collapse treatment and aversive molding has additionally been utilized in patients with Obsessive Compulsive Disorder. In conduct treatment, patients should be really dedicated to progress.

3. Psychotherapy

Without sufficient investigations of understanding focused psychotherapy for Obsessive Compulsive Disorder, any substantial speculations about its adequacy are difficult to make, despite the fact that there are recounted reports of victories. Singular experts have seen striking and enduring improvements in patients with over the top urgent behavioral condition, particularly when they can deal with the forceful motivations lying behind their person characteristics. Moreover, investigators and powerfully arranged therapists have noticed stamped indicative improvement in patients with Obsessive Compulsive Disorder over the span of examination or delayed knowledge psychotherapy. Strong psychotherapy without a doubt has its place, particularly for those Obsessive Compulsive Disorder patients who, in spite of side effects of changing levels of seriousness, can work and make social changes. With nonstop and standard contact with an intrigued, thoughtful, and empowering proficient individual, patients might have the option to work by ethicalness of this assistance, without which their side effects would cripple them. Incidentally when fixation ceremonies and uneasiness arrive at a painful force, it is important to hospitalize patients until the haven of an organization and the expulsion from outer natural burdens reduce side effects to an average level. A patient's relatives are frequently headed to the skirt of depression by the patient's conduct. Any Psychotherapeutic undertakings should incorporate regard for the relatives through arrangement of enthusiastic help, consolation, clarification, and exhortation on the best way to oversee and react to the patient.

4. Group Therapy

Treating patients in a social environment is here and there attempted for different conditions. For instance, patients with disturbing social tension are regularly treated in friendly abilities gatherings. In some new treatment software engineers, patients experiencing impulses have been effectively treated in gatherings; patients whose principle issues are fixations are bound to profit with singular treatment. Care groups for patient have been discovered to be of some advantage when utilized as a subordinate to singular treatment. Relatives may likewise be remembered for the Obsessive Compulsive Disorder family support gatherings. Lately, self-improvement associations have been running care groups for patients and families, and many have discovered these to be useful.

5. Different Therapies

Family treatment is frequently valuable in supporting the family, decreasing conjugal disagreement coming about because of the disorder, and building a treatment partnership with the relatives to benefit the patient. Gathering treatment is helpful as an emotionally supportive network for certain patients. For outrageous cases that are therapy safe and constantly weakening, electro convulsive treatment (ECT) and psychosurgery might be thought of. ECT isn't just about as powerful as psychosurgery, yet it ought to be attempted before a medical procedure. The most well-known psychosurgical technique for Obsessive Compulsive Disorder is cingulotomy, which is fruitful in getting 25 30 percent of in any case treatment-lethargic patients. The most well-known intricacy of psychosurgery is the improvement of seizures, which are quite often constrained by treatment with phenytoin (Dilantin). A few patients who don't react to psychosurgery alone and who didn't react to pharmacotherapy or conduct treatment before the activity do react to pharmacotherapy or conduct treatment after psychosurgery.

6. Cognitive Behavioural Therapy

Cognitive conduct treatment is a commonsense, active methodology that helps individual's changes the manner in which they feel by assessing and changing the manner in which they think and act. It is the blend of two distinct kinds of treatment: conduct treatment and cognitive treatment.

7. Cognitive Therapy

Cognitive treatment was at first evolved during the 1960s by Aaron Beck as a momentary strategy for getting melancholy by showing individuals perceive their broken reasoning and think all the more objectively. Different analysts have made varieties of cognitive treatment. Today, cognitive treatment and its variations are utilized to treat conditions including Obsessive Compulsive Disorder, alarm disorder, posttraumatic stress disorder, the dietary issues, and behavioural conditions (Beck, J. S., & Beck, A. T., 1995).

8. Conduct Therapy

This therapy was crafted by Professor Hans Eysenck (1916-97) in London added to the turn of events and acknowledgment of conduct treatment as a significant way to deal with certain mental issues. Fundamentally, he said that cycles of learning procure numerous un-adaptive social issues – and what a realizing interaction has gained can be untaught. Un-adaptive conduct falls into two classifications: instances of defective un-adaptive learning, like silly apprehensions, or issues that emerge on account of an inability to learn versatile conduct. Regardless, it ought to be feasible to address matters by applying the standards of learning. The broken learning can be fixed, and new learning can be advanced.

Along these lines, conduct treatment focused on the issue of conduct itself. It didn't expect, as the then predominant psychoanalytical methodology did, that patient's troubles are indications of more profound oblivious buildings. Maybe than endeavoring to unwind the putative profound causes, conduct advisors worked straightforwardly on the issue conduct. They focused more on the issue as it is presently, and what variables are as of now connected with it, instead of its previous history. Obviously, specialists need to know from the patient when the issue began, how it created, etc., yet the fundamental spotlight is on the issue as it is currently, and advisor's endeavors are equipped towards adjusting this issue.

NORMAL COGNITIVE ERRORS

We as a whole have examples of reasoning, and this might affect our enthusiastic state and conduct. In some cases our examples are not exactly precise. These are cognitive mistakes or cognitive contortions, and they commonly fall into specific classifications. Figuring out how to perceive our own cognitive blunders builds our capacity to disregard the negative idea or effectively change it, which empowers us to deliberately change our feelings and our practices. Coming up next is a rundown of the most widely recognized cognitive contortions.

Win Big or Bust Thinking

Placing encounters in one of two classifications Examples: 1) People are for the most part great or all terrible. 2) Projects are awesome or disappointments. 3) I am a delinquent, or I am a holy person.

Over Summing Up

Accepting that, something will consistently happen in light of the fact that it happened once. Examples: 1) I won't ever have the option to make companions at a gathering since I once offered an off-kilter expression to somebody, and they would not like to be my companion. 2) I won't ever have the option to talk in open since I once had a fit of anxiety prior to giving a discourse.

Limiting the Positive

Concluding that if something to be thankful for occurs, it should not be significant or doesn't tally Examples: 1) I breezed through the test this time, however it was an accident. 2) I didn't have a fit of anxiety today, however it's simply because I was too occupied to ever be concerned.

Making Hasty Judgments

Concluding how to react to a circumstance without having all the data Examples: 1) the man/lady I am keen on never got back to me since he believes I'm inept. 2) That individual cut me off in rush hour gridlock since he/she is a jerk!

Clairvoyance

Accepting that you know how another person is feeling for sure they are thinking with no proof. Examples: 1) I realize she despises my guts. 2) That individual believes I'm a failure.

Fortune Telling

Accepting that, you can anticipate a future result, while disregarding different choices Examples: 1) I will bomb this test. 2) I will have a fit of anxiety on the off chance that I go out in the open.

Catastrophizing

Twisting the significance of positive and adverse occasions. Examples: 1) I said some unacceptable thing so I won't ever have a sweetheart. 2) My nose is large to such an extent that nobody will at any point love me. 3) It doesn't make any difference in case I'm brilliant in light of the fact that I won't ever be alluring, athletic, well known, rich, and so on 4) Making a mountain out of a molehill.

Passionate Reasoning

Accepting something to be valid on the grounds that it feels valid. Models: 1) I am a disappointment since I feel like a disappointment. 2) I am useless on the grounds that I feel useless.

Personalization

Assuming fault for some contrary occasion despite the fact that you were not mindful, you were unable to have known to do another way, there were uncontrollable issues at hand, or others were included. Models: 1) It's my deficiency he hits me. 2) My mom is miserable as a result of me.

Cognitive Behavioral Therapy and Pharmacotherapy

The pharmacotherapy capacities like water wings do in assisting a kid with figuring out how to swim: It diminishes the dread and makes it simpler to "skim along" while you're learning the strokes. The relationship appears to be especially well-suited in light of the fact that similarly as youngsters who are figuring out how to swim can work with less and less air in the water wings and ultimately manage without them, individuals with Obsessive Compulsive Disorder who utilize Cognitive Behavior treatment can get by with lower and lower dosages of pharmacotherapy as the weeks pass by and they continue to chip away at their conduct treatment. In the end a considerable lot of them end up on low portions or no medicine by any means. In the beginning the patient has expanded uneasiness level, less adjustment to go through Cognitive Behavior Therapy consequently first with the assistance of pharmacotherapy the nervousness decreases and set up for Cognitive conduct Therapy. In Obsessive Compulsive Disorder, one of the successful medicines is Cognitive Behavior Therapy and Pharmacotherapy supporting these medicines it was found in this examination that necessity of pharmacotherapy is progressively decreased, it has great adequacy this medicines patient can help himself for lifetime.

Funding: NIL

REFERENCES

Agüero-Torres, H., Thomas, V. S., Winblad, B., & Fratiglioni, L. (2002). The impact of somatic and cognitive disorders on the functional status of the elderly. *Journal of Clinical Epidemiology*, *55*(10), 1007–1012. doi:10.1016/S0895-4356(02)00461-4 PMID:12464377

Andersen, C. K., Wittrup-Jensen, K. U., Lolk, A., Andersen, K., & Kragh-Sørensen, P. (2004). Ability to perform activities of daily living is the main factor affecting quality of life in patients with dementia. *Health and Quality of Life Outcomes*, *2*(1), 1–7. doi:10.1186/1477-7525-2-52 PMID:15383148

Barberger-Gateau, P., Fabrigoule, C., Helmer, C., Rouch, I., & Dartigues, J. F. (1999). Functional impairment in instrumental activities of daily living: An early clinical sign of dementia? *Journal of the American Geriatrics Society*, *47*(4), 456–462. doi:10.1111/j.1532-5415.1999.tb07239.x PMID:10203122

Beck, J. S., & Beck, A. T. (1995). Cognitive therapy: Basics and beyond (No. Sirsi). New York: Guilford Press.

Costafreda, S. G., Dinov, I. D., Tu, Z., Shi, Y., Liu, C. Y., Kloszewska, I., Mecocci, P., Soininen, H., Tsolaki, M., Vellas, B., Wahlund, L.-O., Spenger, C., Toga, A. W., Lovestone, S., & Simmons, A. (2011). Automated hippocampal shape analysis predicts the onset of dementia in mild cognitive impairment. *NeuroImage*, *56*(1), 212–219. doi:10.1016/j.neuroimage.2011.01.050 PMID:21272654

Evans, C. (2007). Cognitive–behavioural therapy with older people. *Advances in Psychiatric Treatment*, *13*(2), 111–118. doi:10.1192/apt.bp.106.003020

Hartman-Maeir, A., Harel, H., & Katz, N. (2009). Kettle Test—A brief measure of cognitive functional performance: Reliability and validity in stroke rehabilitation. *The American Journal of Occupational Therapy*, *63*(5), 592–599. doi:10.5014/ajot.63.5.592 PMID:19785258

Karno, M., Golding, J. M., Sorenson, S. B., & Burnam, M. A. (1988). The epidemiology of obsessive-compulsive disorder in five US communities. *Archives of General Psychiatry*, *45*(12), 1094–1099. doi:10.1001/archpsyc.1988.01800360042006 PMID:3264144

Khanna, T. (1990). *Foundations of neural networks*. Addison-Wesley Longman Publishing Co., Inc.

Kiernan, R. J., Mueller, J., Langston, J. W., & Van Dyke, C. R. A. I. G. (1987). The Neurobehavioral Cognitive Status Examination: A brief but differentiated approach to cognitive assessment. *Annals of Internal Medicine*, *107*(4), 481–485. doi:10.7326/0003-4819-107-4-481 PMID:3631786

Musallam, S., Andersen, R. A., Corneil, B. D., Greger, B., & Scherberger, H. (2010). *U.S. Patent No. 7,826,894*. Washington, DC: U.S. Patent and Trademark Office.

Palmer, K., Fratiglioni, L., & Winblad, B. (2003). What is mild cognitive impairment? Variations in definitions and evolution of nondemented persons with cognitive impairment. *Acta Neurologica Scandinavica*, *107*, 14–20. doi:10.1034/j.1600-0404.107.s179.2.x PMID:12603245

Perneczky, R., Wagenpfeil, S., Komossa, K., Grimmer, T., Diehl, J., & Kurz, A. (2006). Mapping scores onto stages: Mini-mental state examination and clinical dementia rating. *The American Journal of Geriatric Psychiatry*, *14*(2), 139–144. doi:10.1097/01.JGP.0000192478.82189.a8 PMID:16473978

Petersen, R. C., Caracciolo, B., Brayne, C., Gauthier, S., Jelic, V., & Fratiglioni, L. (2014). Mild cognitive impairment: A concept in evolution. *Journal of Internal Medicine*, *275*(3), 214–228. doi:10.1111/joim.12190 PMID:24605806

Rockwood, K., Howard, K., MacKnight, C., & Darvesh, S. (1999). Spectrum of disease in vascular cognitive impairment. *Neuroepidemiology*, *18*(5), 248–254. doi:10.1159/000026219 PMID:10461050

Shafto, M. A., & Tyler, L. K. (2014). Language in the aging brain: The network dynamics of cognitive decline and preservation. *Science*, *346*(6209), 583–587. doi:10.1126cience.1254404 PMID:25359966

Tabert, M. H., Albert, S. M., Borukhova-Milov, L., Camacho, Y., Pelton, G., Liu, X., Stern, Y., & Devanand, D. P. (2002). Functional deficits in patients with mild cognitive impairment: Prediction of AD. *Neurology*, *58*(5), 758–764. doi:10.1212/WNL.58.5.758 PMID:11889240

Winblad, B., Palmer, K., Kivipelto, M., Jelic, V., Fratiglioni, L., Wahlund, L. O., Nordberg, A., Backman, L., Albert, M., Almkvist, O., Arai, H., Basun, H., Blennow, K., de Leon, M., DeCarli, C., Erkinjuntti, T., Giacobini, E., Graff, C., Hardy, J., ... Petersen, R. C. (2004). Mild cognitive impairment–beyond controversies, towards a consensus: Report of the International Working Group on Mild Cognitive Impairment. *Journal of Internal Medicine*, *256*(3), 240–246. doi:10.1111/j.1365-2796.2004.01380.x PMID:15324367

KEY TERMS AND DEFINITIONS

Catastrophizing: Twisting the significance of positive and adverse occasions.

CDT (Clock Drawing Test): Is a short test and requires 5 minutes to control. The CDT measures visuospatial and chief capacities.

Clairvoyance: Accepting that you know how another person is feeling for sure they are thinking with no proof.

Cognitive Behavioral Therapy: Cognitive conduct treatment is a common sense, active methodology that helps individuals changes the manner in which they feel by assessing and changing the manner in which they think and act.

Cognitive Disorders: Disorders that significantly impairs the cognitive function of a person to the point everyday life in society is impossible without treatment.

Cognitive Impairments: It is the trouble in remembering, concentrating, learning new things, or making decisions in everyday life.

Cognitive Therapy: Momentary strategy for getting melancholy by showing individuals perceive their broken reasoning and think all the more objectively.

Dementia: It can be characterized as an aggravation in scholarly capacities, and it is normal joined by changes in the individual's conduct and character.

Group Therapy: Treating patients in a social environment is here and there attempted for different conditions.

Mini Mental State Examination (MMSE): The MMSE is the most regularly utilized test worldwide for evaluating cognitive capacity.

Chapter 4
A Brief Discussion on Acute Disseminated Encephalomyelitis (ADEM) and Agenesis of the Corpus Callosum (ACC)

Mohammed Junaid Mouda
University of Technology and Applied Sciences, Oman

Dinamani M.
Dayananda Sagar College of Engineering, India

Jyothi M. S.
AMC College of Engineering, India

Sangmesh D.
Madanjeet School of Green Energy Technologies, Pondicherry University, India

ABSTRACT

The word "cognitive disorder" is assigned to behavioral and personality changes leading to a gradual decline of various cognitive realms which further disturbs the day-to-day social as well as professional activities. Acute disseminated encephalomyelitis (ADEM) and agenesis of the corpus callosum (ACC) are the irreversible and growing brain conditions destroying the memory and thinking ability causing dementia. Though there exists an exponential increase in both the patients, they are well demarcated clinically with various biomarkers. However, the limited efficiency of the available therapeutic agents for treating AD is a spotlight to develop novel drugs. Herein, the chapter deals with the basic information on symptoms, stages, causes, and even treatment methods for ADEM and ACC.

DOI: 10.4018/978-1-7998-9534-3.ch004

ACUTE DISSEMINATED ENCEPHALOMYELITIS (ADEM)

Acute disseminated encephalomyelitis (ADEM) is considered as a loss or destruction of myelin in nerve tissue disease of the central nervous system (CNS). Most commonly affected are Young and adolescent children (Anil Apak et al., 1999; Anlar et al., 2003; Dale et al., 2000; Hynson et al., 2001; Leake et al., 2004; S. K. Murthy, Faden, Cohen, & Bakshi, 2002). ADEM followed common childhood infections such as measles, smallpox, and chickenpox were associated with significant mortality and morbidity. The estimated incidence is 0.8 per 100 000 populations per year (Leake et al., 2004). Huge numbers of cases among adults and even elderly patients have been reported (Schwarz, Mohr, Knauth, Wildemann, & Storch–Hagenlocher, 2001); however, the incidence may be considerably lower. In contrast with cases of multiple sclerosis (MS), there appears to be no sex preponderance in ADEM (Dale et al., 2000; Leake et al., 2004). 50% to 75% of all cases, the clinical onset of disease is preceded by viral or bacterial infections, mostly nonspecific upper respiratory tract infections (Hynson et al., 2001; Leake et al., 2004; S. K. Murthy et al., 2002). Acute disseminated encephalomyelitis may also develop following a vaccination (post immunization encephalomyelitis). ADEM is a relatively rare disorder, but it is of real concern for several reasons. The reasons are

(i) Vaccination schedules, particularly for children, have expanded over the past years.
(ii) ADEM may result in permanent neurological disability appears very early in life.

Vaccination-associated ADEM is most commonly observed after measles, mumps, or rubella vaccinations. It also reported after polio and European tick-borne encephalitis vaccinations (Schattenfroh, 2004; Tenembaum, Chamoles, & Fejerman, 2002). It is significant that the incidence of a measles vaccination–associated ADEM is about 10 to 20 per 100 000 vaccinated individuals and thus considerably lower than the incidence of ADEM after a wild-type measles encephalitis (100 per 100 000 infected individuals). A number of infectious agents, mainly viruses, have been associated with ADEM. Clinical signs and symptoms of ADEM may show themselves para infectiously or post infectiously.

Figure 1. Representative picture of ADEM

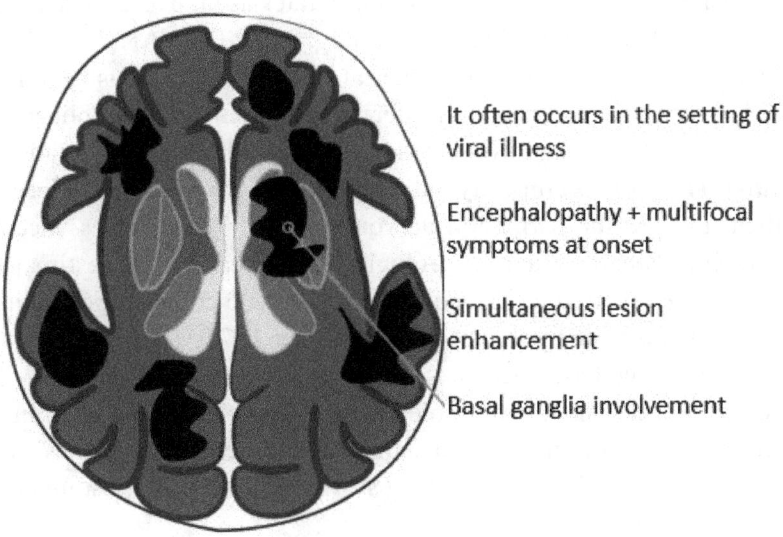

Typically, there is a lag period of 7 to 14 days between a feverish type of illness and the onset of neurological symptoms. In the case of vaccination-associated ADEM, this lag period may be longer. The recognition of the temporary association between a vaccination or infection and the appearance of neurological signs and symptoms is critical and complex. The Collaborating Center for Reference and Research on Viral Hepatitis of the World Health Organization (Geneva, Switzerland), for instance, has estimated a maximum period of 3 months to diagnose a vaccination-associated ADEM. Such a long lag period may be helpful for the recognition of vaccination associated ADEM because individual vaccinations are always separated by months and even years and can be easily identified in careful history records. Conversely, a widely accepted general rule for the latent period between infections and the occurrence of ADEM has not been firmly established. One reason for this may be that it is statistically challenging to establish a causal link between a feverish illness and neurological sequelae. In children who were diagnosed with ADEM, a history of a febrile event can be established in 50% to 75% of all cases (Hynson et al., 2001; Leake et al., 2004).

The actual incidence of ADEM is unknown. Earlier, ADEM was observed in childhood infections (like measles, smallpox, and chickenpox) and was associated with considerable mortality and morbidity. Owing to the advances in infectious disease control, ADEM in developed countries is now seen most frequently after non-specific upper respiratory tract infections and the disease causing agent remains unknown. In a recent study by Murthy et al, despite vigorous attempts to identify microbial pathogens in 18 patients, only one patient had Epstein-Barr virus isolated as the definite microbial cause of ADEM. Of the other two patients with rotavirus disease, in one patient infection was considered as possibly associated with ADEM. Failure to identify a viral agent suggests that the inciting agents are unusual or cannot be recovered by standard laboratory procedures (S. K. Murthy et al., 2002). In developing and poor countries, because of poor implementation of immunization programs, measles and other viral infections are still widely prevalent and account for frequent occurrences of post infectious demyelinating diseases. ADEM in developing countries is much more frequent than reported (J. Murthy, Yangala, Meena, & Reddy, 1999). In the past it had been observed that ADEM occurred in one out of 1000 measles infections. ADEM was relatively uncommon after varicella infection and the incidence that had been reported was about one per 10 000 patients. The incidence of ADEM after rubella infection was approximately one per 500 infections. Mortality and major neurological sequelae of ADEM after varicella and rubella infections were much lower in comparison with ADEM after measles infection. ADEM found after measles was associated with mortality rates as high as 25% and 25%–40% of survivors were left with permanent neurological sequelae (Garg, 2003; LITVAK, SANDS, & GIBEL, 1943; J. Murthy et al., 1999). Mycoplasma The main bacterial infection, which has been implicated with the occurrence of ADEM. Other viral and bacterial infections that have been implicated with ADEM are listed in box 2. Another common variant of ADEM is that which follows vaccination (post immunization encephalomyelitis). This form is clinically indistinguishable from the post infectious variety except the former more often involves the peripheral nervous system. When rabies vaccine was generated from virus grown in rabbit brain, the rate of neurological complications was estimated to be as high as one in 400 vaccinations. The reported incidence of neuroparalytic complications with the Simple type of anti-rabies vaccine varied between one per 600 to one per 1575 vaccinations. Such complications are now rare as non-neural tissue based vaccines are being used. An incidence rate of one per 25 000 vaccinations occurred with duck embryo anti rabies vaccine, a preparation containing minimal amount of neural tissue. Introduction of the non-neural human diploid cell vaccine has virtually eliminated neuroparalytic complications of rabies vaccinations (Stüv & Zamvil, 1999; Swamy et al., 1984). When smallpox vaccination was a part of a universal immunization program, encephalomyelitis followed one in 4000 vaccinations. Currently, post immunization encephalomyelitis is most commonly associated with measles, mumps, and rubella vaccinations. The incidence is 1–2 per million for live measles vaccine immunisations, which is significantly lower than that for post infectious encephalomyelitis from measles itself. The risk of occurrence of ADEM is 20 times lower after vaccination than ADEM after natural measles virus infection (Chakravarty, 2001).

Preceding Infectious Illnesses

1. **Infections**
   a. Viral
      i. Measles.
      ii. Mumps.
      iii. Influenza A or B.
      iv. Hepatitis A or B.
      v. Herpes simplex.
      vi. Human herpes virus E.
      vii. Varicella, rubella.
      viii. Epstein-Barr virus.
      ix. Cytomegalovirus.
      x. HIV.
   b. Others
      i. Mycoplasma pneumonia.
      ii. Chlamydia.
      iii. Legionella.
      iv. Campylobacter.
      v. Streptococcus.
2. **Vaccines**
   a. Rabies.
   b. Diphtheria, tetanus, pertussis.
   c. Smallpox.
   d. Measles.
   e. Japanese B encephalitis.
   f. Polio.
   g. Hepatitis B.
   h. Influenza.

Extensive experimental data shows that both primary autoimmune responses and immune responses secondary to an infection may contribute to CNS inflammation with subsequent demyelination. Two animal models closely resemble ADEM clinically and histopathologically. First, experimental autoimmune encephalomyelitis is widely used to study underlying disease mechanisms of ADEM (Rivers, Sprunt, & Berry, 1933). After immunization with CNS homogenate or encephalitogenic myelin peptides emulsified in Freund complete adjuvant, susceptible animals present with a monophasic disease with tetraparesis, weight loss, and incontinence. Histopathologically, inflammatory demyelinating lesions are detectable in the brains and spinal cords of affected animals. Second, Theiler murine encephalomyelitis, which was established as an animal model in the 1930s, was used to specifically study infectious and para infectious mechanisms that may contribute to the pathogenesis of ADEM (Lipton, 1975). Susceptible mouse strains present with sub-acute encephalitis and extensive demyelination after direct injection of a cerebral hemisphere with the Theiler murine encephalomyelitis virus. The disease found to be triggered by a major histocompatibility complex class 1 restricted CD8 T-cell response against viral epitopes, while the ongoing inflammation is sustained by major histocompatibility complex class 2 restricted CD4T-cell responses against myelin determinants. Extensive research with these animal models has led to the development of two current pathogenic concepts. The inflammatory cascade concept implies a direct CNS infection with a neurotropic pathogen, resulting in CNS tissue damage and systemic leakage of CNS-confined auto antigens into the systemic circulation through a disintegrated blood-brain barrier. These auto antigens, once processed in systemic lymphatic organs, will lead to tolerance breakdown and to a self-reactive and encephalitogenic T-cell response. Such activated T cells are capable of invading the CNS and sustaining CNS inflammation even further. The molecular mimicry concept proposes a structural or partial amino-acid sequence homology between the injected pathogen and myelin proteins of the host (Fujinami & Oldstone, 1985). This structural homology is not enough for a pathogen to be recognized as "self," which would result in immune tolerance. Antigen-presenting cells such as B cells or dendritic cells process the pathogen at the site of injection, leading to T-cell activation. Activated T cells may in turn cross activate antigen-specific B cells. Both activated T cells and B cells are quite capable of entering the CNS for routine immune observation. Thus, even after clearance of the pathogen, these antigen-specific cells may encounter the homologue myelin protein during their physiologic surveillance of the CNS. They may become reactivated by local antigen-presenting cells such as microglia, causing an inflammatory immune reaction against the presumed foreign antigen; thus, the initially physiological immune response leads to destructive autoimmunity. Some of the vaccine-associated ADEM cases can be directly attributed to the contamination of the specific vaccine with CNS tissue. This contamination may explain the substantial 0.15% incidence of ADEM after immunization with a live attenuated rabies virus vaccine (Semple vaccine) in developing countries, which is propagated in cultures of rabbit or goat CNS tissue. In this regard, antibodies against myelin antigens are detectable in patients with Semple vaccine–associated ADEM (Hemachudha et al., 1987). Newer rabies vaccines are propagated in human diploid cells and do not cause this particular adverse effect. A similar mechanism may account for ADEM observed after vaccination against Japanese B encephalitis, where certain vaccine strains are propagated in mouse brains (Plesner, Arlien-Søborg, & Herning, 1998).

Treatment

Controlled clinical trials that would meet the type A or type B criteria proposed by the American Academy of Neurology, Saint Paul, Minn, and the MS Council for Clinical Practice Guidelines have not yet been conducted in ADEM. At this time, intravenous high-dose corticosteroids are, based on empirical evidence (type C recommendation), widely accepted as first-line treatment (Shahar, Andraus, Savitzki, Pilar, & Zelnik, 2002). The aim is to reduce the CNS inflammatory reaction as soon as possible and to achieve an increased clinical improvement. A number of various other anti-inflammatory and immunosuppressant therapies may also be quite effective. Several case studies have reported beneficial effects of plasmapheresis (Keegan et al., 2002) and intravenous immunoglobulin therapies (Keegan et al., 2002; Shahar et al., 2002). Immunosuppressive agents, such as mitoxantrone or cyclophosphamide, should be considered as alternative therapies if corticosteroid treatment shows no clinical effect (Apak, Anlar, & Saatci, 1999; Nishikawa, Ichiyama, Hayashi, Ouchi, & Furukawa, 1999) or if relative and absolute contraindications for corticosteroids exist. As a pragmatic and clinical practical approach, the following treatment scheme was proposed. For therapeutic interventions in MS relapses, an initial regime of high-dose intravenous methylprednisolone with a cumulative dose of 3 to 5 g, followed by a prolonged oral prednisolone taper of 3 to 6 weeks was proposed. Should a patient not respond adequately to corticosteroids, therapy should be escalated, preferentially with intravenous immunoglobulin (0.4 g/kg of body weight over 5 days) (Keegan et al., 2002; Shahar et al., 2002) alternatively, or if this approach fails, plasmapharesis was considered [28]. In very severe cases, immunosuppression with cyclophosphamide or mitoxantrone should be attempted. In general, treatment should be initiated as early as possible and as aggressive as necessary.

As most children shows meningism with fever, and an acute encephalopathy, with evidence of inflammation in blood and CSF, they should be covered initially with cefotaxime or other appropriate antibiotic and acyclovir until a diagnosis can be established. Once the diagnosis of ADEM is established, treatment usually commences with 3–5 days of intravenous methylprednisolone (20–30 mg/kg/day), with or without a following course of oral prednisolone commencing at 2 mg/kg/day and tapering over 4–6 weeks, depending on resolution of clinical signs. In children who have early relapses or in whom there has been a delay in diagnosis, a tapering course of intravenous methylprednisolone over two weeks after the initial course was used; for example, single dose intravenous methylprednisolone 10 mg/kg, one week after the last dose, followed by another single dose of 5 mg/kg a week later. Other treatment options include dexamethasone, intravenous immunoglobulins (Sahlas, Miller, Guerin, Veilleux, & Francis, 2000), and plasmapheresis (Kanter et al., 1995), but little evidence exists for their effectiveness.

AGENESIS OF THE CORPUS CALLOSUM (ACC)

Agenesis of the corpus callosum (ACC) is one of several disorders of the corpus callosum, the structure that connects the two hemispheres (left and right) of the brain. In ACC the corpus callosum is partially or completely absent. It is caused by a disruption of brain cell migration during fetal development. ACC can occur as an isolated condition or in combination with other cerebral abnormalities, including Arnold-Chiari malformation, Dandy-Walker syndrome, schizencephaly (clefts or deep divisions in brain tissue), and holoprosencephaly (failure of the forebrain to divide into lobes.) Girls may have a gender-specific condition called Aicardi syndrome, which causes severe cognitive impairment and developmental delays, seizures, abnormalities in the vertebra of the spine, and lesions on the retina of the eye. ACC can also be associated with malformations in other parts of the body, such as midline facial defects. The effects of the disorder range from subtle or mild to severe, depending on associated brain abnormalities. Children with the most severe brain malformations may have intellectual impairment, seizures, hydrocephalus, and spasticity. Other disorders of the corpus callosum include dysgenesis, in which the corpus callosum is developed in a malformed or incomplete way, and hypoplasia, in which the corpus callosum is thinner than usual. Individuals with these disorders have a higher risk of hearing deficits and cardiac abnormalities than individuals with the normal structure. Impairments in social interaction and communication in individuals having a disorder of the corpus callosum may overlap with autism spectrum disorder behaviors. It is estimated that at least one in 4,000 individuals has a disorder of the corpus callosum.

There is no standard course of treatment for ACC. Treatment usually involves management of symptoms and seizures if they occur. Associated difficulties are much more manageable with early recognition and therapy, especially therapies focusing on left/right coordination. Early diagnosis and interventions are currently the best treatments to improve social and developmental outcomes.

Signs and symptoms of ACC and other callosal disorders vary greatly among individuals. However, some characteristics common in individuals with callosal disorders include vision impairments, low muscle tone (hypotonia), poor motor coordination, delays in motor milestones such as sitting and walking, delayed toilet training and dysautonomic symptoms such as low perception of pain or chewing and swallowing difficulties.

Figure 2. Representative picture for ACC

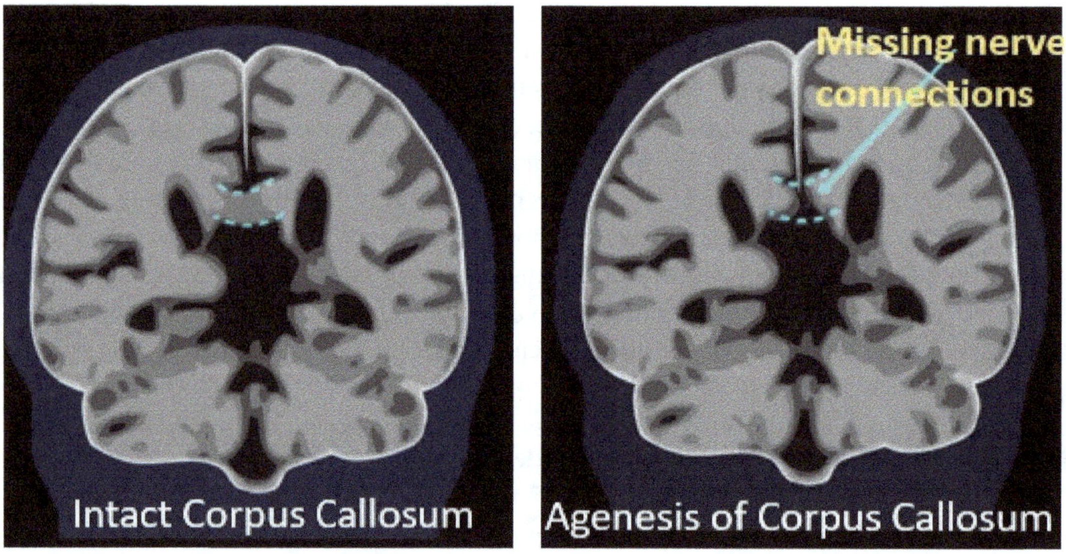

Laboratory research has demonstrated that individuals with ACC have difficulty transferring more complex information from one hemisphere to the other (Staff, 2011). They also have been shown to have some cognitive disabilities (difficulty in complex problem solving) and social difficulties (missing subtle social cues), even when their intelligence quotient is normal. Recent research suggests that specific social difficulties may be a result of impaired face processing (Aldinger & Doherty, 2016). The unusual social behavior in childhood often resembles that of an autism spectrum disorder.

Other characteristics sometimes associated with callosal disorders include seizures, spasticity, early feeding difficulties and/or gastric reflux, hearing impairments, abnormal head and facial features, and intellectual disability (Hueber et al., 2012).

Signs and Symptoms

Agenesis of corpus callosum (ACC) may initially become evident through the onset of epileptic seizures during the first weeks of life or within the first two years. However, not all individuals with ACC have seizures. (For more information on these types of seizures choose “epilepsy” as your search term in the Rare Disease Database).

Other symptoms that may begin early in life are feeding problems and delays in holding the head erect. Sitting, standing and walking may also be delayed. Impairment of mental and physical development, and/or an accumulation of fluid in the skull (hydrocephalus) are also symptomatic of the early onset type of this disorder. (For more information, choose “hydrocephalus” as your search term in the Rare Disease Database.) Non-progressive mental retardation, impaired hand-eye coordination and visual or auditory (hearing) memory impairment can be diagnosed through neurological testing of patients with ACC.

In some mild cases, symptoms may not appear for many years. Older patients are usually diagnosed during tests for symptoms such as seizures, monotonous or repetitive speech, or headaches. In mild cases it may be overlooked due to lack of obvious symptoms during childhood. Some patients may have deep-set eyes and a prominent forehead. An abnormally small head (microcephaly), or sometimes an unusually large head (macrocephaly), may be present. Tags of skin in front of the ears (pre-auricular skin tags), one or more bent fingers (camptodactyly), and delayed growth have also been associated with some cases of agenesis of corpus callosum. In other cases wide-set eyes (telecanthus), a small nose with upturned (anteverted) nostrils, abnormally shaped ears, excessive neck skin, short hands, diminished muscle tone (hypotonia), abnormalities of the larynx, heart defects, and symptoms of Pierre-Robin syndrome may be present. (For more information choose “Pierre-Robin” as your search term in the Rare Disease Database).

Aicardi syndrome, thought to be inherited as an X-linked dominant disorder, consists of agenesis of corpus callosum, infantile spasms, and abnormal eye structure. This disorder is an extremely rare congenital disorder in which frequent seizures, striking abnormalities of the eye’s middle coat (choroid) and retinal layers, and the absence of the structure linking the two cerebral hemispheres (the corpus callosum), accompany severe mental retardation. Only females are affected. (For more information on this disorder, choose “Aicardi” as your search term in the Rare Disease Database).

Andermann syndrome, identified in 1972, is a genetic disorder characterized by a combination of agenesis of corpus callosum, mental retardation, and progressive sensorimotor nervous system disturbances (neuropathy). All known cases of this disorder originate from Charlevois County and the Saguenay-Lac St. Jean area of Quebec, Canada. The gene causing this rare form of ACC was recently identified and testing for this gene (SLC12A6) is currently available. XLAG (X linked lissencephaly with ambiguous genitalia is a rare genetic disorder in which males have small and smooth brains (lissencephaly), small penis, severe mental retardation and intractable epilepsy. This is caused by mutations in the ARX gene. In females, these same mutations can cause ACC alone, whereas less severe mutations in males can cause mental retardation. Testing for this disorder is also clinically available.

Causes

In most cases, the cause of ACC is not known. However, agenesis of corpus callosum can be inherited as an autosomal recessive trait or an X-linked dominant trait. This disorder may also be due in part to an infection during pregnancy (intrauterine) leading to abnormal development of the fetal brain. Genetic diseases are determined by the combination of genes for a particular trait that are on the chromosomes received from the father and the mother.

Recessive genetic disorders occur when an individual inherits the same abnormal gene for the same trait from each parent. If an individual receives one normal gene and one gene for the disease, the person will be a carrier for the disease, but usually will not show symptoms. The risk for two carrier parents to both pass the defective gene and, therefore, have an affected child is 25% with each pregnancy. The risk to have a child who is a carrier like the parents is 50% with each pregnancy. The chance for a child to receive normal genes from both parents and be genetically normal for that particular trait is 25%. The risk is the same for males and females.

In X-linked dominant disorders, a female with only one X chromosome with an abnormal gene will develop the disease. However, the affected male always has a more severe condition. Sometimes, affected males die before birth so that only female patients survive. This seems to be true for one form of agenesis of corpus callosum known as Aicardi syndrome. The majority of patients diagnosed so far have been females. Aicardi syndrome has been seen occasionally in males with an extra X chromosome.

Agenesis of the corpus callosum is caused by disruption to development of the fetal brain between the 3rd and 12th weeks of pregnancy (Paul, Corsello, Kennedy, & Adolphs, 2014). In most cases, it is not possible to know what caused an individual to have ACC or another callosal disorder. However, research suggests that some possible causes may include chromosome errors, inherited genetic factors, prenatal infections or injuries, prenatal toxic exposures, structural blockage by cysts or other brain abnormalities and metabolic disorders (Hueber et al., 2012). Ciliopathies: rare genetic disorders

Until recently, the medical literature did not indicate a connection among many genetic disorders, both genetic syndromes and genetic diseases that are now being found to be related. As a result of new genetic research, some of these are, in fact, highly related in their root cause despite the widely varying symptoms apparent on clinical examination. Agenesis of the corpus callosum is one such disease, part of an emerging class of diseases called ciliopathies. The underlying cause may be a dysfunctional molecular mechanism in the primary cilia structures of the cell organelles that are present in many cellular types throughout the human body. The cilia defects adversely affect "numerous critical developmental signaling pathways" essential to cellular development and thus offer a plausible hypothesis for the often multi-symptom nature of a large set of syndromes and diseases. Known ciliopathies include primary ciliary dyskinesia, Bardet–Biedl syndrome, polycystic kidney and liver disease, nephronophthisis, Alström syndrome, Meckel–Gruber syndrome and some forms of retinal degeneration (Edwards, Sherr, Barkovich, & Richards, 2014).

Diagnosis

Callosal disorders can be diagnosed through brain imaging studies or during autopsy (Ahearne et al., 1992). They may be diagnosed through an MRI, CT scan, Sonography, prenatal ultrasound, or prenatal MRI.

Treatment

There are currently no specific medical treatments for callosal disorders, but individuals with ACC and other callosal disorders may benefit from a range of developmental therapies, educational support, and services. It is important to consult with a variety of medical, health, educational, and social work professionals. Such professionals include neurologists, neuropsychologists, occupational therapists, physical therapists, speech and language pathologists, pediatricians, recreation therapists, music therapists, geneticists, social workers, special educators, early childhood intervention specialists, and caregivers for adults. Treatment is symptomatic and supportive. Anti-seizure medications, special education, physical therapy, and related services may be of benefit depending upon the range and severity of symptoms. When hydrocephalus is present it may be treated with a surgical shunt to drain the fluid from the brain cavity, thereby lowering the increased pressure on the brain. Genetic counseling may also be of benefit to families with this disorder.

Prognosis varies depending on the type of callosal abnormality and associated conditions or syndromes. It is not possible for the corpus callosum to regenerate (Ahearne et al., 1992). Neuropsychological testing reveals subtle differences in higher cortical function compared to individuals of the same age and education without ACC, although some individuals with callosal disorders have average intelligence and live normal lives.

Prognosis depends on the extent and severity of malformations. Intellectual impairment does not worsen. Individuals with a disorder of the corpus callosum typically have delays in attaining developmental milestones such as walking, talking, or reading; challenges with social interactions; clumsiness and poor motor coordination, particularly on skills that require coordination of left and right hands and feet (such as swimming, bicycle riding, and driving; and mental and social processing problems that become more apparent with age, with problems particularly evident from junior high school into adulthood.

The possibility that in autism, smaller neurons may produce fewer long-range connections, including interhemispheric callosal axons, might be explained by a significantly smaller neuronal body in 4- to 8-year-old autistic children in 13 of the examined subcortical structures, archicortex, cerebellum, and brainstem (Courchesne et al., 2011), superior and middle frontal gyrus (Wegiel et al., 2015), inferior frontal cortex (Casanova et al., 2006), anterior mid-cingulate (Uppal et al., 2014), and cingulate cortex (Simms, Kemper, Timbie, Bauman, & Blatt, 2009), and in other brain structures (Bauman & Kemper, 1985).

The risk of fetal and postnatal distortion of CC development appears to be very high because of the extremely dynamic process of CC growth during fetal life, with an increase in the number of axons by 1.8×10^6 per day in the last 100 days of rhesus fetal life, and CC reorganization, with the loss of 4.4×10^6 axons per day during the first 3 weeks of postnatal life (LaMantia & Rakic, 1990). One may speculate that even a short exposure of the human fetus or infant to noxious factors may permanently distort CC structure and function and contribute to the autism phenotype. However, it is still not known whether defects in axonal pruning affect CC size and contribute to callosal hypoplasia in humans.

STUDY LIMITATIONS

The results of clinical studies (based on brain MRI) of hundreds of individuals with autism and typically developing control subjects, may provide partially different results than postmortem studies, which are usually limited to much fewer brains of subjects diagnosed with autism and a similar number of age-matched control cases. One of the causes of these differences might be a higher mortality rate in the population diagnosed with autism, epilepsy, and intellectual disabilities than in the general population (Pickett, Xiu, Tuchman, Dawson, & Lajonchere, 2011), resulting in higher prevalence and more severe developmental anomalies in postmortem than in clinical studies. The presence of partial agenesis in 3 of 10 examined subjects, as well as ectopias and dysplastic changes in other brain regions, appears to be a reflection of this higher prevalence of multiregional and diverse developmental anomalies detected in the postmortem-examined group (Wegiel et al., 2013; Wegiel et al., 2012). The concentration of focal agenesis in the youngest subjects (5, 8, and 11 years of age), but its absence in examined postmortem adults might be an effect of a small group or may indicate that CC partial agenesis is a sign of a more complex and severe developmental pathology that increases the risk of death, especially related to epilepsy. Another factor contributing to the lower prevalence of CC developmental anomalies in clinical studies might be the limited resolution of routine clinical imaging in comparison to macroscopic and microscopic examination of hundreds of serial 200-µm-thick sections in this postmortem study.

REFERENCES

Ahearne, P. M., Baillie, J. M., Cotton, P. B., Baker, M. E., Meyers, W. C., & Pappas, T. N. (1992). An endoscopic retrograde cholangiopancreatography (ERCP)-based algorithm for the management of pancreatic pseudocysts. *American Journal of Surgery*, *163*(1), 111–116. doi:10.1016/0002-9610(92)90262-P PMID:1733357

Aldinger, K. A., & Doherty, D. (2016). *The genetics of cerebellar malformations.* Paper presented at the Seminars in Fetal and Neonatal Medicine.

Anil Apak, R., Kose, G., Topaloglu, H., Anlar, B., Turanh, G., & Özdirim, E. (1999). Acute disseminated encephalomyelitis in childhood: Report of 10 cases. *Journal of Child Neurology*, *14*(3), 198–201. doi:10.1177/088307389901400312 PMID:10190272

Anlar, B., Basaran, C., Kose, G., Guven, A., Haspolat, S., Yakut, A., ... Karaagaoglu, E. (2003). Acute disseminated encephalomyelitis in children: Outcome and prognosis. *Neuropediatrics*, *34*(04), 194–199. doi:10.1055-2003-42208 PMID:12973660

Apak, R. A., Anlar, B., & Saatci, I. (1999). A case of relapsing acute disseminated encephalomyelitis with high dose corticosteroid treatment. *Brain & Development*, *21*(4), 279–282. doi:10.1016/S0387-7604(99)00011-X PMID:10392753

Bauman, M., & Kemper, T. L. (1985). Histoanatomic observations of the brain in early infantile autism. *Neurology*, *35*(6), 866–866. doi:10.1212/WNL.35.6.866 PMID:4000488

Casanova, M. F., van Kooten, I. A., Switala, A. E., van Engeland, H., Heinsen, H., Steinbusch, H. W., Hof, P. R., Trippe, J., Stone, J., & Schmitz, C. (2006). Minicolumnar abnormalities in autism. *Acta Neuropathologica*, *112*(3), 287–303. doi:10.100700401-006-0085-5 PMID:16819561

Chakravarty, A. (2001). Neurologic illness following post-exposure prophylaxis with purifiled chick embryo cell antirabies vaccine. *The Journal of the Association of Physicians of India*, *49*, 927–928. PMID:11837768

Courchesne, E., Mouton, P. R., Calhoun, M. E., Semendeferi, K., Ahrens-Barbeau, C., Hallet, M. J., Barnes, C. C., & Pierce, K. (2011). Neuron number and size in prefrontal cortex of children with autism. *Journal of the American Medical Association*, *306*(18), 2001–2010. doi:10.1001/jama.2011.1638 PMID:22068992

Dale, R., De Sousa, C., Chong, W., Cox, T., Harding, B., & Neville, B. (2000). Acute disseminated encephalomyelitis, multiphasic disseminated encephalomyelitis and multiple sclerosis in children. *Brain*, *123*(12), 2407–2422. doi:10.1093/brain/123.12.2407 PMID:11099444

Edwards, T. J., Sherr, E. H., Barkovich, A. J., & Richards, L. J. (2014). Clinical, genetic and imaging findings identify new causes for corpus callosum development syndromes. *Brain, 137*(6), 1579–1613. doi:10.1093/brain/awt358 PMID:24477430

Fujinami, R. S., & Oldstone, M. (1985). Amino acid homology between the encephalitogenic site of myelin basic protein and virus: Mechanism for autoimmunity. *Science, 230*(4729), 1043–1045. doi:10.1126cience.2414848 PMID:2414848

Garg, R. K. (2003). Acute disseminated encephalomyelitis. *Postgraduate Medical Journal, 79*(927), 11–17. doi:10.1136/pmj.79.927.11 PMID:12566545

Hemachudha, T., Griffin, D. E., Giffels, J. J., Johnson, R. T., Moser, A. B., & Phanuphak, P. (1987). Myelin basic protein as an encephalitogen in encephalomyelitis and polyneuritis following rabies vaccination. *The New England Journal of Medicine, 316*(7), 369–374. doi:10.1056/NEJM198702123160703 PMID:2433582

Hueber, W., Sands, B. E., Lewitzky, S., Vandemeulebroecke, M., Reinisch, W., Higgins, P. D., ... Karczewski, M. (2012). Secukinumab, a human anti-IL-17A monoclonal antibody, for moderate to severe Crohn's disease: Unexpected results of a randomised, double-blind placebo-controlled trial. *Gut, 61*(12), 1693–1700. doi:10.1136/gutjnl-2011-301668 PMID:22595313

Hynson, J., Kornberg, A., Coleman, L., Shield, L., Harvey, A., & Kean, M. (2001). Clinical and neuroradiologic features of acute disseminated encephalomyelitis in children. *Neurology, 56*(10), 1308–1312. doi:10.1212/WNL.56.10.1308 PMID:11376179

Kanter, D., Horensky, D., Sperling, R., Kaplan, J., Malachowski, M., & Churchill, W. (1995). Plasmapheresis in fulminant acute disseminated encephalomyelitis. *Neurology, 45*(4), 824–827. doi:10.1212/WNL.45.4.824 PMID:7723979

Keegan, M., Pineda, A., McClelland, R., Darby, C., Rodriguez, M., & Weinshenker, B. (2002). Plasma exchange for severe attacks of CNS demyelination: Predictors of response. *Neurology, 58*(1), 143–146. doi:10.1212/WNL.58.1.143 PMID:11781423

LaMantia, A., & Rakic, P. (1990). Axon overproduction and elimination in the corpus callosum of the developing rhesus monkey. *The Journal of Neuroscience: The Official Journal of the Society for Neuroscience, 10*(7), 2156–2175. doi:10.1523/JNEUROSCI.10-07-02156.1990 PMID:2376772

Leake, J. A., Albani, S., Kao, A. S., Senac, M. O., Billman, G. F., Nespeca, M. P., Paulino, A. D., Quintela, E. R., Sawyer, M. H., & Bradley, J. S. (2004). Acute disseminated encephalomyelitis in childhood: Epidemiologic, clinical and laboratory features. *The Pediatric Infectious Disease Journal, 23*(8), 756–764. doi:10.1097/01.inf.0000133048.75452.dd PMID:15295226

Lipton, H. L. (1975). Theiler's virus infection in mice: An unusual biphasic disease process leading to demyelination. *Infection and Immunity, 11*(5), 1147–1155. doi:10.1128/iai.11.5.1147-1155.1975 PMID:164412

Litvak, A. M. (1943). Encephalitis complicating measles: Report of fifty-six cases with follow-up studies in thirty-two. *American Journal of Diseases of Children, 65*(2), 265–295. doi:10.1001/archpedi.1943.02010140073006

Murthy, J., Yangala, R., Meena, A., & Reddy, J. J. (1999). Acute disseminated encephalomyelitis: Clinical and MRI study from South India. *Journal of the Neurological Sciences*, *165*(2), 133–138. doi:10.1016/S0022-510X(99)00094-5 PMID:10450798

Murthy, S. K., Faden, H. S., Cohen, M. E., & Bakshi, R. (2002). Acute disseminated encephalomyelitis in children. *Pediatrics*, *110*(2), e21–e21. doi:10.1542/peds.110.2.e21 PMID:12165620

Nishikawa, M., Ichiyama, T., Hayashi, T., Ouchi, K., & Furukawa, S. (1999). Intravenous immunoglobulin therapy in acute disseminated encephalomyelitis. *Pediatric Neurology*, *21*(2), 583–586. doi:10.1016/S0887-8994(99)00042-9 PMID:10465150

Paul, L. K., Corsello, C., Kennedy, D. P., & Adolphs, R. (2014). Agenesis of the corpus callosum and autism: A comprehensive comparison. *Brain*, *137*(6), 1813–1829. doi:10.1093/brain/awu070 PMID:24771497

Pickett, J., Xiu, E., Tuchman, R., Dawson, G., & Lajonchere, C. (2011). Mortality in individuals with autism, with and without epilepsy. *Journal of Child Neurology*, *26*(8), 932–939. doi:10.1177/0883073811402203 PMID:21471551

Plesner, A. M., Arlien-Søborg, P., & Herning, M. (1998). Neurological complications to vaccination against Japanese encephalitis. *European Journal of Neurology*, *5*(5), 479–485. doi:10.1046/j.1468-1331.1998.550479.x PMID:10210877

Rivers, T. M., Sprunt, D., & Berry, G. (1933). Observations on attempts to produce acute disseminated encephalomyelitis in monkeys. *The Journal of Experimental Medicine*, *58*(1), 39–53. doi:10.1084/jem.58.1.39 PMID:19870180

Sahlas, D., Miller, S., Guerin, M., Veilleux, M., & Francis, G. (2000). Treatment of acute disseminated encephalomyelitis with intravenous immunoglobulin. *Neurology*, *54*(6), 1370–1372. doi:10.1212/WNL.54.6.1370 PMID:10746613

Schattenfroh, C. (2004). Acute disseminated encephalomyelitis after active immunization against early summer encephalitis. *Der Nervenarzt*, *75*(8), 776–779. PMID:15309308

Schwarz, S., Mohr, A., Knauth, M., Wildemann, B., & Storch–Hagenlocher, B. (2001). Acute disseminated encephalomyelitis: A follow-up study of 40 adult patients. *Neurology*, *56*(10), 1313–1318. doi:10.1212/WNL.56.10.1313 PMID:11376180

Shahar, E., Andraus, J., Savitzki, D., Pilar, G., & Zelnik, N. (2002). Outcome of severe encephalomyelitis in children: Effect of high-dose methylprednisolone and immunoglobulins. *Journal of Child Neurology*, *17*(11), 810–814. doi:10.1177/08830738020170111001 PMID:12585719

Simms, M. L., Kemper, T. L., Timbie, C. M., Bauman, M. L., & Blatt, G. J. (2009). The anterior cingulate cortex in autism: Heterogeneity of qualitative and quantitative cytoarchitectonic features suggests possible subgroups. *Acta Neuropathologica*, *118*(5), 673–684. doi:10.100700401-009-0568-2 PMID:19590881

Stüv, O., & Zamvil, S. S. (1999). Pathogenesis, diagnosis, and treatment of acute disseminated encephalomyelitis. *Current Opinion in Neurology*, *12*(4), 395–401. doi:10.1097/00019052-199908000-00005 PMID:10555827

Swamy, H. S., Shankar, S., Chandra, P. S., Aroor, S. R., Krishna, A. S., & Perumal, V. K. (1984). Neurological complications due to beta-propiolactone (BPL)-inactivated antirabies vaccination: Clinical, electrophysiological and therapeutic aspects. *Journal of the Neurological Sciences*, *63*(1), 111–128. doi:10.1016/0022-510X(84)90113-8 PMID:6699651

Tenembaum, S., Chamoles, N., & Fejerman, N. (2002). Acute disseminated encephalomyelitis: A long-term follow-up study of 84 pediatric patients. *Neurology*, *59*(8), 1224–1231. doi:10.1212/WNL.59.8.1224 PMID:12391351

Uppal, N., Wicinski, B., Buxbaum, J. D., Heinsen, H., Schmitz, C., & Hof, P. R. (2014). Neuropathology of the anterior midcingulate cortex in young children with autism. *Journal of Neuropathology and Experimental Neurology*, *73*(9), 891–902. doi:10.1097/NEN.0000000000000108 PMID:25101703

Wegiel, J., Flory, M., Kuchna, I., Nowicki, K., Ma, S. Y., Imaki, H., ... Wierzba-Bobrowicz, T. (2015). Neuronal nucleus and cytoplasm volume deficit in children with autism and volume increase in adolescents and adults. *Acta Neuropathologica Communications*, *3*(1), 1–17. doi:10.118640478-015-0183-5 PMID:25595448

Wegiel, J., Kuchna, I., Nowicki, K., Imaki, H., Wegiel, J., Ma, S. Y., ... Cohen, I. L. (2013). Contribution of olivofloccular circuitry developmental defects to atypical gaze in autism. *Brain Research*, *1512*, 106–122. doi:10.1016/j.brainres.2013.03.037 PMID:23558308

Wegiel, J., Schanen, N. C., Cook, E. H., Sigman, M., Brown, W. T., Kuchna, I., ... Ma, S. Y. (2012). Differences between the pattern of developmental abnormalities in autism associated with duplications 15q11. 2-q13 and idiopathic autism. *Journal of Neuropathology and Experimental Neurology*, *71*(5), 382–397. doi:10.1097/NEN.0b013e318251f537 PMID:22487857

Chapter 5
A Brief Discussion on Depression, Schizophrenia, and Obsessive Compulsive Disorder

Venkatesh Andavar
Salale University, Ethiopia

Shweta Gupta
Jain University, Bengaluru, India

ABSTRACT

This chapter describes three types of cognitive diseases: depression, obsessive-compulsive disorder (OCD), and schizophrenia. Depression is a frequent kind of mental illness. More than 264 million individuals of all ages suffer from depression across the world. Women are more likely than males to suffer from depression. Suicide can be caused by depression. For mild and severe depression, there are effective psychological and pharmaceutical therapies. Obsessive-compulsive disorder (OCD) or obsessive-compulsive ailment is an anxiety disorder. It is divided into two parts: obsessions and compulsions. Obsessions are recurring thoughts, ideas, visions, or impulses that are unpleasant and distressing. Compulsions are behaviors, routines, or mental acts that you engage in to relieve the distress brought on by your obsessions. Schizophrenia is a severe mental illness in which patients have distorted perceptions of reality. Schizophrenia can include hallucinations, delusions, and severely disorganized thought and behavior, which can make it difficult to operate on a daily basis.

INTRODUCTION

Depression is a frequent kind of mental illness. More than 264 million individuals of all ages suffer from depression across the world. Depression is a primary cause of disability globally and contributes significantly to the global illness burden. Women are more likely than males to suffer from depression. Suicide can be caused by depression. Depression is distinct from normal mood swings and short-term

DOI: 10.4018/978-1-7998-9534-3.ch005

emotional reactions to ordinary stresses. For mild and severe depression, there are effective psychological and pharmaceutical therapies.

A person's grief might be exacerbated by the death of a loved one, the loss of a career, or the termination of a relationship. It's natural to experience melancholy or grief in reaction to such circumstances. Those who have suffered a loss may describe themselves as *depressed.*

However, sadness is not the same as depression. Grief is a normal and individual process that shares some of the same characteristics as depression. Grief and depression can both cause extreme sadness and a withdrawal from daily activities.
They're also distinct in a number of ways:

- In sorrow, painful emotions come in waves, frequently intermingled with happy recollections of the departed.
- Self-esteem is generally preserved during bereavement. Feelings of worthlessness and self-loathing are frequent in severe depression.
- When thinking about or daydreaming about joining a departed loved one, thoughts of death may arise. The goal of serious depression is to terminate one's life because one feels worthless or undeserving of live, or because one is unable to cope with the anguish of despair.

BACKGROUND

Le HN, Boyd RC (2006), Online social media makes it difficult to identify non-depressed people. Their emotional state will be fluid and unpredictably variable. World Health Organization (2013) described that emotional states of an individual will be revealed through their social interactions, awareness, and internet posting.

Halfin A. (2007 Nov), Broadband transmission is inescapable internationally, and social media networks are enticing individuals to connect with one another from any distance within their domain. Picardi, A (2016) described that in many developing nations, Google, Facebook and Instagram, Twitter, Linkdin and Snapchat are perhaps the most popular social media platforms. It will also be utilized to assist people in sharing their thoughts, sentiments, emotions, desires, accomplishments, and so on.

Cameron, I., Cardy et.al (2011) provided a variety of subjects to debate and react to in any forum in an open and unrestricted manner. As a result, individuals are freely generating chances to operate in social networks and engage in dispute resolution with one another. It will gradually impact the mental condition of every individual who wishes to respond to someone else's shared ideas.

Smarr, K et.al (2011), Losada, Det. Al (2017), Park, M. at. el (2013) described that these social media networks will soon cause mental health problems, indicating that it is a form of addiction. Finally, it will aid any emotional individual in society in suicidal ideation.

Wongkoblap, A., et.al (2017), Aladag, A (2018), Rice, S. (2015), Balani, S (2015) stated that emotions are dealing with mental state. Among all online social media, the mental states are reading with some things happiness, sadness, anxiety, anger, and depression.

Grief and depression are two emotions that may coexist. The death of a loved one, the loss of a career, or being the victim of a physical attack or a catastrophic tragedy can all contribute to depression in certain people. Grief that is accompanied by depression is more acute and lasts longer than grief that is not accompanied by sadness.

Ustun G. (2021) categorized different levels of depression that a person underwent during COVID19. Female participants between the ages of 18 and 29, who were unmarried, students, and had less income than their costs had greater depression ratings than others. When compared to other individuals, those who were afraid of becoming sick and infecting others, had a cleanliness preoccupation, concern about the future, melancholy, and nervousness had lower levels of depression. Loneliness, dread of death, hopelessness, sleep issues, feelings of worthlessness, starting to smoke and consume alcohol, and mild depression were all reported by participants who had to relocate their place of residence during the quarantine.

Kleanthi, G., & Maria, G. (2021) described women with a lower educational background who were not married had greater mean values of alexithymia, anxiety, and depressive symptomatology than women with a higher educational background who were married. Infertile women also exhibited similar levels of alexithymia, anxiety, and depressive symptomatology as women who did not have reproductive issues.

Gupta, S. and Kant, V., (2020) presents a comparative study of genetic algorithm (GA) and genetic programming (GP) techniques by calculating weights for each criterion in a system, to aggregate criteria ratings for forecasting user preferences in MCRS. The efficacy of genetic programming and genetic algorithm techniques in multi-criteria rating systems are compared.
Symptoms of depression range from moderate to severe, and include:

- Sadness or a gloomy mood o Loss of interest or pleasure in previously liked activities
- Appetite changes — weight loss or increase that is unrelated to dieting
- Inability to sleep or excessive sleeping
- Excessive tiredness or a loss of energy
- Increased involuntary physical activity (e.g., difficulty to sit still, pacing, and handwringing) or slower motions or speech (these actions must be severe enough to be observable by others)
- A sense of worthlessness or shame
- Difficulty focusing, thinking, or making decisions
- Suicide or death thoughts

Depression can be caused by a variety of circumstances, including:

- Environmental factors: People who are constantly exposed to violence, neglect, abuse, or poverty may be more susceptible to depression.
- Genetics: Depression is a condition that can run in families. If one identical twin suffers depression, the other has a 70% probability of developing the disorder at some point in their lives.
- Biochemistry: Differences in some substances in the brain may play a role in depressive symptoms.
- Personality: People who have low self-esteem, are quickly overwhelmed by stress, or are gloomy in general appear to be more likely to suffer from depression.

TREATMENTS OF DEPRESSION

Depression is one of the most easily treated mental illnesses.

- Antidepressants may be prescribed to assist change a person's brain chemistry.
- Psychotherapy, often known as "talk therapy," is sometimes used alone to treat minor depression; however, it is frequently used in conjunction with antidepressant drugs to treat moderate to severe depression.
- CBT teaches a person to notice distorted/negative thinking and to change their ideas and behaviors so that they can respond to situations in a more positive way.
- Electroconvulsive Therapy (ECT) is a medical treatment used to treat individuals with severe major depression who have failed to respond to conventional treatments. While the patient is sedated, a brief electrical stimulation of the brain is performed. ECT is usually administered two to three times each week for a total of six to twelve treatments.

TYPES OF DEPRESSION

- **Premenstrual Dysphonic Disorder (PMDD)**: About a week before menstruation, a woman with PMDD has extreme depression, irritability, and stress. Mood swings, impatience or rage, depression, and worry or tension are all common symptoms. Other signs and symptoms include a loss of interest in typical activities, difficulties concentrating, a lack of energy or easy exhaustion, changes in appetite with specific food cravings, problems sleeping or sleeping too much, and a feeling of being overwhelmed or out of control. Breast discomfort or swelling, joint or muscle pain, a feeling of bloating, or weight gain are all possible physical signs. Every year, between 1.8 percent and 5.8 percent of menstruation women are thought to suffer from premenstrual dysphoric disorder.

Antidepressants, birth control pills, and nutritional supplements can all be used to treat PMDD. Reducing coffee and alcohol consumption, getting enough sleep and exercise, and practicing relaxation techniques can all help.

- **Disruptive Mood Dysregulation Disorder**: It affects children and adolescents aged 6 to 18. It is characterized by persistent and extreme irritation, as well as frequent and violent temper outbursts. Temper tantrums can be verbal or violent in nature, resulting in aggressiveness toward people or property. Disruptive mood dysregulation disorder can have a major impact on a child's capacity to function as well as the family's ability to operate. Psychotherapy (cognitive behavior therapy) and/or medicines are commonly used in treatment.
- **Persistent Depressive Disorder**: For at least two years, a person with persistent depressive illness (formerly known as dysthymic disorder) is depressed for the majority of the day, on more days than not. The mood in children and teenagers might be irritated or melancholy, and it must last at least one year. Symptoms include: Decreased appetite or overeat, Difficulty sleeping, Low energy or tiredness, Low self-esteem, Difficulty concentrating or difficulties making decisions, Low self-esteem and a sense of despair.

OBSESSIVE-COMPULSIVE DISORDER (OCD)

Obsessive-compulsive disorder (OCD) or obsessive-compulsive ailment is an anxiety disorder. It is divided into two parts: obsessions and compulsions. Obsessions are recurring thoughts, ideas, visions, or impulses that are unpleasant and distressing. Compulsions are behaviours, routines, or mental acts that you engage in to relieve the distress brought on by your obsessions. For example, you are always anxious that you will forget to switch off all of the appliances before leaving the house, so you double-check everything before leaving. You may be worried that if you fail to switch off an item, the house will burn down. Your fear is obsessive, and you get it on a regular basis.

Figure 1. Viscous cycle of OCD

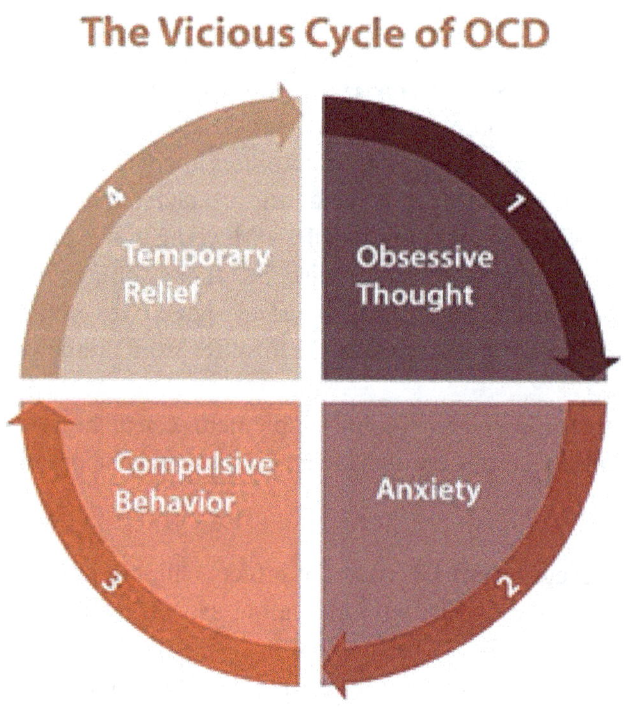

Common things that a person does due to obsession are listed below.

- Washing: Do you spend a lot of time cleaning or sanitizing your home? Do you have to follow a specific washing, cleaning, or grooming procedure all of the time?
- Counting/Touching: Doing things a given number of times or counting to a certain number of times? Do you have a certain style of touching objects?
- Hoarding: Keeping things that other people throw away, such as old newspapers?
- Mental Routines: Staying away from anything that has to do with an unlucky number. Saying a prayer or visualizing an image every time you have a negative thought?

- Confessing Is Necessary: Confessing to friends or family a nasty notion like shoving someone into traffic and requesting frequent reassurance that you're not a bad person?

The Viscous Cycle of OCD

The majority of OCD sufferers fit into one of the following groups:

- Washers are concerned about cross-contamination. Cleaning or hand-washing compulsions are common in them.
- Checkers repeatedly check objects they link with injury or risk (oven switched off, door secured, etc.).
- Doubters and sinners fear that if everything isn't flawless or done correctly, something bad will happen to them or they will be punished.
- Counters and arrangers are obnoxious about symmetry and order. They could be afraid of certain numbers, colors, or configurations.
- Hoarders are afraid that if they throw anything away or hoard stuff they don't need or use, something awful will happen. There are differences, however, between OCD-related hoarding and hoarding disorder. Hoarders with OCD are less likely to amass so many belongings that their homes become untenable.

OCD Signs and Symptoms

Figure 2. Anatomy of brain

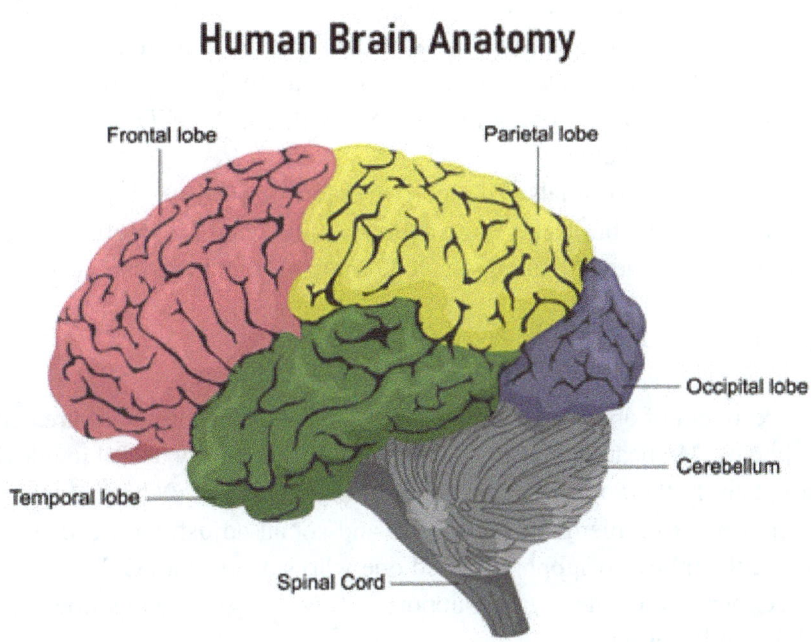

Obsessions and compulsions are common in people with obsessive-compulsive disorder; however, some people only have one or the other.
Common obsessive thoughts in OCD are:

- Fear of being infected by microbes or dust, or of infecting others,
- Anxiety of losing control and injuring yourself or others.
- Sexually explicit or violent thoughts and pictures that are intrusive.
- An overabundance of religious or moral notions.
- Fear of misplacing or losing important items.
- Symmetry and order: the belief that everything must be in its proper place.
- Superstitions are when people pay too much attention to something that is deemed lucky or unlucky.

Common compulsive thoughts in OCD are:

- An excessive amount of double-checking of items like locks, appliances, and switches.
- Checking in on loved ones on a regular basis to ensure their safety.
- Reducing anxiousness by counting, tapping, repeating particular words, or performing other inane things.
- Washing or cleaning for an extended period of time.
- Getting things "just right" in terms of order or arrangement.
- Excessive praying or rituals induced by religious apprehension.
- Amassing trash such as old newspapers or empty food cans.

A person's genes, like many other health issues, have a part in whether or not they develop OCD. That is why OCD is so common in families. Genes can influence the chemistry, structure, and function of several brain regions. The brain anatomy is as shown in figure 2. These differences cause undesired ideas to become 'stuck,' rather than moving on, in those with OCD. OCD develops when someone inherits genes that make it more likely.

However, OCD persists due to rituals. The more people that perform rituals, the more severe OCD become. This occurs because our brains get more adept at doing what we practice. In addition, our brains learn to do more of what is rewarded. Rituals in OCD 'reward' the brain with a sense of relief.

OCD Treatments

Medication: In the treatment of obsessive-compulsive disorder, antidepressants are occasionally used in conjunction with therapy. Medication alone, on the other hand, is rarely useful in alleviating symptoms.

Family Therapy: Family therapy can assist enhance knowledge of OCD and lessen family disputes because it frequently causes problems in family life and social adjustment. It can also inspire family members and educate them how to support a loved one who suffers from OCD.

Group Therapy: Group treatment provides support and encouragement to fellow OCD sufferers while also reducing feelings of isolation.

Obsessive-Compulsive Disorder (OCD) in Children

It is unknown what causes OCD. It appears to be a neurological issue, according to research. In the brains of people with OCD, a neurotransmitter called serotonin is deficient.

OCD is a condition that runs in families. As a result, it's possible that it's hereditary. It can, however, happen without a familial history of OCD. Streptococcal infections can cause or worsen OCD in certain people.

OCD treatment usually consists of a mix of the following:

- Cognitive-behavioral and cognitive-behavioral therapy: Cognitive approaches assist a youngster in recognizing and comprehending his or her worries. They also educate a child with new techniques for dealing with or reducing their worries. Behavioral approaches assist the child and family in making agreements or guidelines to regulate or change behavior. Setting a limit on how many times a compulsive hand washer can wash his or her hands is one example.
- Family counseling: In any therapeutic process, parents play a critical role. The school of a child may also be included in the child's care.
- Serotonin reuptake inhibitors that are selective (SSRIs): These drugs work by increasing serotonin levels in the brain.
- Antibiotics: Teens with OCD are more likely to develop one or more eating disorders. These, too, will require therapy.

SCHIOPHRENIA

Schizophrenia is a serious mental illness that affects a person's ability to think, act, express emotions, perceive reality, and interact with others. Schizophrenia is the most persistent and devastating of the major mental diseases, despite its rarity. This chronic illness cannot be cured, but it can be managed with the right medication.

It is characterized by psychosis, a mental condition in which a person is unable to distinguish between what is real and what is imagined. People suffering from psychotic disorders can lose contact with reality at times. The world may appear to be a tangle of perplexing ideas, images, and noises. Their actions could be unusual and even alarming. A psychotic episode is a sudden change in personality and behavior that occurs when those who have it lose touch with reality.

Early symptoms

Men in their late teens or early twenties are more likely to develop the illness. It primarily affects women in their early twenties and thirties. The prodromal interval is the time between the onset of symptoms and the onset of complete psychosis. It can linger for days, weeks, or even years at a time. Because there is usually no precise trigger, it might be difficult to detect. It's possible that you'll only notice minor behavioral changes, especially in teenagers.

This includes the following:

- A drop in grades
- Withdrawal from social situations
- Concentration issues
- Flares of temper
- Sleeping problems

Psychotic symptoms of Schizophrenia include:

- Delusions: These are erroneous, muddled, and sometimes odd ideas that a person refuses to give up, even when confronted with facts. A person suffering from delusions may believe, for example, that others can hear their thoughts, that they are God or the devil, or that others are implanting thoughts in their heads or scheming against them.
- Hallucinations: Sensations that aren't genuine are referred to as hallucinations. The most prevalent delusion in patients with schizophrenia is hearing voices. The voices may make observations about the person's actions, insult them, or issue directives. Seeing objects that aren't there, tasting weird aromas, having a peculiar taste in your tongue, and feeling sensations on your skin even when nothing is touching your body are some of the less common forms.
- Catatonia: It is a condition in which a person stops speaking and remains in a single position for an extended period of time.

Positive signs that indicate a person's inability to think clearly or behave appropriately. Here are several examples:

- Making it difficult for the person to converse or conduct a conversation by speaking in illogical sentences or using nonsensical words.
- Rapidly shifting from one thought to the next with no clear or logical links between them
- Slowly moving
- Inability to make judgments
- Excessive writing, but with little meaning
- Forgetting or misplacing items
- Pacing or walking in circles are examples of repetitive motions or gestures.
- Having trouble deciphering ordinary sights, sounds, and sensations.

Negative Symptoms of Schizophrenia

- Emotional numbness or a restricted range of emotions
- Withdrawal from family, friends, and social activities is a common symptom of depression.
- Lack of motivation due to a lack of energy
- Loss of interest or joy in life
- Poor cleanliness and hygiene practices

Cognitive Symptoms of Schizophrenia

- Understanding data and utilizing it to make decisions (a doctor may term this weak cognitive performance)
- Paying attention or focusing
- Using what they've learned as soon as possible
- Discovering that they are suffering from any of these issues

Causes of Schizophrenia

- Genetics (heredity): Schizophrenia can run in families, which implies that a higher risk of developing schizophrenia can be handed down from parents to offspring.
- Brain chemistry and circuits: People with schizophrenia may be unable to manage brain chemicals known as neurotransmitters, which govern particular nerve cell routes, or "circuits," that impact thought and action.
- Brain abnormality: People with schizophrenia have aberrant brain anatomy, according to research. This, however, does not apply to everyone who has this disease. It can impact those who aren't sick.
- Environment: In those whose genes make them more susceptible to develop schizophrenia, things like viral infections, exposure to poisons like marijuana, or very stressful conditions may cause the disease.

Treatment of Schizophrenia

- Medication: Antipsychotics are the most common medicines used to treat schizophrenia. These medications do not cure schizophrenia, but they do assist to alleviate the most distressing symptoms, such as delusions, hallucinations, and cognitive difficulties.
- Coordinated specialty care (CSC): When the initial signs of schizophrenia occur, this is a team approach to treating it. It integrates medical and therapeutic interventions with social assistance, employment, and educational programme. As much as possible, the family is involved. The importance of early therapy in assisting patients in leading a normal life cannot be overstated.
- Psychosocial therapy: It includes Rehabilitation, Cognitive remediation, Individual psychotherapy, Family therapy and Group therapy/support groups.
- Electroconvulsive therapy (ECT): Electrodes are connected to the person's skull during this surgery. Doctors give them a tiny electric stimulation to the brain while they're unconscious under general anaesthesia. ECT therapy generally entails 2-3 sessions per week over a period of several weeks. A controlled seizure occurs after each shock treatment. Over time, a succession of therapies leads to an improvement in mood and thinking. ECT-induced seizures, according to some studies, may alter the release of neurotransmitters in the brain. Because ECT has a lower success

rate in treating schizophrenia than depression or bipolar illness, it isn't utilized as frequently when mood symptoms aren't present. It can assist when medicines are no longer effective.

- Research: To treat schizophrenia, researchers are looking into a method known as deep brain stimulation (DBS). Electrodes are surgically attached in particular brain regions that are supposed to influence thinking and perception. Though DBS is a proven treatment for severe Parkinson's disease and essential tremor, it is still considered experimental in the treatment of psychiatric illnesses.
- Hospitalization

CONCLUSION

Depression is a frequent kind of mental illness. More than 264 million individuals of all ages suffer from depression across the world. Depression is a primary cause of disability globally and contributes significantly to the global illness burden. Women are more likely than males to suffer from depression. Suicide can be caused by depression. Depression is distinct from normal mood swings and short-term emotional reactions to ordinary stresses. For mild and severe depression, there are effective psychological and pharmaceutical therapies. Obsessive-compulsive disorder (OCD) is a form of anxiety condition. Obsessive thoughts are unwanted by a youngster with OCD. They're tied to phobias like touching filthy stuff. To cope with his or her concerns, the kid engages in compulsive rituals such as handwashing. The person performing the ritual may find it sensible or irrational. It's possible that the child has no idea why they perform these routines. They may be embarrassed that the actions happen and that they are unable to control them. OCD's exact cause is uncertain. A neurotransmitter called serotonin is deficient in the brains of children with OCD. Repeated doubts and an obsession with filth or germs are examples of obsessive symptoms. Schizophrenia patients frequently struggle in society, at job, in education, and in relationships. They may appear fearful and withdrawn, as if they have lost contact with reality. This chronic illness cannot be cured, but it can be managed with the right medication.

REFERENCES

Aladag, A., Muderrisoglu, S., Akbas, N., Zahmacioglu, O., & Bingol, H. (2018). Detecting Suicidal Ideation on Forums: Proof-of-Concept Study. *Journal of Medical Internet Research, 20*(6), e215. doi:10.2196/jmir.9840 PMID:29929945

Balani, S., & De Choudhury, M. (2015). Detecting and Characterizing Mental Health Related Self-Disclosure in Social Media. *Proceedings of the 33Rd Annual ACM Conference Extended Abstracts on Human Factors in Computing Systems*. 10.1145/2702613.2732733

Brain Anatomy and How the Brain Works. (2021). Retrieved 9 October 2021, from https://www.hopkinsmedicine.org/health/conditions-and-diseases/anatomy-of-the-brain

Cameron, I., Cardy, A., Crawford, J., du Toit, S., Hay, S., Lawton, K., Mitchell, K., Sharma, S., Shivaprasad, S., Winning, S., & Reid, I. C. (2011). Measuring depression severity in general practice: Discriminatory performance of the PHQ-9, HADS-D, and BDI-II. *The British Journal of General Practice, 61*(588), e419–e426. doi:10.3399/bjgp11X583209 PMID:21722450

Gupta, S., & Kant, V. (2020). A Comparative Analysis of Genetic Programming and Genetic Algorithm on Multi-Criteria Recommender Systems. *2020 5th International Conference on Communication and Electronics Systems (ICCES)*.

Halfin, A. (2007, November). Depression: The benefits of early and appropriate treatment. *The American Journal of Managed Care*, *13*(4, Suppl), S92–S97. PMID:18041868

Kleanthi, G., & Maria, G. (2021). Alexithymia, Stress and Depression in Infertile Women: A Case Control Study. *Materia Socio-Medica*, *33*(1), 70–74. doi:10.5455/msm.2021.33.70-74 PMID:34012355

Le, H. N., & Boyd, R. C. (2006). Prevention of major depression: Early detection and early intervention in the general population. *Clin Neuropsychiatry*, *3*(1), 6–22.

Losada, D., Crestani, F., & Parapar, J. (2017). eRISK 2017: CLEF Lab on Early Risk Prediction on the Internet: Experimental Foundations. *Lecture Notes in Computer Science*, *10456*, 346–360. doi:10.1007/978-3-319-65813-1_30

Obsessive-Compulsive Disorder. (2021). Retrieved 9 October 2021, from https://www.helpguide.org/articles/anxiety/obssessive-compulsive-disorder-ocd.htm

Park, M., McDonald, D., & Cha, M. (2013) Perception differences between the depressed and nondepressed users in Twitter. In *International AAAI Conference on Web and Social Media (ICWSM)*. The AAAI Press.

Picardi, A., Lega, I., Tarsitani, L., Caredda, M., Matteucci, G., Zerella, M., Miglio, R., Gigantesco, A., Cerbo, M., Gaddini, A., Spandonaro, F., & Biondi, M.The SET-DEP Group. (2016). A randomised controlled trial of the effectiveness of a program for early detection and treatment of depression in primary care. *Journal of Affective Disorders*, *198*, 96–101. doi:10.1016/j.jad.2016.03.025 PMID:27015158

Rice, S., Goodall, J., Hetrick, S., Parker, A., Gilbertson, T., Amminger, G., Davey, C. G., McGorry, P. D., Gleeson, J., & Alvarez-Jimenez, M. (2014). Online and Social Networking Interventions for the Treatment of Depression in Young People: A Systematic Review. *Journal of Medical Internet Research*, *16*(9), e206. doi:10.2196/jmir.3304 PMID:25226790

Smarr, K., & Keefer, A. (2011). Measures of depression and depressive symptoms: Beck Depression Inventory-II (BDI-II), Center for Epidemiologic Studies Depression Scale (CES-D), Geriatric Depression Scale (GDS), Hospital Anxiety and Depression Scale (HADS), and Patient Health Questionna. *Arthritis Care and Research*, *63*(S11), S454–S466. doi:10.1002/acr.20556 PMID:22588766

Ustun, G. (2021). Determining depression and related factors in a society affected by COVID-19 pandemic. *The International Journal of Social Psychiatry*, *67*(1), 54–63. doi:10.1177/0020764020938807 PMID:32605422

Wongkoblap, A., Vadillo, M., & Curcin, V. (2017). Researching Mental Health Disorders in the Era of Social Media: Systematic Review. *Journal of Medical Internet Research*, *19*(6), e228. doi:10.2196/jmir.7215 PMID:28663166

World Health Organization. (2013). *Comprehensive mental health action plan 2013-2020*. https://www.who.int/ mental_health/action_plan_2013/en/

Chapter 6
Parkinson's Disease:
Neuro-Cognitive Perspective

Soumya Jacob P.
Jain University (Deemed), India

ABSTRACT

Parkinson's disease is a neurodegenerative disorder characterized by severe cognitive impairments. This is a condition of degeneration of substantia nigra of basal ganglia. Parkinsonism adversely influences the mental health of the person too. Parkinson's disease was first described in 1817 by James Parkinson. Parkinsonism patients may get severe complications like cognitive deficiency, which include loss of memory, attention difficulties, visual abnormalities, slow thinking, problems with word finding, and motor symptoms. Symptoms of this disease range from Parkinson's disease mild cognitive impairment (PD-MCI) to Parkinson's disease dementia (PDD). The primary motor symptoms are trembling in hands, arms, legs, jaw, and face; rigidity or stiffness of the limbs and trunk; slowness of movement; postural instability; and impaired balance and coordination. Studies on treatments of Parkinson's disease are progressing to prevent complications and sustain the normal functions of patients.

INTRODUCTION

Parkinson's disease (PD) can be considered as the most complex neurologic disease, which pertains to severe cognitive deficits. Parkinson's disease was first described by James Parkinson in 1817. James Parkinson was a British physician who had published a research paper on a disease with some classical symptoms called, shaking palsy. Later the disease was named by his name and became popular in this new name Parkinson's disease (Lee et al, 2009). Vigorous researches on this disease paved the way for unfolding the mystery behind the disease for implementing better treatment modalities. In the early 1960s, researchers identified the fundamental brain defect that is a hallmark of the disease: degeneration of brain cells that produce chemicals responsible for direct muscle activities. This discovery was a turning point in medical field to devise new and even more successful therapies for Parkinson's disease (Williams-Gray & Worth, 2016).

DOI: 10.4018/978-1-7998-9534-3.ch006

BACKGROUND

General Review on Parkinson's Disease

Parkinson's disease is a chronic, slow, progressive disorder characterized by degeneration of neurons that produce Dopamine in the Substantia Nigra near to the Basal Ganglia. It is also found that the presence of Lewy bodies and Lewy neuritis can also be the reason for Parkinsonism (Berg et al, 2014). The disease is characterized by a group of symptoms: tremors, bradykinesia or slowness of movement and postural instability or impaired balance and coordination (Armstrong & Okun, 2020). It is an unfortunate thing that PD can worsen as year goes on and reach to a stage of severe cognitive deficits and even psychosis. This leads to morbidity of patients, increased care giver burden and decreased prognosis. When patients develop cognitive impairment they may feel worthless and develop signs of depression. Later patients develop some signs of psychosis especially hallucinations and delusions. Finally there is a stage of disease where the patient will lose his or her insight completely. This is the most complex scenario of a patient with Parkinson's disease (Zahodne& Fernandez, 2010).

Related Anatomy and Physiology

In order to study Parkinson's disease we need to have a brief look on anatomy and physiology of Basal Ganglia. Deep within the each cerebral hemisphere there are three nuclei collectively called Basal ganglia, which is inter-connected with the Cerebral cortex, Thalamus and Brainstem. Basal ganglia have variety of functions like motor control, cognition, emotions and learning. The nearby structures functionally connected to the Basal ganglia are the Substantia Nigra of the mid brain and sub-thalamic nuclei of the Diencephalon. Substantia Nigra is a core structure of the Basal ganglia which has cells responsible for producing Dopamine (Kordower et al, 2013). In addition to this the dopaminergic cells inside the Substantia Nigra may possess some aggregation of protein called Lewy bodies which may pre dispose Parkinsonism (Goedert et al, 2012). De-pigmentation or degeneration of Substantia Nigra can obviously result in drop in Dopamine and motor and non-motor symptoms responsible for Parkinson's disease.

Epidemiology

Parkinsonism is the second commonest neurological disorder after Alzheimer's disease that affects almost 1% of individuals older than 60 years with the prevalence of 0.5 -1% and rising to 1-3% among people older than 80 years (Kalia & Lang, 2015). Among elderly population, both the prevalence and incidence of Parkinson's disease are expected to increase by more than 30% by 2030. Prevalence of this disease is more in Europe, North America and South America compared with African, Asian and Arabic countries (Kouli et al, 2018).

Etiology

The causes of Parkinsonism Disease are multi-factorial. There are both genetic and environmental factors which plays major role in Parkinson's disease. The exact cause of Parkinsonism is unknown. Thus it has considered as an idiopathic disease. It was found that there is minority of cases (10-15%) that report a family history. About 5% of people with Parkinson's disease have Mendelian inheritance (Deng et al,

2018). The genes that have been found potential for causing Parkinson's disease are coined as PARK genes. Till date there are 23 PARK genes believed to be responsible for Parkinson's disease (Subtle & Gasser, 2011). Other most important genetic risk factors responsible for pre disposing Parkinson's disease are mutations to genes especially GBA1, a gene encoding Beta Glucocerebrosides (Nichols et al, 2009). The commonest cause of autosomal dominant form Parkinson's disease is mutation of Leucine –rich repeat kinase 2 (LRRK2). Autosomal recessive Parkinson's disease is mainly pre-disposed by a link between three PARK designed genes and mitochondrial homeostasis (Healy et al, 2008, Simon-Sanchez et al, 2009 & Moon & Paek, 2015).

Neuropathology of Parkinson's Disease

Idiopathic Parkinson's disease is macroscopically characterized by mild atrophy of the frontal cortex and ventricular dilation in some cases only. The most common pathological changes observed in Parkinson's disease are loss of the darkly pigmented area in the Substantia Nigra pars compacta (SNpc) and Locus coeruleus (Dickson, 2012). The loss of pigmentation always related to the necrosis of the dopaminergic neuromelanin-containing neurons named A9 neurons in the SNpc and noradrenergic neurons in the locus coeruleus. Apart from this, several cell losses can also be seen in several sub-cortical nuclei, dorsal motor nuclei of vagus nerve, the raphe nuclei, hypothalamus and olfactory bulb (Giguere et al, 2018). Thus there are involvement of multiple noradrenergic systems such as the cholinergic, adenosinergic, glutamatergic, GABAergic, noradrenergic, serotonergic and histaminergic (Kalia et al, 2013). Hence Parkinson's disease has some non motor symptoms especially cognitive deficiency which cannot be treated well with Dopamine replacement therapies (Chaudhuri, 2006). Microscopic evaluations reveal that, there is presence of Lewy bodies in the neuronal cell bodies. Lewy bodies are the aggregation of pathologic proteins or intra cytoplasmic inclusions with a granular and fibrillar core with a surrounding halo. More than one Lewy bodies can be seen in a single neuron. Presence of Lewy bodies is usually accompanied by dystrophic neuritis predominantly axonal (Spillantini et al 1997). Braak and colleagues proposed 6 stages of Parkinson's disease. According to Bark et al as Parkinsonism progresses there is involvement of the entire neo cortex and high-order areas. Clinically patients manifest with severe gait problems and dementia (Braak et al, 2003). Later Braak hypothesis was revised to propose that α-synuclein-associated pathology of Parkinsonism (Hawkes et al., 2007). Phosphorylated α-synuclein histopathology has observed not only inside brain but also outside brain especially in the spinal cord, cervical and sympathetic ganglia, in several peripheral organs especially retina, uterus, bladder, skin parts, parts of the cardio vascular system and gastrointestinal system (Beach et al., 2010 & Beach et al., 2014).

Clinical Features

The classical clinical manifestations of Parkinson's disease are the triad of motor symptoms commonly seen in patients namely tremor, rigidity and bradykinesia with postural instability. However this disease is also associated with several non-motor symptoms; often precede the motor symptoms as years pass. Evidenced based practices revealed that, Parkinson's disease may begin in the peripheral autonomic system before involving the substantia nigra. Hence pre-motor or prodromal phase of PD may begin 12-14 years before diagnosing the disease (Katzenschlager, 2008). Due to this, patient complains hyposmia, constipation and rapid eye movement sleep disorders before the onset of motor symptoms of PD. One research study showed that people who developed symptoms like tremor, balance problems, depression, constipation, fatigue and urinary dysfunctions had gradually diagnosed with PD after 5 years. People with constipation and tremor are in risk of developing PD (Schrag, 2015). Motor symptoms like tremor, rigidity and bradykinesia worsen over time. If patients on Dopamine replacement therapy, there are chances of complications like dyskinesia, non-motor fluctuations and psychosis that are most difficult situations to manage. When disease advances, it's difficult to manage both motor and non-motor symptoms as patients become resistant to Dopamine replacement therapies. Postural instability and freezing of gait may lead to falls and fractures and special care is essential for those people who develop cognitive deficiency like dementia, attention problems, difficulty in concentration and hallucination. PD has significant impact on the quality of life of patients as patient may also suffer with impaired olfactory ability, autonomic dysfunctions, pain, fatigue, and sleep disorders, cognitive and psychiatric disturbances (Martinez-Martin et al., 2011).

RECENT ADVANCEMENTS IN DIAGNOSIS AND TREATMENT OF PARKINSON'S DISEASE

Even though the causes of Parkinson's are evident from Medical researchers, there is no specific test for Parkinson's disease (Levin et al, 2015). Usually Neurologist diagnoses the disease by physical examination and clinical history. Single Photon Emission Computerized Tomography (SPECT) scan and Dopamine Transporter scan help to support diagnosing Parkinson's disease. MRI (Magnet Resonance Imaging), Ultra sound of the brain and PET (Proton Emission Tomography) scan can also useful for diagnosing Parkinson's disease. Till now there are no gene markers for identifying Parkinson's disease (Jankovic, 2008).

For treating Parkinson's disease Dopamine replacement therapy had introduced about 5 decades ago. L- dopa and Carbi-dopa were the drug of choice for Parkinsonism. Still it goes on. Along with Dopamine therapy Parkinsonism patients are treated with Anti-inflammatory medicines like Silmaryn, Berberine and Mucina prurins to prevent neuroinflammation and neurodegeneration, (Niranjan, 2014) Cholesterol lowering agent named Statin has major role to protect neurons (Aguirre-Vidal et al, 2015). By 1950's neurologists had come up with Neurotrophic factors or Neurotrophins a subset of growth factors which is essential for maintenance of specific neurons of Nervous system. The family of Neurotrophins consisted of NGF (Nerve Growth Factors), BDNF (Brain-derived neurotrophic factors), GDNF (Glial cell line-derived neurotrophic factors) and so on. For treating Parkinson's disease there are numerous Neurotrophic factors have been advanced and under investigation (Hegarty et al, 2014).

Deep Brain Stimulation (DBS) has found effective for reducing symptoms like tremor, rigidity and Bradykinesia. In case of Parkinsonism, DBS focuses on Subthalamic Nucleus and Globus Pallidus. The major clinical indicators for DBS are dystonia, essential tremor, depression, dyskinesia, that is not effectively controlled by medical therapy (Williams and Okun, 2013).

Clinical trials on Stem cell therapy had proven effective for treating Parkinson's disease. This is indicated when pharmacological therapy fails (Gonzalez et al, 2015). Gene therapy is also in advancement to give good prognosis for Parkinson's disease. Here viral vectors are in demand for faster and long term gene expression. Gene therapy mainly aims on augmentation of dopamine level through increased neurotransmitter production, modulation of neuronal phenotype and neural protection (Coune etal, 2012). Nano-technology, artificial intelligence and newer sophisticated approaches in medical sciences are progressing to come up with advanced diagnostic and treatment options. It was found that Artificial

Intelligence could be successfully used in the diagnosis of Parkinson's disease from Ioflupane-123 SPECT (Single-photon Emission Computed Tomography) dopamine transporter scan using transfer-learning (Kim et al, 2018).

PARKINSON'S DISEASE AND COGNITION

Cognition refers to the ability of a person to think, memorize, learn, concentrate, attend on stimulus, judgment, evaluate, and make decisions and so on. When a person has cognition difficulties there is a risk of poor self esteem and self concept. More over this can affect social life too. Some patients start to sit inside the home and like to live isolated and lonely life. If the disease condition hit the patient in his or her early life, this cognitive impairment challenges the economic balance of the whole family due to loss of lob and morbidity. If family members are not able to accept the PD patients as a whole, the client will face a disrupted and altered family process. Thus unlike motor symptoms of the disease, cognitive symptoms are something which is penetrating to the different dimensions of a person's life like physiological, psychological, social, emotional, and economic and so on.

Parkinsonism is a devastating disease which will affect the cognition of people like Alzheimer's disease. This is the most disappointing period of Parkinson's disease where mental health of the person will be in question. Cognitive deficiency can vary from mild cognitive deficiency to severe stage of illness with Dementia. Due to this, people used to go for depression in their later period. Mild cognitive impairment (MCI) is a pre dementia stage or a transitory stage between normal cognition and Dementia where patients report slight changes in memory, concentration and attention. Patients with subjective cognitive decline (SCD) are more likely to develop MCI within two years of first diagnosis of Parkinsonism. Neurotransmitter deficits are always associated with cognitive impairment in Parkinson's disease. Deficiency of Dopamine, Nor-adrenalin and cholinergic deficiencies may result in cognitive deficiency and severe Dementia. Dementia associated with Parkinsonism is known as Parkinson's disease Dementia (PDD). Noradrenergic locus coeruleus has Neuromelanin pigment responsible for cognition. Reduction in neuromelanin pigment can result in deterioration of attention, concentration, working and long term memory. Gradually patients reached to a stage of PDD and severe cognitive impairment (Aarsland et al, 2021).

Tempero- parietal atrophy on MRI was the first biomarker for diagnosing cognitive impairment (Reginold et al, 2014). In addition to this basal forebrain atrophy is associated with cognitive deficiency of Parkinson's disease. More recent MRI technique named Diffusion tensor Image is a promising biomarker to map the extent of cognitive impairment among patients with Parkinsonism. Neuropsychological testing popular for Parkinson's disease has five domains of testing: attention and working memory, executive, language, memory and visuospatial functions. Mattis Dementia Rating Scale 2nd edition (MDRS-2), Parkinson's disease- Cognitive rating scale (PD-CRS), Mini – Mental Parkinson (MMP) and Scale for outcomes in Parkinson's disease-cognition (SCOPA-COG) are some major cognitive scales for assessing patients with Parkinson's disease. Computerized tests are on demand to see the changes in cognition from remote. Medical management for cognition mainly focuses on balance in Neurotransmitters to enhance global cognition and memory. Unfortunately cognitive deficiency associated with Parkinson's disease is a major reason for decreased health related quality of life and increased global burden (Aarsland et al, 2021).

Thus Parkinson's disease can be viewed as the serious neuro-cognitive illness. It's a neurological disorder as it affects the brain cells at the same time it is a motor illness as it has tremor, bradykinesia and rigidity as the major symptoms. There is plethora of evidence which depicts the cognitive involvement of Parkinsonism. Newer research studies must focus on preventing complications of PD which affect the higher order thinking, attention, concentration, memory, learning and other major dimensions of a personal life. Cognition impairment is the reason for major morbidity of patients with Parkinson's disease.

PARKINSON'S DISEASE AND PSYCHOSIS

Psychosis is the major reason for nursing home placement of patients with Parkinsonism. Approximately 20% to 40% of patients with PD will develop psychotic symptoms like Hallucinations, illusions, paranoid delusions and so on. The most common delusions found among PD patients are visual hallucinations. As years pass, patients will reach to a stage of complete loss of insight. In initial period the patients experience vivid dreaming and misperceptions, later it develops to hallucinations and delusions and finally florid psychosis and dementia. Parkinson Psychosis is the predisposing factor for increased care giver distress, nursing home placement and mortality. Neuro transmitter imbalance linked with dopaminergic drugs and other treatment regimen is the major risk factor for Parkinson's disease psychosis. Addition of an anti psychotic drug named Clozapine or Quetiapine or Risperidone is essential for treating and preventing Parkinson's disease Psychosis (Zahodne& Fernandez, 2010).

ROLE OF ARTIFICIAL INTELLIGENCE FOR DIAGNOSING AND TRTEATING PARKINSON'S DISEASE

Artificial Intelligence, especially machine learning has wide applications in diagnosing, monitoring and treating several neurodegenerative disorders especially Parkinson's disorder. The main attraction of these sophisticated techniques is nothing but precise in the diagnosis of the disease as well as accurate delivery of drugs. Current machine learning algorithms are excellent for assessing patient with Parkinson's disease along with diagnosing the specific type of Parkinsonism. Different machine learning algorithms have been demonstrated promising effect on early diagnosis of Parkinsonism. However we could not reach to a level of full application of Artificial Intelligence and machine learning in the field of treating Parkinson's disease for complete cure by exploiting Artificial Intelligence and Machine learning. Hence further collaborative researches advancing among medical institutions, clinicians and researchers to put some light on various aspects of this neuro degenerative disorder (Belic et al, 2019).

SCOPE OF FUTURE RESEARCHES IN PARKINSON'S DISEASE

Parkinson's disease is a one of the neurodegenerative disorder which is striving for more accurate diagnosis and treatment. Medical researchers are successful to elicit the specific genes responsible for this disease but till now no diagnostic tests are available for detecting biomarkers or gene markers to diagnose the exact cause and extent of Parkinson's disease. Longitudinal research studies are on demand to determine which specific biomarker is most useful for early diagnosis of Parkinson's disease. Presently potential diagnostic imaging or biofluid assays are confined to clinical assessment only; instead these techniques can be compared with gold standards of neuropathology. In addition to this, novel biomarkers and analytic method should be identified for better clarity in the diagnosis of Parkinson's disease. Research studies on imaging techniques for detecting Alfa-synuclein in brain cells can be fastened to map the extent of the disease. Parkinson's disease researches collaborating with Artificial Intelligence and machine learning are the need of the moment to unfold the mysteries associated with Parkinson's disease (Goldman & Patel, 2015).

Even though the science has progressed to find solutions for many disorders, there is no complete cure for neurodegenerative disorders especially Parkinsonism. Stem cell therapy and genetic therapy are progressing in their pace but newer researches are welcoming to find treatment for preventing mortality and morbidity among patients with Parkinsonism. Surgical implantation of dopaminergic cells in the Substantia Nigra can be an option for recovery of Parkinson's disease. Likewise much more studies are expecting in this field to prevent complications of Dopamine replacement therapies too. Patients are suffering not only with the severity of disorders but also with the complications related to treatment of the disease. Thus future researches must keep this in mind to introduce complex therapeutic approaches. Deep Brain stimulation is very effective for treating motor symptoms of Parkinson's disease but it cannot alter the course of the disease. Thus researches on disease modifying treatments are urgently needed to minimize the neurodegenerative symptoms and course of the disease. Moreover researches on different non invasive Deep Brain Stimulation techniques are needed to ensure patient safety and comfort. Thus much more research studies on gene therapy, immune therapy, cell transplantation and circuit Neuromodulation are essential in this field for accurate diagnosis and treatment (Lee & Lozano, 2018).

CONCLUSION

Parkinson's disease has considered as an irreversible neuro- degenerative disorders from years back. De pigmentation of basal ganglia and corresponding depletion in the dopaminergic neurons are responsible for severe cognitive impairment and motor deficits in patients with PD. Parkinson's disease Dementia is the most complex stage of Parkinson's disease where patients face severe memory loss. Thus the life of patients with PD is questionable in relation to health related quality of life. Moreover the patients are prone to develop depression due to cognitive deficiency. Newer researches are progressing to present a complete remedy for Parkinsonism with sophisticated computerized techniques. Future researches should also focus on preventing severe complications of PD especially cognition of clients. Cognition of a person is most valuable to live as a complete man or woman. Researches on Parkinsonism can utilize all advanced technologies to prevent the complications of this illness and promote health in all dimensions. Even though the world is in the finger tips of digitalization, we could not find satisfying results in certain areas of health sector. Diagnosis of many diseases has become easy for health professionals with modern technologies present today but early diagnosis and treatment of Parkinsonism is still in challenging situation. We can see that specific gene markers or biomarkers tests are available for most complicated carcinomas and many patients had survived from this illness as they could diagnose the disease little earlier. In case of Parkinson's disease it's treatment: dopamine replacement therapy itself contributes severe complication in the neuro cognitive centers of brain. Hence the numerous people in this world are anticipating for newer treatment modalities with promising results to cure the disease completely. As Artificial Intelligence and machine learning are fast growing sector in medical field, let us hope for the best in Parkinson's disease diagnosis and management.

REFERENCES

Aarsland, D., Batzu, L., Halliday, G. M., Geurtsen, G. J., Ballard, C., Ray Chaudhuri, K., & Weintraub, D. (2021). Parkinson disease-associated cognitive impairment. *Nature Reviews. Disease Primers*, *7*(1), 47. doi:10.103841572-021-00280-3 PMID:34210995

Aguirre-Vidal, Y., Montes, S., Tristan-López, L., Anaya-Ramos, L., Teiber, J., Ríos, C., Baron-Flores, V., & Monroy-Noyola, A. (2015). The Neuroprotective Effect of Lovastatin on MPP+-In- duced Neurotoxicity Is Not Mediated by PON2. *Neurotoxicology*, *48*, 166–170. doi:10.1016/j.neuro.2015.03.012 PMID:25842176

Armstrong, M. J., & Okun, M. S. (2020). Diagnosis and Treatment of Parkinson Disease: A Review. *Journal of the American Medical Association*, *323*(6), 548–560. doi:10.1001/jama.2019.22360 PMID:32044947

Beach, T.G., Adler, C.H., Sue, L.I., Vedders, L., Lue, L., White, C.L. (2010). Multi-organ distribution of phosphorylated α-synuclein histopathology in subjects with Lewy body disorders. *Acta Neuropathol*, *119*(6), 689–702. .95 doi:10.1007/s00401-010-0664-3

Beach, T. G., Carew, J., Serrano, G., Adler, C. H., Shill, H. A., Sue, L. I., Sabbagh, M. N., Akiyama, H., & Cuenca, N. (2014). Phosphorylated α-synuclein-immunoreactive retinal neuronal elements in Parkinson's disease subjects. *Neuroscience Letters*, *571*, 34–38. doi:10.1016/j.neulet.2014.04.027 PMID:24785101

Berg, D., Postuma, R. B., Bloem, B., Chan, P., Dubois, B., Gasser, T., Goetz, C. G., Halliday, G. M., Hardy, J., Lang, A. E., Litvan, I., Marek, K., Obeso, J., Oertel, W., Olanow, C. W., Poewe, W., Stern, M., & Deuschl, G. (2014). Time to redefine PD? Introductory statement of the MDS Task Force on the definition of Parkinson's disease. *Movement Disorders*, *29*(4), 454–462. doi:10.1002/mds.25844 PMID:24619848

Braak, H., Del Tredici, K., Rüb, U., de Vos, R. A., Steur, E. N. J., & Braak, E. (2003). Staging of brain pathology related to sporadic Parkinson's disease. *Neurobiology of Aging*, *24*(2), 197–211. doi:10.1016/S0197-4580(02)00065-9 PMID:12498954

Chaudhuri, K. R., Healy, D. G., & Schapira, A. H. (2006). Non-motor symptoms of Parkinson's disease: Diagnosis and management. *Lancet Neurology*, *5*(3), 235–245. doi:10.1016/S1474-4422(06)70373-8 PMID:16488379

Chaudhuri, K. R., & Schapira, A. H. (2009). Non-motor symptoms of Parkinson's disease: Dopaminergic pathophysiology and treatment. *Lancet Neurology*, *8*(5), 464–474. doi:10.1016/S1474-4422(09)70068-7 PMID:19375664

Coune, P. G., Schneider, B. L., & Aebischer, P. (2012). Parkinson's Disease: Gene Therapies. *Cold Spring Harbor Perspectives in Medicine*, *4*(4), a009431. Advance online publication. doi:10.1101/cshperspect.a009431 PMID:22474617

Deng, H., Wang, P., & Jankovic, J. (2018). The genetics of Parkinson disease. *Ageing Research Reviews*, *42*, 72–85. doi:10.1016/j.arr.2017.12.007 PMID:29288112

Dickson, D. W. (2012). Parkinson's disease and Parkinsonism: Neuropathology. *Cold Spring Harbor Perspectives in Medicine*, *2*(8), a009258. Advance online publication. doi:10.1101/cshperspect.a009258 PMID:22908195

Elobeid, A., Libard, S., Leino, M., Popova, S. N., & Alafuzoff, I. (2016, April). Altered proteins in the aging brain. *Journal of Neuropathology and Experimental Neurology*, *75*(4), 316–325. doi:10.1093/jnen/nlw002 PMID:26979082

Goedert, M., Spillantini, M. G., Del Tredici, K., & Braak, H. (2012). 100 years of Lewy pathology. *Nature Reviews. Neurology*, *9*(1), 13–24. doi:10.1038/nrneurol.2012.242 PMID:23183883

Goldman, J., & Patel, R. (2015). Diagnosis of Parkinson's disease: Progress and future prospects. *Journal of Parkinsonism and Restless Legs Syndrome*, *19*, 19. Advance online publication. doi:10.2147/JPRLS.S62065

Gonzalez, C., Bonilla, S., Flores, A. I., Cano, E., & Liste, I. (2016). An Update on Human Stem Cell-Based Therapy in Parkinson's Disease. *Current Stem Cell Research & Therapy*, *11*(7), 561–568. Advance online publication. doi:10.2174/1574888X10666150531172612 PMID:26027681

Hawkes, C. H., Tredici, K. D., & Braak, H. (2007). Parkinson's disease: A dual-hit hypothesis. *Neuropathology and Applied Neurobiology*, *33*(6), 599–614. doi:10.1111/j.1365-2990.2007.00874.x PMID:17961138

Healy, D. G., Falchi, M., O'Sullivan, S. S., Bonifati, V., Durr, A., Bressman, S., Brice, A., Aasly, J., Zabetian, C. P., Goldwurm, S., Ferreira, J. J., Tolosa, E., Kay, D. M., Klein, C., Williams, D. R., Marras, C., Lang, A. E., Wszolek, Z. K., Berciano, J., ... Wood, N. W. (2008). Phenotype, genotype, and worldwide genetic penetrance of LRRK2-associated Parkinson's disease: A case-control study. *Lancet Neurology*, *7*(7), 583–590. doi:10.1016/S1474-4422(08)70117-0 PMID:18539534

Hegarty, S. V., O'Keeffe, G. W., & Sullivan, A. M. (2014). Neurotrophic Factors: From Neurodevelopmental Regulators to Novel Therapies for Parkinson's Disease. *Neural Regeneration Research*, *9*, 1708–1711. doi:10.4103/1673-5374.143410 PMID:25422631

Jankovic, J. (2008). Parkinson's disease: Clinical features and diagnosis. *Journal of Neurology, Neurosurgery, and Psychiatry*, *79*(4), 368–376. doi:10.1136/jnnp.2007.131045 PMID:18344392

Jankovic, J., McDermott, M., Carter, J., Gauthier, S., Goetz, C., Golbe, L., Huber, S., Koller, W., Olanow, C., Shoulson, I., Stern, M., Tanner, C., & Weiner, W. (1990). Variable expression of Parkinson's disease: A base-line analysis of the DATATOP cohort. The Parkinson Study Group. *Neurology*, *40*(10), 1529–1534. doi:10.1212/WNL.40.10.1529 PMID:2215943

Kalia, L. V., Brotchie, J. M., & Fox, S. H. (2013). Novel nondopaminergic targets for motor features of Parkinson's disease: Review of recent trials. *Movement Disorders*, *28*(2), 131–144. doi:10.1002/mds.25273 PMID:23225267

Kalia LV, Lang AE. (2015), Parkinson's disease. *Lancet*, *386*(9996), 896–912. . doi:10.1016/S0140-6736(14)61393-3

Katzenschlager, R. (2014). Parkinson's disease: Recent advances. *Journal of Neurology.*

Katzenschlager, R., Head, J., Schrag, A., Ben-Shlomo, Y., Evans, A., & Lees, A. J. (2008). Fourteen-year final report of the randomized PDRG-UK trial comparing three initial treatments in PD. *Neurology, 71*(7), 474–480. doi:10.1212/01.wnl.0000310812.43352.66 PMID:18579806

Kim, D. H., Wit, H., & Thurston, M. (2018). Artificial intelligence in the diagnosis of Parkinson's disease from ioflupane-123 single-photon emission computed tomography dopamine transporter scans using transfer learning. *Nuclear Medicine Communications, 39*(10), 887–893. doi:10.1097/MNM.0000000000000890 PMID:30080748

Kobilecki, C. (2020). Update on the diagnosis and management of Parkinson's disease. *Clinical Medicine, 20*(4), 393–398. doi:10.7861/clinmed.2020-0220 PMID:32675145

Kordower, J. H., Olanow, C. W., Dodiya, H. B., Chu, Y., Beach, T. G., Adler, C. H., Halliday, G. M., & Bartus, R. T. (2013). Disease duration and the integrity of the nigrostriatal system in Parkinson's disease. *Brain, 136*(8), 2419–2431. doi:10.1093/brain/awt192 PMID:23884810

Kouli, A., Torsney, K. M., & Kuan, W. L. (2018). Parkinson's Disease: Etiology, Neuropathology, and Pathogenesis. In *Parkinson's Disease: Pathogenesis and Clinical Aspects.* doi:10.15586/codonpublications.parkinsonsdisease.2018.ch1

Lee, D., & Lozano, A. (2018). The Future of Surgical Treatments for Parkinson's Disease. *Journal of Parkinson's Disease, 8*(s1), S79–S83. doi:10.3233/JPD-181467 PMID:30584156

Lees, A. J., Hardy, J., & Revesz, T. (2009). Parkinson's disease. *Lancet, 373*(9680), 2055–2066. doi:10.1016/S0140-6736(09)60492-X PMID:19524782

Levin, J., Hasan, A., & Höglinger, G. U. (2015). Psychosis in Parkinson's disease: Identification, prevention and treatment. *Journal of Neural Transmission (Vienna, Austria).* Advance online publication. doi:10.100700702-015-1400-x PMID:25894288

Martinez-Martin, P., Rodriguez-Blazquez, C., Kurtis, M.M., & Chaudhuri, K.R. (2011). The impact of non-motor symptoms on health-related quality of life of patients with Parkinson's disease. *Mov Disord, 26*(3), 399–406. . doi:10.1002/mds.23462

Moon, H. E., & Paek, S. H. (2015). Mitochondrial dysfunction in Parkinson's disease. *Experimental Neurobiology, 24*(2), 103–116. doi:10.5607/en.2015.24.2.103 PMID:26113789

Nichols, W. C., Pankratz, N., Marek, D. K., Pauciulo, M. W., Elsaesser, V. E., Halter, C. A., Rudolph, A., Wojcieszek, J., Pfeiffer, R. F., & Foroud, T. (2009). Mutations in GBA are associated with familial Parkinson disease susceptibility and age at onset. *Neurology, 72*(4), 310–316. doi:10.1212/01.wnl.0000327823.81237.d1 PMID:18987351

Niranjan, R. (2014). The Role of Inflammatory and Oxidative Stress Mechanisms in the Pathogenesis of Parkinson's Disease: Focus on Astrocytes. *Molecular Neurobiology, 49*(1), 28–38. doi:10.100712035-013-8483-x PMID:23783559

Reginold, W., Lang, A. E., Marras, C., Heyn, C., Alharbi, M., & Mikulis, D. J. (2014). Longitudinal quantitative MRI in multiple system atrophy and progressive supranuclear palsy. *Parkinsonism & Related Disorders, 20*(2), 222–225. doi:10.1016/j.parkreldis.2013.10.002 PMID:24239142

Schrag, A., Horsfall, L., Walters, K., Noyce, A., & Petersen, I. (2015). Prediagnostic presentations of Parkinson's disease in primary care: A case-control study. *Lancet Neurology*, *14*(1), 57–64. doi:10.1016/S1474-4422(14)70287-X PMID:25435387

Schulte, C., & Gasser, T. (2011). Genetic basis of Parkinson's disease: Inheritance, penetrance, and expression. *The Application of Clinical Genetics*, *1*(4), 67–80. PMID:23776368

Simon-Sanchez, J., Schulte, C., Bras, J. M., Sharma, M., Gibbs, J. R., Berg, D., Paisan-Ruiz, C., Lichtner, P., Scholz, S. W., Hernandez, D. G., Krüger, R., Federoff, M., Klein, C., Goate, A., Perlmutter, J., Bonin, M., Nalls, M. A., Illig, T., Gieger, C., ... Gasser, T. (2009). Genome-wide association study reveals genetic risk underlying Parkinson's disease. *Nature Genetics*, *41*(12), 1308–1312. doi:10.1038/ng.487 PMID:19915575

Spillantini, M. G., Crowther, R. A., Jakes, R., Hasegawa, M., & Goedert, M. (1998). α-Synuclein in filamentous inclusions of Lewy bodies from Parkinson's disease and dementia with Lewy bodies. *Proceedings of the National Academy of Sciences of the United States of America*, *95*(11), 6469–6473. doi:10.1073/pnas.95.11.6469 PMID:9600990

Spillantini, M. G., Schmidt, M. L., Lee, V. M., Trojanowski, J. Q., Jakes, R., & Goedert, M. (1997). Alpha-synuclein in Lewy bodies. *Nature*, *388*(6645), 839–840. doi:10.1038/42166 PMID:9278044

StokerT. B.BarkerR. A. (2020). Recent developments in the treatment of Parkinson's Disease. *F1000Research*, 862, doi:10.12688/f1000research.25634.1

Williams, N. R., & Okun, M. S. (2013). Deep Brain Stimulation (DBS) at the Interface of Neurology and Psychiatry. *The Journal of Clinical Investigation*, *123*(11), 4546–456. doi:10.1172/JCI68341 PMID:24177464

Williams-Gray, C. H., & Worth, P. F. (2016). Parkinson's disease. *Medicine*, *44*(9), 542–546. doi:10.1016/j.mpmed.2016.06.001

Zahodne, L. B., & Fernandez, H. H. (2010). Parkinson's psychosis. *Current Treatment Options in Neurology*, *12*(3), 200–211. doi:10.100711940-010-0072-y PMID:20842582

ADDITIONAL READING

Bor-Seng-Shu, E., Felicio, A. C., & Braga-Neto, P. (2014). Dopamine transporter imaging using 99mTc-TRODAT-1 SPECT in Parkinson's disease. *Medical Science Monitor*, *20*, 1413–1418. doi:10.12659/MSM.890522 PMID:25109468

Cheng, H.-C., Ulane, C. M., & Burke, R. E. (2010). Clinical progression in Parkinson's disease and the neurobiology of axons. [*Annals of Neurology*, *67*(6), 715–725. doi:10.1002/ana.21995 PMID:20517933

Giguère, N., Burke Nanni, S., & Trudeau, L.-E. (2018). On cell loss and selective vulnerability of neuronal populations in Parkinson's disease. *Frontiers in Neurology*, *9*, 455. doi:10.3389/fneur.2018.00455 PMID:29971039

Lautier, C., Goldwurm, S., Dürr, A., Giovannone, B., Tsiaras, W. G., Pezzoli, G., Brice, A., & Smith, R. J. (2008). Mutations in the GIGYF2 (TNRC15) gene at the PARK11 locus in familial Parkinson disease. *American Journal of Human Genetics*, *82*(4), 822–833. doi:10.1016/j.ajhg.2008.01.015 PMID:18358451

Mirabella, G. (2015). Is art therapy a reliable tool for rehabilitating people suffering from brain/mental diseases? *Journal of Alternative and Complementary Medicine (New York, N.Y.)*, *21*(4), 196–199. doi:10.1089/acm.2014.0374 PMID:25848886

Nalls, M. A., Pankratz, N., Lill, C. M., Do, C. B., Hernandez, D. G., Saad, M., DeStefano, A. L., Kara, E., Bras, J., Sharma, M., Schulte, C., Keller, M. F., Arepalli, S., Letson, C., Edsall, C., Stefansson, H., Liu, X., Pliner, H., Lee, J. H., ... Singleton, A. B. (2014). Large-scale meta-analysis of genome-wide association data identifies six new risk loci for Parkinson's disease. *Nature Genetics*, *46*(9), 989–993. doi:10.1038/ng.3043 PMID:25064009

Noyce, A. J., Bestwick, J. P., Silveira-Moriyama, L., Hawkes, C. H., Giovannoni, G., Lees, A. J., & Schrag, A. (2012). Meta-analysis of early nonmotor features and risk factors for Parkinson disease. *Annals of Neurology*, *72*(6), 893–901. doi:10.1002/ana.23687 PMID:23071076

Perez-Pardo, P., Kliest, T., Dodiya, H. B., Broersen, L. M., Garssen, J., Keshavarzian, A., & Kraneveld, A. D. (2017). The gut-brain axis in Parkinson's disease: Possibilities for food-based therapies. *European Journal of Pharmacology*, *15*(817), 86–95. doi:10.1016/j.ejphar.2017.05.042 PMID:28549787

Takahashi, T., Tamura, M., Osabe, K., Tamiya, T., Miki, K., Yamaguchi, M., Akira, K., Kamei, S., & Takasu, T. (2014). A rare case of Parkinson's disease with severe neck pain owing to crowned dens syndrome. *Case Reports in Neurology*, *6*(2), 149–155. doi:10.1159/000362514 PMID:24926265

KEY TERMS AND DEFINITIONS

Autosomal: A specific gene located in the non sex chromosome.

Atrophy: A medical condition of wasting away or shrinking of the cells or muscles often occurs due to prolonged immobility or disuse.

Bradykinesia: A physical state of impairment of voluntary motor control characterized by slow movement.

Degeneration: A process of deterioration of tissues and loss of function.

Dementia: Impaired ability to recall, think or make decisions which influence the activities of daily living.

Dyskinesia: Involuntary movements that is difficult to control or cannot control.

Dystonia: A neurological state characterized by muscle contractions responsible for slow repetitive movements or abnormal postures.

Idiopathic: Unknown cause.

Morbidity: A condition of prolonged suffering with a disease that disrupts the quality of life of a person.

Necrosis: Death of the cells.

Rigidity: A condition of increased muscle tone with stiffness or inflexibility of the muscles.

Tremor: An involuntary, rhythmic muscle contraction leading to shaking movements in one or more parts of the body.

Chapter 7
Neuropsychological and Cognitive Control Deficits in Depression

Meenakshi Banerjee
O. P. Jindal Global University, India

ABSTRACT

The chapter explores the research done so far on neuropsychological deficits in major depressive disorder (MDD). The most prominent deficits have been reported in executive function and the cognitive control networks. These deficits have also been shown to affect various cognitive aspects of a patient, such as metacognitions and emotional regulation. They are also predictors of socio-occupational functioning and of recovering and relapse in patients. This makes it pertinent that these newer treatments for MDD account for these deficits and work on ameliorating them for long-term gains.

INTRODUCTION

Major Depressive Disorder (MDD) is a chronic disease prevalent worldwide. It impairs daily functioning, induces depressive thoughts, and reduces the quality of life. It has also shown to increase risks of acquiring cardiovascular disease, increase morbidity and mortality (Seligman & Nemeroff, 2015). More than 300 million individuals in the world are estimated to be affected by depression. The World Health Organisation (WHO) recognises it as a major public health crisis (Ferrari et al., 2013) and as the largest factor contributing to global disability (Smith et al., 2014).

Liu et al. (2019) found that the number of cases of depression worldwide increased by 49.86% from 1990 to 2017. It affects 16% of the global population (Kessler et al., 2003). WHO has predicted that by 2030, MDD will become the leading cause of disability in the world (Yang et al., 2015). In India, the National Mental Health Survey 2015-16 revealed that approximately one in every 20 Indians suffers from depression. It is estimated that in 2012, India had over 258,000 suicides, with the age-group of 15-49 years being most affected.

DOI: 10.4018/978-1-7998-9534-3.ch007

BACKGROUND

MDD is an illness characterized by low mood, loss of interest, difficulty in concentration and easy fatigability. Whilst depressed mood and loss of interest are one of the key features, other cognitive symptoms indicate the severity and character of the episode and contribute to significant functional impairment and impact recovery. Neurocognitive dysfunction is now understood to be central to depression. Deficits are reported mainly in cognitive control functions such as, attention, working memory and other executive functions (EF), which are harbingers of cognitive biases and metacognitive deficits (Shallice, 1996; Vinogradov, Fisher, & De Villers-Sidani, 2012).

Though depression is characterized as an episodic illness, prospective studies have found that most patients have a recurrence (Mueller et al., 1999). Researchers have noted a distinct ruminative form of thinking in patients suffering from MDD. Ruminations are defined as focused attention on symptoms of one's distress, and on its possible causes and consequences, as opposed to its solutions (Nolen-Hoeksema, 1991). From a neuropsychological perspective rumination may be understood as a result of failure to generate an adaptive response by the executive, top down systems controlling limbic activations (Marchetti et al., 2012; Pisner, 2018).

Cognitive control is the ability to control the contents of working memory (WM), which therefore might play an important role in recovery from negative affect. It involves the WM's ability to maintain what is currently of importance, allow response inhibition (RI) to filter what is less relevant and mental flexibility to change a line of thought/action to suit the goal. Reduced cognitive control over attention plays a major role in the diagnosis of depression (Dean & Keshavan, 2018).

EF ability is also linked to metacognition and emotional strategy selection (Ochsner & Gross, 2005). Activation of prefrontal control mechanisms have specifically been linked with attenuation of emotional responses (Siegle, Ghinassi, & Thase, 2007). These are known to persist after episodic recovery of depression disorder. Effective emotional and self-control has been linked to metacognition (Manser, Cooper, & Trefusis, 2012; Pennequin, Questel, Delaville, Delugre, & Maintenant, 2019). Both EF and Metacognition are now assumed to regulate deliberate, goal directed, and self-regulated information processing (Blair, Clancy & Diamond, 2008). When a need is created, the hot/emotional system urges the individual to approach desirable stimuli and the cool, cognitive system executes top-down control over the hot system and works towards achieving the desired goal (Metcalfe & Mischel, 1999). Normally, the cool system helps a person to maintain pursuit of his/her initial goal by refraining from impulses, delaying gratification. Thus it is this cool system that overlaps EF.

Cognitive Control

Cognitive control refers to mental processes that allow behaviour to vary adaptively depending on current goals. It is multifaceted, with one of its core functions being to override, restrain, or inhibit unwanted yet dominant response tendencies (Miyake et al., 2000). Cognitive control is recruited during low-level reaction time tasks, but also during complex self-regulatory behaviours (Hofmann, Schmeichel, & Baddeley, 2012). For example, cognitive control could involve inhibiting consistent reading responses on the Stroop test, limiting one's wish for unhealthy foods, or overcoming stereotypical associations of an ethnic community. Hence, cognitive control and its related aspects of self-regulation help us to hold on to long term goals in presence of counterproductive short term distractors. This mechanism is beneficial for individuals and society as it helps generate better outcomes.

The cognitive control network has been shown to regulate emotions and support the inhibitory role of lateral and dorsal regions of the prefrontal cortex (PFC) and dorsal anterior cingulate cortex (dACC) in modulating neural activity in emotional appraisal systems (Inzlicht, Legault, & Teper, 2014). In particular, cognitive reappraisal studies have demonstrated increased activation in prefrontal regions including the orbitofrontal cortex (OFC), dorsolateral prefrontal cortex (DLPCF), lateral prefrontal cortex (LPFC) and medial prefrontal cortex (MPFC) alongside decreased activation in subcortical regions (e.g. amygdala). These subcortical regions are known to embody certain types of emotional information (Ochsner & Gross, 2005). Also, PFC is known to generate and preserve alternate ways of thinking about a situation (Izard, 2010). Further, as a part of this constellation is MPFC which is exclusively implicated in self-monitoring processes and supervises the internal emotional responses to outside stimuli (Wright, Carver, & Scheier, 2000). MPFC may also be the link between DLPFC and limbic regions as they do not have a direct connection (Inzlicht et al., 2014). The dACC monitors the interference between top-down reappraisals (that counterbalance the emotional reaction) and bottom-up assessment of the stimulus that keeps eliciting an emotional response (Barrett & Lindquist, 2012), hence playing the role of conflict monitoring and inhibition (Carver & Scheier, 1998).

Early research posited cognition and emotion to be opposed elements as emotion reduced the capacity to regulate behaviour (Metcalfe & Mischel, 1999). Contemporary research, however, has found these two constructs to be integrated, and not found evidence for a clear distinction between the two in the brain (Barrett & Lindquist, 2012). In recent years there has been a large amount of research on emotion–cognition interactions (Robinson, Watkins, & Harmon-Jones, 2013), not only the effect of emotion on control but also how that control can be comprehended as an emotional process (Inzlicht, Bartholow, & Hirsh, 2015). Given this context, that there are two kinds of emotions that influence cognitive control: integral and incidental (Schmeichel & Inzlicht, 2013). Incidental emotion can be seen as secondary, caused by some unrelated task or mood manipulation whereas integral emotion, is caused by aspects of the proximal task itself (such as the experience of conflict) and hence is crucial for signalling the need for more control. These are different, such that, emotion arising as an extrinsic factor may moderate self-control, but operates separately from task (e.g. fear of failure, low self-perception, high distress). These incidental emotions can have varying effects on control dynamics (Proudfit, Inzlicht, & Mennin, 2013) either working together with control, contending control, or not having any effect on it (Gray, 2004; Pessoa, 2009).

Figure 1. Valence of affective cue is judged to be high at the sensory thalamic level, then it goes through the reactive system and is quickly responded to without going through the scrutiny of the frontal systems. If it is not threatening, then the information goes from the brainstem and sensory thalamus to the prefrontal and limbic systems which work together to determine an appropriate response. The default mode is minimally engaged, with some inputs in from autobiographical memory of previously handled situations but largely central executive is involved in assessing response cost-benefits in terms of desired future outcome

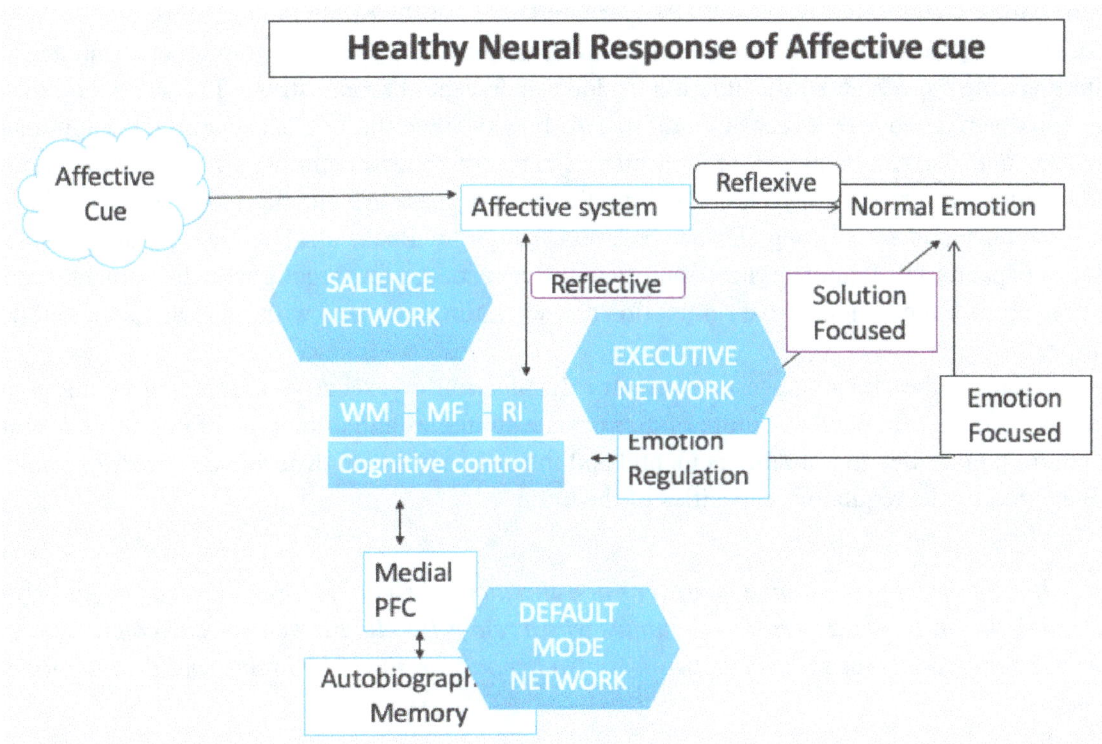

Cognitive Control and Neurobiological Underpinnings of Depression

Multiple pathways have been known to be involved in the neurocircuitry of depression (Mayberg, 2007). In current understanding, depression is viewed as a progressive illness. The Sequenced Treatment Alternatives to Relieve Depression (STAR*D) project reported that out of 1500 participants 74% experienced more than one episode (Madhoo & Levine, 2015) and they concluded that these were driven by neurobiological vulnerabilities. The Kindling Hypothesis (Post, 1992) proposes that depressive episodes are more easily triggered over time. The tendency for an increase in the number of episodes is predicted more by duration of the previous episodes rather than by life stressors (Post, 2007). As the number of episodes increases the probability of recovery decreases. Also, as the length of episodes increase the chances of recovery fall drastically (Monroe & Harkness, 2005). Large numbers of studies have shown that even when individuals are not in an episode of depression, they show residual cognitive deficits (Lebowitz et al., 1997). It has also been noted that these residual deficits are predictive of a greater probability of future episodes (Gotlib & Joormann, 2010), specifically cognitive vulnerabilities (Mongrain

& Blackburn, 2005). A large sample study with a sample of 3000 adolescents and young adults showed that 90% patients with recurrent MDD reported having "very much" impairment, which limited their work productivity and social interactions (Wittchen, Nelson, & Lachner, 1998).

Research regarding depressive cognitions implicates working memory, attention, processing speed and executive dysfunction (Papazacharias & Nardini, 2012). Recent literature primarily implicates the Cognitive Control Network (CCN) of the EF system as the dysfunction in Depression (Fales et al., 2008; Hwang et al., 2015; Wang, Yang, Sun, Shi, & Duan, 2016). This cognitive dysfunction continues even after remission of depressive symptoms (Reppermund et al., 2009; Smith et al., 2006).

In depression, these CCNs are shown to be affected due to excessive bottom up emotion activated signalling arising from high stress situation or due to persistent chronic stress. The stress disrupts the frontal 'top down' control by overwhelming it. This breaks down the PFC's capacity for reappraisal of the situation and also results in lack of inhibition of certain incidental emotions consequently resulting in failed regulation. The neuropsychological implications of these are impaired capacity for inhibition, working memory and set shifting (Disner, Beevers, Haigh, & Beck, 2011). This manifests clinically as reduced capacity for deliberate direction of cognitive resource for target goal achievement, reduced capacity to come out of a depressive rumination and work through plans with more adaptive emotional regulation.

To summarise, the above suggests a primary dysfunction of executive control on emotions. The dysfunction may be examined as failure of appropriate strategies and allocation of cognitive resources to the required goals due to both the incidental and intrinsic emotional disturbances overwhelming the control exerted by the regulatory capacities of the brain.

Figure 2. Biased threat perception a neutral or non-threatening signal is also perceived negatively and goes through the brain stem to sensory thalamus which relays it to limbic system. The cognitive control systems are suboptimal and salience network is also hypoactive since the limbic and default mode are hyper active

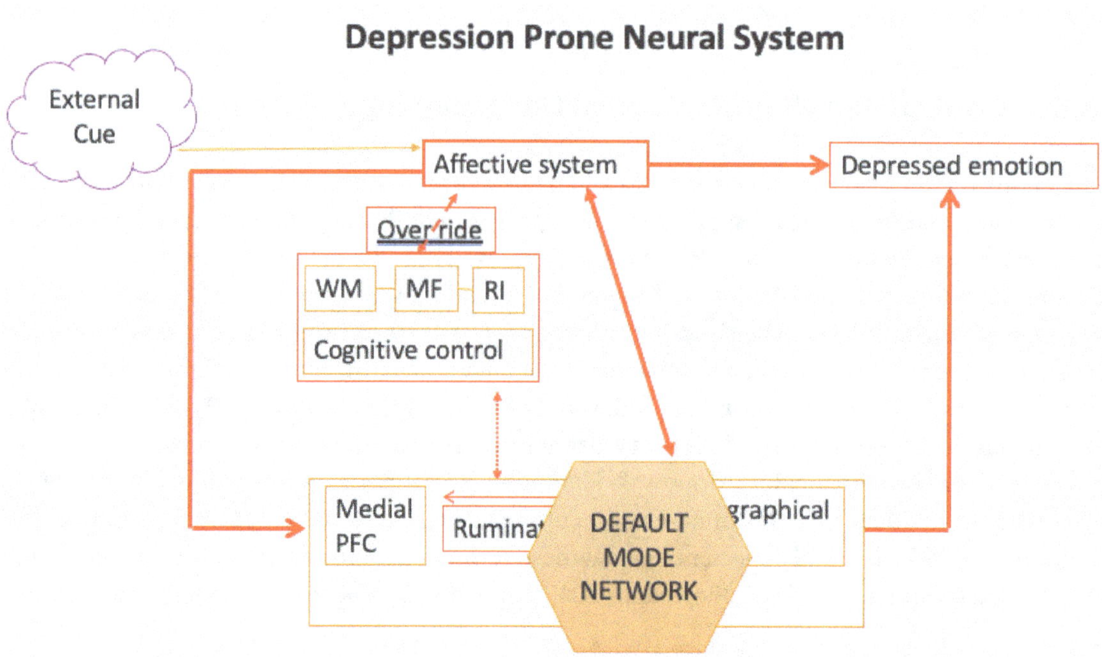

This causes misinterpretation and high reliance on negatively biased autobiographical memories, which furthers the low mood. Restricts adequate uptake and assimilation of new information/assessment of situation and perpetuation biased schema formation.

Studies on Neuropsychological and Cognitive Control in Depression

Attention and concentration difficulties in Depression are well acknowledged and are also used as somatic markers to indicate the severity of the condition in Diagnostic Statistical Manual and International Classification of Disease. Decision making is another cognitive deficit faced by individuals suffering from depression, this is used as a cognitive marker to assess severity in Beck's Depression Inventory (BDI), one of the most widely used scales to assess depression severity. Other deficits like working memory, mental flexibility, response inhibition, memory and learning are less understood. Research in this area started a few decades ago facilitated by the advent of structural and functional imaging. It is now well accepted that Major Depression Disorder is associated with multiple cognitive deficits which exist before an active episode/diagnosis and continue even after recovery.

Neuropsychological studies in depression have shown specific deficits during episodes and after symptomatic recovery, with attention, EF and memory being specially implicated. These studies found that unipolar patients presented deficits in visuospatial sequencing, immediate memory and attention compared to healthy controls (HCs). These impairments also persisted during post symptomatic recovery. These impairments have been associated with symptom severity, with hospitalised patients exhibiting more intense deficits. Memory abnormalities were also associated with dysregulation in hypothalamus-pituitary-adrenal axis, with stress hormones affecting the hippocampus (Rozenthal, Laks, & Engelhardt, 2004).

Depressed patients display recall deficits in tasks that involve the spontaneous use of strategies compared to controls, implying deficits in cognitive initiative. They specifically show deficits in recalling material which is "tiring" to process, because of reduced capacity to execute these procedures, however not due to reduction in the amount of material remembered. Hence indicating that the memory difficulties in depression maybe more related to executive function than memory per se. These deficits are hence seen in tasks contingent on additional automatic processing (Hertel & Hardin, 1990).

Studies have found that nearly 25– 50% MDD patients had deficits that are higher than 1 *SD* below the mean on minimum one cognitive domain. Also, 48% score more than 2 *SD* below the mean. Indicating that cognitive deficits in MDD are consistent, replicable, nonspecific, clinically significant, and of small to medium in effect size (McIntyre et al., 2013; Rock et al., 2014; Snyder, 2014) .

The systematic reviews demonstrate that most affected areas of cognition are attention, EF and WM. Somewhat inconsistent findings regarding other areas like memory and motor speed maybe because they are more state markers than trait markers. Earlier reviews have shown mixed results, probably because of heterogenous tests and population chosen. The more recent reviews show more consistent findings. The studies also show that cognitive impairment persists before and after symptomatic recovery and represents a core feature of depression.

Many studies have specifically explored EF deficits called the 'Depression-executive dysfunction syndrome' (Alexopoulos et al., 2002). The executive dysfunction is linked with difficulties in daily life and the prognosis of these cases. This phenomenon happens in MDD because the person is biased on emotional material which is negative. The competing emotional material takes precedence when the supervisory system allocates resources. Hence, even when the limbic region is overactive over redundant material, cognitive resources continue to be drained out to maintain that activity. This depletes the resources available for task/s at hand (Pessoa, 2009).

Impairments in Cognitive Control

Recent literature has identified specific deficits in depression to be related to Cognitive Control Networks (CCN). These networks are primarily related to the ability to override pre-potent responses and to inhibit the processing of irrelevant or previously relevant information. "These abilities are related to the functioning of executive control processes, such as inhibition, switching, and updating in working memory" (Miyake et al., 2000).

Effect of deficits of cognitive control for emotional information on rumination and depressive symptoms have been studied through prospective designs and follow up of patients (Demeyer et al., 2012). Mediation analyses reveal significant effect of dysfunction of cognitive control for emotional information on depressive symptoms, at baseline. This effect was mediated by rumination. These findings emphasize the importance of cognitive control abilities as a process underlying rumination and as a vulnerability aspect for depression. This understanding should motivate translational research that will advance the effectiveness of interventions, which aim to reduce susceptibility, by targeting cognitive control.

When studying the role of CC, it is also important to delineate whether MDD patients show an overall CC deficit or a deficit specific to emotional information. Murphy, Michael, & Sahakian, (2012) studied whether the set-shifting deficit in MDD is more apparent on emotional relative to non-emotional CC tasks. They compared the performance of patients with MDD with matched HC participants on neutral and emotional variants of a dynamic CC task. The task involved shifting attention and response from one category to another. MDD patients were found to have deficit in performance accuracy in the two tasks. However, the MDD patients had preserved ability to flexibly shift attention and respond to different stimuli on neutral go/no-go task. It was on the emotional go/no-go task where they showed slower response rate on blocks of trials where shifting of attention was required between different emotional categories. The authors concluded that deficits of cognitive flexibility and control related deficits were evident on tasks that involve processing of relevant emotional material rather than on neutral tasks.

In a more recent study Zuckerman et al. (2018) conducted a narrative review of studies exploring cognition as a relevant aspect of MDD. Observational studies, clinical trials, and review articles pertaining to cognition and cognitive impairment in MDD were incorporated. They also manually reviewed related terms and citations from the references. The authors classified 'hot' and 'cold' cognitions; "hot" cognition denoted affective-laden cognitive processes impacted by the person's emotional state such as negative attentional bias, emotion-linked recall or rumination.

They concluded that neuropsychological testing shows critical inferences into altered pathophysiology of neural brain networks with direct effects on "cold" cognitive functioning. Neural networks including the prefrontal cortex and cingulate gyrus, subcortical regions in the striatum and thalamus, and temporal lobe structures including the amygdala and hippocampus are functionally modified in depression. More explicitly, deficits in EF have been associated with pathophysiology in the lateral aspects of the prefrontal cortex. Also, memory impairment was shown to be linked with decrease in hippocampal volume which could be gradual result of MDD (Clark, 2009).

Researchers have also tried to understand whether overall psychosocial functioning in MDD is mediated by scores on specific cognitive domains, namely- EF, attention, immediate memory, delayed memory, spatial cognition, semantic fluency and if specific cognitive domains mediate the adverse outcome of a current episode of MDD on specific psychosocial issues, namely- autonomy, occupational functioning, interpersonal relationships, financial issues, subjective cognitive dysfunction, leisure time. A recent study (Knight & Baune, 2018) has shown that overall psychosocial functioning analysis has found that spatial cognition and EF partially mediated the negative effect of current MDD on psychosocial functioning. However, only spatial cognition mediated deficits in IPR, while only EF mediated difficulties in leisure time. This a unique study and the findings offer evidence that executive and spatial cognition have significant part in the pathology of specific psychosocial issues in MDD.

The author explains the role of EF in autonomy by the use of EF in a range of behavioural and cognitive abilities like planning ahead, problem-solving and managing functional independence. Spatial cognition may influence autonomy by worsening spatial errors and oversights which could further affect self-confidence in maintaining autonomy specially for those who are prone to hypersensitive internalization of errors. The spatial and EF failures may also influence subjective cognitive deficits by augmenting cognitive failures such as forgetting appointments/names and deficits in solving problems. These are further associated with reduced cognitive functioning and worsen self-perception of cognitive deficit.

Figure 3. Low mood even in the absence of a trigger as the hyperactive default mode continues to feed in negatively biased memories. Ruminative thoughts keep the limbic system hyperactive. Exhausted EF networks continue to work at suboptimal level and unable to generate better coping strategies

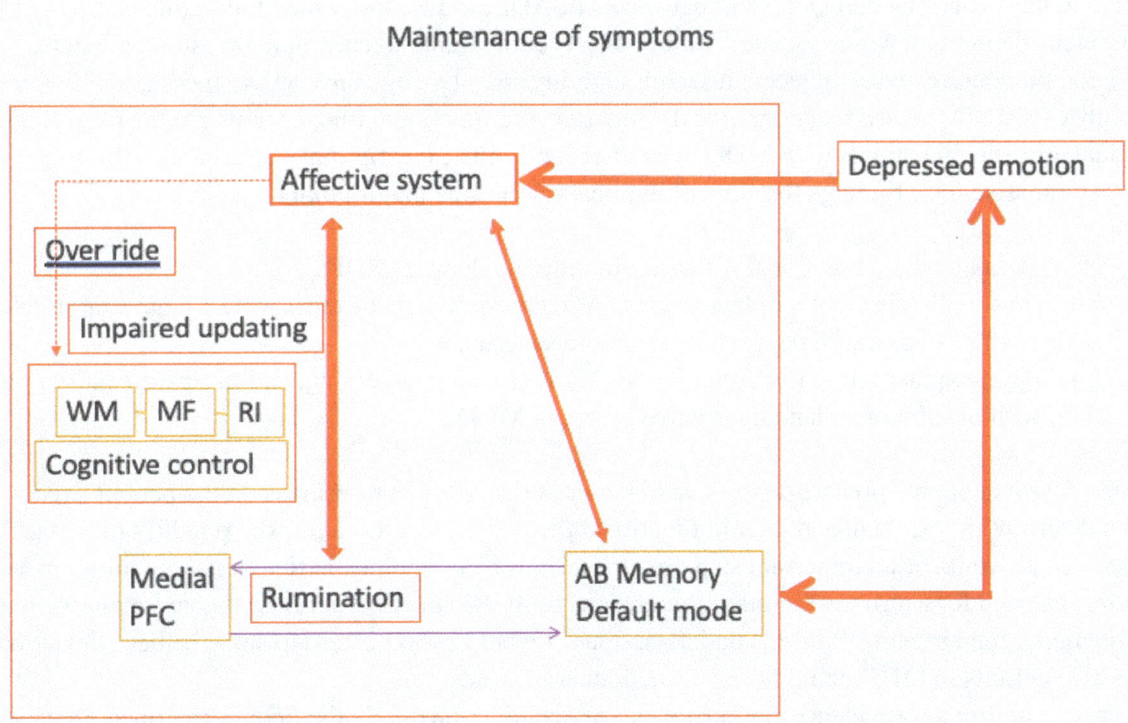

Neurocognitive Deficits and Functional Recovery in Depression

Neurocognitive (NC) deficits affect the socio-occupational function in depression including general/ life functioning (GF/LF), employment and integration into community. In other psychiatric conditions, NC deficits have proven to affect LF in different ways such as obtaining and keeping employment, educational and career progress, managing a household, and social and familial associations (Gold et al.,2002). Problem solving ability relies directly on NC, dysfunctional neurocognitions may heighten disability in a vulnerable population (Wilder-Willis et al., 2002). It has also been noted that persistent LF disability adds to the burden of families, friends and co- workers (Judd et al., 1998) which often leads to withdrawal of their support and augments the patient's dependence on poor PS ability to maintain LF, adding to stress. Research has shown that these NCs play a role in improvement by other interventions.

The link between NC deficits, work performance and depression is an important one. Studies have reported that current depression worsened cognitive performance in all domains (Baune et al., 2010). They also found that participants with previous depression had continuing cognitive impairments in immediate memory and attention compared to HCs. Patients with current depression had lesser scores in total score than ones with previous depression. The currently unemployed patients group overall performed significantly worse in all domains. Some of the other findings from the study were that individuals with current depression performed poorer in the visuospatial/constructional and attention tasks and had worse total score compared with patients with previous depression; they did not find NC to be related to physical or mental QoL or impairments of ADL, IADL; lastly they found that unemployment in previous depression was associated with poor NC comparable to current depression patients.

A comprehensive review of recent research studying cognitive dysfunction as a mediator of functional disability in MDD showed that cognitive dysfunction and functional impairments are the most frequent residual ailments in patients with MDD even after remission of symptoms (Lam et al., 2014).
They summarise their findings for clinical implication in three major points:

- NC deficits mediate functional disability in individuals with MDD.
- Mechanistically different antidepressants (ADs) seem to benefit measures of cognition unrelated to their effects on overall depression symptom severity.
- It is suggested that future research may work on screening, assessing, and mitigating NC dysfunction, with the aim of enhancing improvements in MDD.

NC deficits not only predate depressive disorder but persist to cause stress on the patient's recovery. It is a deterrent in treatment and later in functional recovery. Thus, for a holistic rehabilitation, tackling these deficits would be an important step. Insufficiencies in symptom and functional outcomes in MDD call for the need for a turn toward other dimensions of MDD (like NC deficits) that are main mediators of functional impairment. With this understanding, it would be important to see whether alleviation of cognitive deficits in MDD could benefit functional outcomes.

There is preliminary evidence that current pharmacologic and psychotherapeutic treatments have some effect on NC functioning in MDD. However, they do not have much effect on their effect on psychosocial functioning and on residual symptoms. Newer cognitive remediation approaches may address these.

Social functioning is another area which is as important as occupational functioning in determining overall recovery and quality of life. Comparison of social cognitive functioning of patients with MDD with HC (Air, Weightman, & Baune (2015) has shown that Depression severity and anxiety symptoms were predictive of score on all social cognition subscales in currently depressed patients. They assessed one hundred and eight individuals with MDD (66 remitted and 42 current) and 52 HCs on Wechsler Advanced Clinical Solutions: Social Perception Subtest. This test measures facial affect recognition alone and in groups with prosody and body language. However they did not find any association between symptom severity and the WAIS ACS in individuals with remitted depression. Higher severity of depression and comorbid anxiety symptoms were associated with worse performance on complex social cognitive tasks. The author suggests that patients with MDD may have difficulty in allocating cognitive resources to attend to and process social information and that currently depressed patients with higher somatic symptoms had poorer scores on affect recognition task.

This section has highlighted typical cognitive deficits in depression which points towards a primary decline in cognitive control abilities. Some studies have specifically pointed towards more WM and SS deficits and some have pointed to specific difficulties in these domains when the stimulus is emotional rather than neutral (non-emotional). These CC deficits seem to be tied to rumination and mediate depression psychopathology. They have also found to be trait like characters of individuals who have tendency towards depression. More recent studies also point out the role of neuropsychological functions in functional recovery. More that 60 percent of the patients (Madhoo & Levine, 2015) continue to have significant disability even after achieving full remission and some get worse overtime. A common finding is the involvement of visuospatial and EF in continued employment, post recovery. Sustained attention and working memory were found to be more related to social competence and recreational quality whereas EF was linked to more adaptive competence tasks. Some limitation of studies so far has been pointed out in terms of heterogeneity of samples and assessments used, cross-sectional designs in most studies and lack of adequately matched control groups.

Some studies point to the issue of allocation of cognitive resources rather than actual depletion of the resource, as seem in difficulties depressed patients have in solving complex social tasks rather than IQ based tasks. This, points to the involvement of supervisory EF, which is often linked to metacognitions. Next section looks at studies that have found connections between these two concepts and their role in depression.

Metacognition, Executive Control and Emotional Regulation in Depression

"Metacognition refers to the aspect of the information-processing system that monitors, interprets, evaluates, and regulates the contents and processes of its organization" (Flavell, 1979; Wells, 2000). Effective emotional and self-control has been linked to metacognition (Manser, Cooper, & Trefusis, 2012; Pennequin et al., 2019). EF and Metacognition have been related in the past (Norman & Shallice, 1986) and recently developmental theorists have shown both to have important links with self-regulation (Roebers, 2017). Both EF and MC are known to regulate deliberate, goal-directed, and self-regulated information processing (Blair, Clancy & Diamond, 2008). When a need is created, the hot/emotional system urges the person to approach a desirable stimulus and the cool cognitive system implements top-down control over this hot system (Metcalfe & Mischel, 1999). Normally, the cool system helps individuals maintain pursuit of her/his initial goal by refraining from impulses, delaying gratification. Hence, this cool system coincides with pure EF.

Perhaps one of the first shifts in cognitive therapy from content-based theories to process based theories was the linking of executive control to metacognition and pathology through attention and rumination by Wells & Matthews (1996) in their "Self-Regulatory Executive Functions System (S-REF)". The multi-level cognitive structure of this model consists of three interrelated levels: first, processing units that run automatically and reflexively; second, attention demanding units which are voluntary; thirdly, stored knowledge or self-beliefs. Wells suggest that in mood disorders, rumination is specifically harmful. Since it is a limited capacity system, ruminating drains processing resources required for execution of plans which could disconfirm the dysfunctional belief. Also, such an activity constantly primes dysfunctional self-beliefs and drives the low-level representations to keep confirming them. This also adds to decreasing thresholds for interruption of congruent information. Eventually, verbal-conceptual type rumination blocks complete emotional processing (Wells & Papageorgiou, 1995).

The S-REF model proposes two types of metacognitive beliefs: positive and negative. The positive beliefs are triggered by internal prompts like negative thoughts and they signal the need for prolonged negative processing by means of rumination or worry to deal with the thought. Then, negative meta-beliefs about the "uncontrollability and danger of rumination and worry" adds to maintaining of and recurrence in episodes of depression.

Neurocognitive correlates of metacognitions have only recently been studied in detail. Spada, Georgiou, & Wells (2010) found that metacognitions about worry were associated with reduced ability to shift and focus attention.

Recently, Kraft et al. (2017) examined this association between metacognitions and executive control. They measured these with objective and standardized neuropsychological tests. The results showed that "negative beliefs about the uncontrollability and danger of worry" and "beliefs about the need to control thoughts" were related to a reduced ability to shift between mental sets. This shifting ability was also related to metacognitions once age, education level, general cognitive function, and depression and anxiety symptoms, were controlled. This indicates that there is a direct association between metacognitions and shifting ability.

It has been previously shown that "negative beliefs about the uncontrollability and danger of worry" and "beliefs about the need to control thoughts" generates a cognitive impasse, which creates more worry (Spada et al., 2008). Kraft's results suggest that this cognitive gridlock is related to reduced ability to shift between mental sets. This explains why individuals having higher metacognitions have more difficulty in stopping rumination and moving to more adaptive coping strategies.

Previously reduced inhibitory control has been linked to negative thought intrusions, and is known to trigger rumination (Daches & Mor, 2014; Koster et al., 2017). Hence, inhibition is important in S-REF model when intrusions from low-level networks activate the supervisory executive. There is a close relationship between metacognitions and rumination (Papageorgiou & Wells, 2009; Solem et al., 2016) and between rumination and inhibition (Yang et al., 2017).

Low cognitive confidence may not be an accurate reflection of actual cognitive performance (Wells, 2000). Kraft's results demonstrate a relationship between cognitive confidence and updating, however this became non- significant once current depression and anxiety were controlled. This is probably because only currently depressed individuals have lower cognitive confidence (Halvorsen et al., 2014).

The author suggests that individual differences in executive control may be central in the individualization of treatment and that cognitive training which targets shifting ability may enhance effectiveness of treatment through increase in ability to stop rumination and reduce metacognitions. It is further suggested that patients with low executive control may benefit from such a training in shifting ability though individuals with better executive control may not need such training.

Neural and Neuropsychological correlates of Emotion Regulation and Ruminations in Depression

Emotion regulation deficits and rumination pose a significant vulnerability factor for depression. Recent literature on depression has focused on cognitive deficits which give rise to disturbed emotion regulation and increased ruminative response to stress which further precipitates or maintains a depressive episode. Previous research has shown that rumination is associated with impaired problem solving, reduced task performance, and with negative affect. Information processing deficits have also been understood to add to ruminative tendencies (De Raedt & Koster, 2010; Koster, 2011). These later models hold that cognitive control deficits increase rumination when the individual is faced with stressful situations. A better understanding of factors which influence rumination will help create targeted interventions for depressive symptoms.

Suboptimal cognitive control has been found to result in larger switch costs. They have also been shown to moderate the association between stress and increased rumination (De Lissnyder et al., 2012).

The study by De Lissnyder examined whether individual differences in cognitive control ability, for non-emotional and emotional material, play a moderating role in the association between the occurrence of a stressful event and the tendency to ruminate. They administered the Internal Switch Task (IST) to assess attentional switching between items WM. After six weeks they administered self-report questionnaires at 4 fixed points to assess measuring stressors, rumination and depressive symptoms.

The most important finding of the study is that reduced switching for emotional material moderates the association between stress and rumination but such a relationship was found for non -emotional material.

Many studies have used the paradigm of inducing rumination or mood to study these variables. Induced internal states provide a good way of tapping mood states and associated features. Park, Goodyer, & Teasdale (2004) investigated the effects of induced rumination as compared to distraction on mood and categoric over general memory in adolescents with first episode Major Depressive Disorder (MDD), and the specificity of any effects to MDD. They used an experimental design and measured "in the moment" depressed mood and categoric over general memory before and after rumination and distraction. In participants with MDD, induced rumination and not distraction increased depressed mood. They did not find significant difference for this between current MDD patients and partially remitted patients. They also found that rumination and not distraction increased over-general memories to negative cues in MDD participants.

Hence, experimentally induced rumination as compared to distraction increases depressed mood and negative categoric memories in adolescents with first episode MDD. The findings suggest that ruminations have a detrimental effect on mood and memory retrieval processes in adolescents with first episode MDD.

Another study that compared ruminators and non-ruminators on the scores on Wisconsin Card Sorting Test (WCST), a measure of cognitive flexibility, found that individuals high on rumination had significantly more perseverative errors and failed to maintain set significantly more times as compared to non-ruminators (Nolen Hoeksema & Davis, 2000). On an advanced section of the WCST designed for this study, male ruminators exhibited significantly greater inflexibility than male non-ruminators. They did not find any relation of these effect to differences in general intelligence or the presence of depressed mood. Hence, the results suggest that tendency for rumination is linked to an inflexible cognitive style.

Nine conceptually different cognitive emotion regulation strategies have been reported: "Self-blame, Other-blame, Rumination, Catastrophizing, Putting into Perspective, Positive Refocusing, Positive Reappraisal, Acceptance and Planning" (Garnefski et al., 2001). Many studies have established that there is a strong link between the use of these strategies and emotional problems (Garnefski et al., 2004; Kraaij et al., 2003). Overall it has been established that use of cognitive styles such as Rumination, Catastrophizing and Self-blame increases vulnerability to emotional problems. On the other hand using strategies such as Positive Reappraisal may reduce these vulnerabilities. To this end Garnefski & Kraaij (2006) studies the relationships between cognitive emotion regulation strategies and depressive symptoms. They compared five different samples (from adolescents to elderly) on their reported use of cognitive emotion regulation strategies. And studied the relationships between these strategies and symptoms of depression.

They found significant differences in strategies across age range, even then, relationships between cognitive emotion regulation strategies and depression symptoms were alike in all. They also hypothesized that psychiatric adults would report highest maladaptive cognitive strategies and lowest adaptive strategies. The results confirmed their hypothesis as MDD group had significantly higher scores on Self- blame, Rumination and Catastrophizing. The results found elderly to be high on acceptance, even the ones in the clinical sample. They argue that a distinction can be made between active Acceptance of self-affirmation and passive Acceptance in sense of submission to negative experiences (Wilson, 1996). In this sample the latter form of Acceptance may be seen, which is a negative adjustment style linked to poor outcomes (Wilson, 1996). Confirming their third hypothesis, it was found that in all groups a substantial percentage of the variance in symptoms of depression was explained by the use of emotion regulation strategies. Rumination, Catastrophizing, reduced Positive Reappraisal and Self-blame were most frequently reported with symptoms of psychopathology.

Having established that maladaptive emotional regulation strategies like rumination are linked to cognitive control and EF some recent researches have tried to look at the neural correlates of such maladaptive emotion regulation strategies. It has been shown previously that during the processing of irrelevant negative material compared to irrelevant positive material, in depressed patients, there is a greater activation of cognitive-control regions such as the prefrontal cortex (PFC) and anterior cingulate cortex (ACC) (Kerestes et al., 2012). Foland-Ross et al. (2013) used functional neuroimaging during an emotional working memory (WM) task to elucidate the neural correlates of difficulties in cognitive control. They hypothesized that depressed patients would also show enhanced activation in these areas while removing negative material from WM. To provide evidence that the ability to update the contents of WM in depression is related to rumination tendency (Joormann & Gotlib, 2008), the authors tested if enhanced activation in these brain regions is associated with higher trait rumination in the depressed. The sample consisted of fourteen individuals diagnosed with MDD and 15 non-depressed control subjects.

They used the modified emotional Sternberg task, in which subjects viewed an encoding display, an instruction cue, and a probe display in each trail. In the encoding display, two lists of three words each were presented simultaneously. One word list was presented in blue, and the other was presented in red. The two lists also differed in word valence: One of the lists contained neutral words only, and the other contained positive, negative, or neutral words. Patients were asked to remember either the red or the blue list depending on which colour they saw after the words. After this cue they were shown a word written in black and they had to respond whether it's from the relevant list or irrelevant list. Trials were separated by an interstimulus interval of varying length. In the WM manipulation involving depressed participants, the dorsal anterior cingulate and parietal and bilateral insular cortices were activated significantly more when negative words were removed from WM than when they were maintained in WM; in contrast, non-depressed participants exhibited stronger neural activations in these regions for positive than for negative material.

The results of this study confirmed that removing relevant negative material from WM is associated in depression with abnormalities in activation of the dACC, a region that is related to cognitive control. More specifically, MDD participants showed a greater increase in activation in these areas when negative material was removed from WM than when it was maintained in WM though this effect did not hold for positive material. This then suggests that they required additional neural and cognitive resources to perform this mental operation.

These findings in the dACC may also relate more specifically to the role of this region in conflict monitoring (Botvinick et al., 1999). During the task presentation of the material in WM, the material encoded earlier interferes and competes for cognitive resources. The role of dACC is to manage this interference by conflict resolution between the two competing WM materials. It does this by controlling maintenance of the previously relevant word list and improving maintenance of the currently relevant material (as recognised by the cue). However, depressed individuals have difficulty disengaging from negative material which has captured their attention (Caseras et al., 2007), and so this material is more likely to continue in the WM for further analysis and is likely facilitated. This may then subsequently demand less activation by the dACC to resolve interference between two competing word lists.

The study has some notable limitations, some participants in the depressed group were on medication or had additional anxiety disorders during scanning, hence these factors may have influenced the results. Though after statistically controlling for them, results did not change. Also the task did not have a separate baseline between the different task periods, it may be that activations observed during the cue period also reflected some residual activity occurring during the encoding time.

Another way of looking at the relation between neurocognitive factors and rumination is by training a cognitive factor to see the effect on rumination. Such a study was done by Cohen, Mor, & Henik (2015) who examined whether training individuals to exert executive control when exposed to negative stimuli can ease rumination. Total of 85 participants were assigned randomly to two trainings. The task was designed such that the experimental group would have to keep shifting between trials and hence train them in recruiting EC when processing emotional stimuli. In addition they were assessed on self -report measures for rumination, anxiety and depression.

The results demonstrated that processing incongruent Flanker stimuli prior to the presentation of emotional stimuli promotes inhibition of irrelevant emotional information and decreased its interference. The results showed that the effect of irrelevant negative stimuli on performance is reduced by the inducing of executive control. The coupling between incongruent stimuli and negative pictures also successfully removed the linked between habitual brooding and sad mood. This was the first study that directed the executive control before presenting emotional information to lower rumination.

The findings indicate that there is specific deficit in engaging inhibitory processes when processing emotional information which direct ruminative thinking. They found that participants in the experimental group showed reduced state rumination compared with those in the control group. The authors argue that training individuals to exert executive control when processing negative stimuli can alleviate ruminative thinking and rumination-related sad mood.

This section of the review points to the role of maladaptive emotion regulation strategies in depression, specifically rumination. Studies conclude that impaired emotional switch mediates stress and rumination, and such a relationship has been seen consistently for emotional switch and rather than for neutral/non affective switching capacity. Studies experimentally inducing rumination in lab settings also show that induced ruminations increase over general memories to negative cues and depressed mood.

This cognitive emotional regulation hence is shown to be result of neurocognitive deficits in cognitive control and related to the dACC.

Studies using single session paradigms to train these patients on exercising executive control through shifting and/or inhibition also not only reduce rumination but also effect the bias for negative material. Hence, most authors proposed that treating the underlying deficits in inflexibility, working memory and shifting in adequately delivered training sessions will improve overall emotional regulation and metacognitive strategy selection, eventually improving depressive symptoms and associated cognitive disability.

The next section elaborates on the neural correlates and networks of the brain involved in triggering/maintaining depressive symptoms. The section also looks at effects and role of autobiographical memory and effects of mood induction on these brain areas.

Impairments in Cognitive Control Networks

Recent literature has identified specific deficits in depression to be related to Cognitive Control Networks (CCN). These networks are primarily related to the ability to override pre-potent responses and to inhibit the processing of irrelevant or previously relevant information. "These abilities are related to the functioning of executive control processes, such as inhibition, switching, and updating in working memory" (Miyake et al., 2000).

When studying the role of CC, it is important to delineate whether MDD patients show an overall CC deficit or specific deficit to emotional information. It has been found that performance of patients with MDD when compared with HC participants on neutral and emotional variants of a dynamic CC task, had preserved ability to flexibly shift attention and respond to different stimuli on neutral go/no-go task (Murphy, Michael, & Sahakian, 2012). It was on the emotional go/no-go task where they showed slower response rate on blocks of trials where shifting of attention was required between different emotional categories. The authors conclude that deficits of cognitive flexibility and control related could be evident on tasks that involve processing of relevant emotional material rather than neutral.

Recent research in imaging has been working towards understanding the discovery of large-scale neural networks encompassing distinct regions across the brain. These networks are functionally linked and inclined to activate in specific patterns (Chen et al., 2013). These functional neural networks seem critical to adaptive functioning of emotions, cognitions, and behaviour. These networks systematize gradually during the critical years when early life situations (ELS) have most influence on functioning.

Neuroimaging has helped understand the supposed neuronal mechanisms which underlie depressed mood and other symptoms such as motivation and cognitive deficits in patients. Specifically, they have worked to understand the changes in interregional connectivity. Though, many different results have been demonstrated which may even seem contradictory. This makes it difficult to draw a general theory. However, some studies have reviewed the findings and we can begin to understand the networks involved in MDD.

One such extensive review was conducted by Kaiser et. al. (2015) who conducted a literature search in Web of Science, PubMed, and EMBASE for articles in press as of June 30, 2014, using the keywords *rest*(-ing), connect*(-ivity),* and *depress*(-ion, -ive)*. They included only original functional magnetic resonance imaging studies which used whole-brain seed-based resting state Functional Connectivity (rsFC) to compare individuals with MDD with a healthy control (HC) group. They contacted the authors who were not able to provide whole-brain effects or seed ROI or peak effect coordinates.

They found lowered connectivity in frontoparietal control systems and disturbed connectivity between control networks involved in internal or external attention. These systems may be responsible for negative biases toward internal thoughts at the cost of engaging with the external world. Deficits in regulating mood may be due to imbalanced connectivity between neural systems involved in cognitive control and those which sustain salience and emotion processing. The authors report that these maybe the empirical basis for a neurocognitive model in which network dysfunction can cause core cognitive and affective abnormalities in depression.

In the same year, Mulders et al., (2015) did a review of the Resting State Functional Connectivity (RSFC) in MDD from 2005-2014, they included total 8 papers using Independent Component (ICA) and 28 papers applying Seed based Correlation Analysis (SCA). They found that all ICA papers studied the DMN, while the CEN and SN were only reported in a subset of studies. In the SCA research, the most commonly chosen seed regions are the ACC, PCC and the amygdala.

One of the most consistent findings was a greater connection strength in the anterior DMN. This increase was between different anterior nodes and in the DMN in general. Another common finding across studies was about the higher in functional connectivity between the anterior DMN and the SN. This has also been observed at the structural level (Fang et al., 2012). It has been pointed out that hyper activity of amygdala is reaction to negative provocation and leads to negativity bias in MDD (Murray et al., 2011). This increased hyperactivity in amygdala is also a result of poor connections with other brain areas for emotional control except sgACC in MDD. A discrepancy in ACC performance and effortful prefrontal recruiting in emotional control in MDD has been reported (Rive et al., 2013). Reduced connectivity of the amygdala with other regions such as insula and lateral PFC is also an important finding in regard to limbic hyperactivity. This also consistent with findings of lateral hypoactivity in resting-state studies in MDD (Northoff, et al., 2011).

These findings also validate another important model by (Mayberg, 1997) which refers to the limbic–cortical dysregulation. The model describes MDD as an inability to control overactive "ventral limbic" regions such as the ventral insula, amygdala, hypothalamus, hippocampus, vmPFC and sgACC, by underactive "dorsal limbic" regions (such as, dACC, PCC, inferior parietal, dorsal frontal areas). Mayberg's model also links the rostral ACC as the major region for pathology and treatment response. The networks between anterior and posterior DMN have also been implicated in many studies. These sub-network within DMN are understood to be essential in self-generated thought. Posterior DMN is also found to have decreased connectivity with CEN in MDD. Posterior DMN is understood to have a role in awareness and selected attention (Leech & Sharp, 2014) and CEN is implicated in higher cognitive operations (Corbetta & Shulman, 2002). This connection difference in MDD and may cause the deficit in switching from a DMN "default-state" primarily internally directed, to a goal directed "executive state" where CEN is active and attention is focussed on outward stimuli (Hamilton et al., 2013).

The most commonly associated networks in MDD are the cortico-limbic network, the default-mode network (DMN), and the affective network. The cortico-limbic network consists of subordinate circuits such as fronto-limbic, the parietal-limbic, and the temporo-limbic network. The DMN includes the ventromedial prefrontal cortex, the posterior cingulate cortex, and the precuneus. Functional magnetic resonance imaging (fMRI) studies have demonstrated that these regions show reduced activity when performing cue-dependent tasks in comparison to resting state.

In another recent systematic review of all neural connectivity in MDD, Helm et al., (2018) report results from studies published between 2002 to 2015. The review supports the previous findings that the limbic cortex has reduced connectivity to other brain regions in MDD. In this system the sgACC is essential in emotional control and so the disturbance could be the reason for the dysregulation seen in MDD. They also report that cerebellum shows reduced connectivity to other brain areas in resting state and in task-related recordings. Unlike the earlier understanding where role of cerebellum was only related to control motor coordination more recent studies have shown its involvement in emotional and cognitive processes. Brains of MDD patients have also found to have reduced cerebellum volume.

The review also reported findings that neuronal connections to the insula were heightened in MDD. The insula is understood to associated with interoceptive awareness and perception. These processes are also intricately linked to processing emotions and decision making. Hence, functionally, insula and other interoception based areas seems to be closely related to depressive symptoms. Insula has also been found to unite with the vagus nerve and stimulating this nerve may hold future opportunity for treatment of MDD.

Another important system found to be active in MDD is the basal ganglia. This system is somewhat overlapping with the limbic areas, such as, in the thalamus and the pallido-striatum. In MDD, the activity and the connections of both regions to other brain regions are enhanced and contribute to the unbalanced cortico- limbic circuits which are essential in mood regulation.

The authors of this review did not support the hypothesis of a dominance of the DMN over other IC, and insufficient support for dysfunction of the SN as the moderator between the DMN and CEN. They found overall reduction within DMN connectivity compared to healthy controls. Same reduced connectivity was also found within the SN and within CEN, they did not find any studies reporting altered connectivity within the CEN when performing tasks.

They found some limitations in the studies reviewed--as none of the studies addressed gender differences. Specially since there has been evidence indicating different neuronal substrates between women and men, in grey matter volumes or resting-state activity. Since this might be another reason for the diverging results in connectivity analyses, this topic should be taken into account in future studies. Also, since it is difficult to draw conclusions, investigation of interhemispheric connectivity may help in understanding the varied results.

CONCLUSION

The evidence is overwhelming that MDD patients show deficits in various neuropsychological measures, most prominent being the executive functions. These deficits are interlinked with deficits in cognitive aspects and socio-occupational functionality in these individuals. The neural network research is also collaborative and shows irregular neuronal connectivity in areas of the medial-, orbito, and lateral-frontal lobe, frontal pole, limbic structures, cerebellum, medial-temporal lobe, basal ganglia, occipital lobe, and the insula in MDD patients. In RS conditions, the connectivity of the medial frontal lobe, medial temporal lobe, and basal ganglia to other regions of the brain is increased, whereas the cerebellum is less connected with other brain regions. While performing tasks, the limbic structures, medial- and lateral-frontal lobe, occipital lobe, cerebellum, and frontal pole are less connected to other brain regions in depressed patients, as compared with HCs. Contrary to this, the medial temporal lobe, the orbitofrontal lobe, and the insula are strongly connected with many other brain regions. More evidence is required to confirm the general understanding of DMN, SN and CEN interconnectivity theory, though there is clear evidence for alteration in and within all three.

It is important to note that since deficits in neuropsychological functions and alterations in neuronal connectivity contribute to the aetiology and to the symptoms of MDD. There have been attempts at such remediations in other neurocognitive conditions such as epilepsy (Gupta, 2020), traumatic brain injury (Banerjee et al., 2021) and attempts at using mood induction to recruit the emotional circuits in MDD (Banerjee & Kumar, 2020). The remedy of these neuropsychological deficits and modulation of neuronal networks may help in the development of effective and sustainable treatments for MDD.

REFERENCES

Air, T., Weightman, M. J., & Baune, B. T. (2015). Symptom severity of depressive symptoms impacts on social cognition performance in current but not remitted major depressive disorder. *Frontiers in Psychology*, *6*(AUG), 1–9. doi:10.3389/fpsyg.2015.01118 PMID:26300814

Alexopoulos, G. S., Buckwalter, K., Olin, J., Martinez, R., Wainscott, C., & Krishnan, K. R. R. (2002). Comorbidity of late life depression: An opportunity for research on mechanisms and treatment. *Biological Psychiatry*, *52*(6), 543–558. doi:10.1016/S0006-3223(02)01468-3 PMID:12361668

Banerjee, M., Hegde, S., Harish, T., Kulkarni, G. B., & Rao, N. (2021). In search of the 'self': Holistic rehabilitation in restoring cognition and recovering the 'self' following traumatic brain injury: A case report. *Neuro Rehabilitation*, 1-12.

Banerjee, M., & Kumar, K. (2020). Mood Induction Can Enhance Cognitive Remediation in Depression. *International Journal of Cognition and Behaviour*, *3*(1). Advance online publication. doi:10.23937/2690-3172/1710008

Baune, B. T., Miller, R., McAfoose, J., Johnson, M., Quirk, F., & Mitchell, D. (2010). The role of cognitive impairment in general functioning in major depression. *Psychiatry Research*, *176*(2–3), 183–189. doi:10.1016/j.psychres.2008.12.001 PMID:20138370

Blair, C., & Diamond, A. (2008). The promotion of self regulation as a means of preventing school failure. *Development and Psychopathology*, *20*(3), 899–911. doi:10.1017/S0954579408000436 PMID:18606037

Botvinick, M., Nystrom, L. E., Fissell, K., Carter, C. S., & Cohen, J. D. (1999). Conflict monitoring versus selection-for-action in anterior cingulate cortex. *Nature*, *402*(6758), 179–181. doi:10.1038/46035 PMID:10647008

Caseras, X., Garner, M., Bradley, B. P., & Mogg, K. (2007). Biases in Visual Orienting to Negative and Positive Scenes in Dysphoria: An Eye Movement Study. *Journal of Abnormal Psychology*, *116*(3), 491–497. doi:10.1037/0021-843X.116.3.491 PMID:17696705

Chen, A. C., Oathes, D. J., Chang, C., Bradley, T., Zhou, Z. W., Williamsa, L. M., Glover, G. H., Deisseroth, K., & Etkin, A. (2013). Causal interactions between fronto-parietal central executive and default-mode networks in humans. *Proceedings of the National Academy of Sciences of the United States of America*, *110*(49), 19944–19949. doi:10.1073/pnas.1311772110 PMID:24248372

Cohen, N., Mor, N., & Henik, A. (2015). Linking executive control and emotional response: A training procedure to reduce rumination. *Clinical Psychological Science*, *3*(1), 15–25. doi:10.1177/2167702614530114

Corbetta, M., & Shulman, G. L. (2002). Control of goal-directed and stimulus-driven attention in the brain. *Nature Reviews. Neuroscience*, *3*(3), 201–215. doi:10.1038/nrn755 PMID:11994752

Daches, S., & Mor, N. (2014). Training ruminators to inhibit negative information: A preliminary report. *Cognitive Therapy and Research*, *38*(2), 160–171. doi:10.100710608-013-9585-5

De Lissnyder, E., Koster, E. H. W., Everaert, J., Schacht, R., Van den Abeele, D., & De Raedt, R. (2012). Internal cognitive control in clinical depression: General but no emotion-specific impairments. *Psychiatry Research*, *199*(2), 124–130. doi:10.1016/j.psychres.2012.04.019 PMID:22578821

De Raedt, R., & Koster, E. H. W. (2010). Understanding vulnerability for depression from a cognitive neuroscience perspective: A reappraisal of attentional factors and a new conceptual framework. *Cognitive, Affective & Behavioral Neuroscience*, *10*(1), 50–70. doi:10.3758/CABN.10.1.50 PMID:20233955

Demeyer, I., De Lissnyder, E., Koster, E. H. W., & De Raedt, R. (2012). Rumination mediates the relationship between impaired cognitive control for emotional information and depressive symptoms: A prospective study in remitted depressed adults. *Behaviour Research and Therapy*, *50*(5), 292–297. doi:10.1016/j.brat.2012.02.012 PMID:22449892

Fang, P., Zeng, L. L., Shen, H., Wang, L., Li, B., Liu, L., & Hu, D. (2012). Increased Cortical-Limbic Anatomical Network Connectivity in Major Depression Revealed by Diffusion Tensor Imaging. *PLoS One*, *7*(9), e45972. Advance online publication. doi:10.1371/journal.pone.0045972 PMID:23049910

Foland-Ross, L. C., Hamilton, J. P., Joormann, J., Berman, M. G., Jonides, J., & Gotlib, I. H. (2013). The Neural Basis of Difficulties Disengaging From Negative Irrelevant Material in Major Depression. *Psychological Science*, *24*(3), 334–344. doi:10.1177/0956797612457380 PMID:23334445

Garnefski, N., & Kraaij, V. (2006). Relationships between cognitive emotion regulation strategies and depressive symptoms: A comparative study of five specific samples. *Personality and Individual Differences*, *40*(8), 1659–1669. doi:10.1016/j.paid.2005.12.009

Garnefski, N., Teerds, J., Kraaij, V., Legerstee, J., & van den Kommer, T. (2004). Cognitive emotion regulation strategies and depressive symptoms: Differences between males and females. *Personality and Individual Differences*, *36*(2), 267–276. doi:10.1016/S0191-8869(03)00083-7

Gold, P. W., Drevets, W. C., Charney, D. S., & Drevets, W. C. (2002). New insights into the role of cortisol and the glucocorticoid receptor in severe depression. *Biological Psychiatry*, *52*(5), 381–385. doi:10.1016/S0006-3223(02)01480-4 PMID:12242053

Gupta, S. (2020). Smartphone based Early Detection of Epileptic Seizures Using Machine Learning. *Proceedings of the 2020 12th International Conference on Bioinformatics and Biomedical Technology.* 10.1145/3405758.3405763

Halvorsen, M., Hagen, R., Hjemdal, O., Eriksen, M. S., Sørli, Å. J., Waterloo, K., Eisemann, M., & Wang, C. E. A. (2014). Metacognitions and Thought Control Strategies in Unipolar Major Depression: A Comparison of Currently Depressed, Previously Depressed, and Never-Depressed Individuals. *Cognitive Therapy and Research*, *39*(1), 31–40. doi:10.100710608-014-9638-4

Helm, K., Viol, K., Weiger, T. M., Tass, P. A., Grefkes, C., Del Monte, D., & Schiepek, G. (2018). *Neuropsychiatric Disease and Treatment Dovepress Neuronal connectivity in major depressive disorder: A systematic review*. doi:10.2147/NDT.S170989

Hertel, P. T., & Hardin, T. S. (1990). Remembering With and Without Awareness in a Depressed Mood: Evidence of Deficits in Initiative. *Journal of Experimental Psychology. General*, *119*(1), 45–59. doi:10.1037/0096-3445.119.1.45 PMID:2141063

Hoorelbeke, K., Koster, E. H. W., Demeyer, I., Loeys, T., & Vanderhasselt, M.-A. (2016). Effects of Cognitive Control Training on the Dynamics of (Mal). *Adaptive Emotion Regulation in Daily Life.*, *16*(August), 945–956. Advance online publication. doi:10.1037/emo0000169 PMID:27177250

John, H. (1979). Metacognition and cognitive monitoring: A new area of cognitive-developmental inquiry. *The American Psychologist*, *34*(10), 906–911. doi:10.1037/0003-066X.34.10.906

Joormann, J., & Gotlib, I. H. (2008). Updating the Contents of Working Memory in Depression: Interference From Irrelevant Negative Material. *Journal of Abnormal Psychology*, *117*(1), 182–192. doi:10.1037/0021-843X.117.1.182 PMID:18266496

Judd, L. L., Akiskal, H. S., Maser, J. D., Zeller, P. J., Endicott, J., Coryell, W., Paulus, M. P., Kunovac, J. L., Leon, A. C., Mueller, T. I., Rice, J. A., & Keller, M. B. (1998). Major depressive disorder: A prospective study of residual subthreshold depressive symptoms as predictor of rapid relapse. *Journal of Affective Disorders*, *50*(2–3), 97–108. doi:10.1016/S0165-0327(98)00138-4 PMID:9858069

Kerestes, R., Ladouceur, C. D., Meda, S., Nathan, P. J., Blumberg, H. P., Maloney, K., Ruf, B., Saricicek, A., Pearlson, G. D., Bhagwagar, Z., & Phillips, M. L. (2012). Abnormal prefrontal activity subserving attentional control of emotion in remitted depressed patients during a working memory task with emotional distracters. *Psychological Medicine*, *42*(1), 29–40. doi:10.1017/S0033291711001097 PMID:21733287

Knight, M. J., & Baune, B. T. (2018). Executive Function and Spatial Cognition Mediate Psychosocial Dysfunction in Major Depressive Disorder. *Frontiers in Psychiatry*, *9*(October), 3–6. doi:10.3389/fpsyt.2018.00539 PMID:30420817

Koster, E. (2011). Understanding depressive rumination. *Dissertation, 32*(0), 1–32.

Koster, E. H. W., Hoorelbeke, K., Onraedt, T., Owens, M., & Derakshan, N. (2017). Cognitive control interventions for depression: A systematic review of findings from training studies. *Clinical Psychology Review*, *53*, 79–92. doi:10.1016/j.cpr.2017.02.002 PMID:28273486

Kraaij, V., Garnefski, N., De Wilde, E. J., Dijkstra, A., Gebhardt, W., Maes, S., & Ter Doest, L. (2003). Negative Life Events and Depressive Symptoms in Late Adolescence: Bonding and Cognitive Coping as Vulnerability Factors? *Journal of Youth and Adolescence*, *32*(3), 185–193. doi:10.1023/A:1022543419747

Kraft, B., Jonassen, R., Stiles, T. C., & Landrø, N. I. (2017). Dysfunctional metacognitive beliefs are associated with decreased executive control. *Frontiers in Psychology*, *8*(APR), 1–6. doi:10.3389/fpsyg.2017.00593 PMID:28469590

Leech, R., & Sharp, D. J. (2014). The role of the posterior cingulate cortex in cognition and disease. *Brain*, *137*(1), 12–32. doi:10.1093/brain/awt162 PMID:23869106

Madhoo, M., & Levine, S. Z. (2015). Initial Severity Effects on Residual Symptoms in Response and Remission: A STAR*D Study during and after Failed Citalopram Treatment. *Journal of Clinical Psychopharmacology*, *35*(4), 450–453. doi:10.1097/JCP.0000000000000354 PMID:26066336

Manser, R., Cooper, M., & Trefusis, J. (2012). Beliefs about Emotions as a Metacognitive Construct: Initial Development of a Self-Report Questionnaire Measure and Preliminary Investigation in Relation to Emotion Regulation. *Clinical Psychology & Psychotherapy*, *19*(3), 235–246. doi:10.1002/cpp.745 PMID:21374759

Marchetti, I., Koster, E. H. W., Sonuga-Barke, E. J., & De Raedt, R. (2012). The Default Mode Network and recurrent depression: A neurobiological model of cognitive risk factors. *Neuropsychology Review*, *22*(3), 229–251. doi:10.100711065-012-9199-9 PMID:22569771

Mayberg, S. (1997). Limbic-Cortical Dysregulation : Depression. *Journal of Neuropsychiatry*, *9*(4), 471–481. PMID:9276848

McIntyre, R. S., Cha, D. S., Soczynska, J. K., Woldeyohannes, H. O., Gallaugher, L. A., Kudlow, P., Alsuwaidan, M., & Baskaran, A. (2013). Cognitive deficits and functional outcomes in major depressive disorder: Determinants, substrates, and treatment interventions. *Depression and Anxiety*, *30*(6), 515–527. doi:10.1002/da.22063 PMID:23468126

Metcalfe, J., & Mischel, W. (1999). A hot/cool-system analysis of delay of gratification: Dynamics of willpower. *Psychological Review*, *106*(1), 3–19. doi:10.1037/0033-295X.106.1.3 PMID:10197361

Miyake, A., Friedman, N. P., Emerson, M. J., Witzki, A. H., Howerter, A., & Wager, T. D. (2000). The Unity and Diversity of Executive Functions and Their Contributions to Complex "Frontal Lobe" Tasks: A Latent Variable Analysis. *Cognitive Psychology*, *41*(1), 49–100. doi:10.1006/cogp.1999.0734 PMID:10945922

Mulders, P. C., van Eijndhoven, P. F., Schene, A. H., Beckmann, C. F., & Tendolkar, I. (2015). Resting-state functional connectivity in major depressive disorder: A review. *Neuroscience and Biobehavioral Reviews*, *56*, 330–344. doi:10.1016/j.neubiorev.2015.07.014 PMID:26234819

Murphy, F. C., Michael, A., & Sahakian, B. J. (2012). Emotion modulates cognitive flexibility in patients with major depression. *Psychological Medicine*, *42*(7), 1373–1382. doi:10.1017/S0033291711002418 PMID:22067530

Murray, E. A., Wise, S. P., & Drevets, W. C. (2011). Localization of dysfunction in major depressive disorder: Prefrontal cortex and amygdala. *Biological Psychiatry*, *69*(12), e43–e54. doi:10.1016/j.biopsych.2010.09.041 PMID:21111403

Nolen Hoeksema, S., & Davis, R. N. (2000). Cognitive inflexibility among ruminators and nonruminators. *Cognitive Therapy and Research*, *24*(6), 699–711. doi:10.1023/A:1005591412406

Norman, D. A., & Shallice, T. (1986). Attention to action: willed and automatic control of behaviour. In Consciousness and self-regulation (4th ed.). Plenum Press. doi:10.1007/978-1-4757-0629-1_1

Northoff, G., Wiebking, C., Feinberg, T., & Panksepp, J. (2011). The "resting-state hypothesis" of major depressive disorder-A translational subcortical-cortical framework for a system disorder. *Neuroscience and Biobehavioral Reviews*, *35*(9), 1929–1945. doi:10.1016/j.neubiorev.2010.12.007 PMID:21192971

Papageorgiou, C., & Wells, A. (2009). A prospective test of the clinical metacognitive model of rumination and depression. *International Journal of Cognitive Therapy*, *2*(2), 123–131. doi:10.1521/ijct.2009.2.2.123

Park, R. J., Goodyer, I. M., & Teasdale, J. D. (2004). *Effects of induced rumination and distraction on mood and overgeneral autobiographical memory in adolescent*. Academic Press.

Pennequin, V., Questel, F., Delaville, E., Delugre, M., & Maintenant, C. (2019). Metacognition and emotional regulation in children from 8 to 12 years old. *The British Journal of Educational Psychology*, *90*(S1), 1–16. doi:10.1111/bjep.12305 PMID:31292954

Pisner, D. A., Shumake, J., Beevers, C. G., & Schnyer, D. M. (2018). A Reproducible Neurobiology of Depressive Rumination. *bioRxiv*.

Rive, M. M., Van Rooijen, G., Veltman, D. J., Phillips, M. L., Schene, A. H., & Ruhé, H. G. (2013). Neuroscience and Biobehavioral Reviews Neural correlates of dysfunctional emotion regulation in major depressive disorder. A systematic review of neuroimaging studies. *Neuroscience and Biobehavioral Reviews*, *37*(10), 2529–2553. doi:10.1016/j.neubiorev.2013.07.018 PMID:23928089

Rock, P. L., Roiser, J. P., Riedel, W. J., & Blackwell, A. D. (2014). Cognitive impairment in depression: A systematic review and meta-analysis. *Psychological Medicine*, *44*(10), 2029–2040. doi:10.1017/S0033291713002535 PMID:24168753

Roebers, C. M. (2017). Executive function and metacognition: Towards a unifying framework of cognitive self-regulation. *Developmental Review*, *45*, 31–51. doi:10.1016/j.dr.2017.04.001

Rozenthal, M., Laks, J., & Engelhardt, E. (2004). Aspectos neuropsicológicos da depressão. *Revista de Psiquiatria Do Rio Grande Do Sul*, *26*(2), 204–212. doi:10.15900101-81082004000200010

Snyder, H. R. (2014). Major Depressive Disorder is Associated with Broad Impairments on Neuropsychological Measures of Executive Function: A Meta-Analysis and Review. *Psychological Bulletin*, *139*(1), 81–132. doi:10.1037/a0028727 PMID:22642228

Solem, S., Hagen, R., Hoksnes, J. J., & Hjemdal, O. (2016). The metacognitive model of depression: An empirical test in a large Norwegian sample. *Psychiatry Research*, *242*, 171–173. doi:10.1016/j.psychres.2016.05.056 PMID:27285952

Spada, M. M., Georgiou, G. A., & Wells, A. (2010). The relationship among metacognitions, attentional control, and state anxiety. *Cognitive Behaviour Therapy*, *39*(1), 64–71. doi:10.1080/16506070902991791 PMID:19735025

Spada, M. M., Mohiyeddini, C., & Wells, A. (2008). Measuring metacognitions associated with emotional distress: Factor structure and predictive validity of the metacognitions questionnaire 30. *Personality and Individual Differences*, *45*(3), 238–242. doi:10.1016/j.paid.2008.04.005

Wells, A. (2000). *Emotional disorders and metacognition: Innovative cognitive therapy*. John Wiley & Sons Ltd.

Wells, A., & Matthews, G. (1996). Modelling cognition in emotional disorders: The S-REF model. *Behaviour Research and Therapy*, *34*(11-12), 881–888. doi:10.1016/S0005-7967(96)00050-2 PMID:8990539

Wells, A., & Papageorgiou, C. (1995). Worry and the incubation of intrusive images following stress. *Behaviour Research and Therapy*, *33*(5), 579–583. doi:10.1016/0005-7967(94)00087-Z PMID:7598681

Wilder-Willis, K. E., Shear, P. K., Steffen, J. J., & Borkin, J. (2002). The relationship between cognitive dysfunction and coping abilities in schizophrenia. *Schizophrenia Research*, *55*(3), 259–267. doi:10.1016/S0920-9964(01)00211-0 PMID:12048149

Wilson, G. T. (1996). Acceptance and change in the treatment of eating disorders and obesity. *Behavior Therapy*, *27*(3), 417–439. doi:10.1016/S0005-7894(96)80025-6

Yang, Y., Cao, S., Shields, G. S., Teng, Z., & Liu, Y. (2017). The relationships between rumination and core executive functions: A meta-analysis. *Depression and Anxiety*, *34*(1), 37–50. doi:10.1002/da.22539 PMID:27378739

Zuckerman, H., Pan, Z., Park, C., Brietzke, E., Musial, N., Shariq, A. S., Iacobucci, M., Yim, S. J., Lui, L. M. W., Rong, C., & McIntyre, R. S. (2018). Recognition and Treatment of Cognitive Dysfunction in Major Depressive Disorder. *Frontiers in Psychiatry*, *9*(December), 1–11. doi:10.3389/fpsyt.2018.00655 PMID:30564155

KEY TERMS AND DEFINITIONS

Cognitive Control: Cognitive control refers to the ability to override pre-potent responses and to inhibit the processing of irrelevant or previously relevant information. These abilities are related to the functioning of executive control processes, such as inhibition, switching, and updating in working memory.

Emotional Regulation: It is defined as the cognitive processes that may assist individuals in regulating their emotions, and gaining control over these without becoming overwhelmed by them.

Metacognition: Metacognition refers to the psychological structures, knowledge, events, and processes that are involved in the control, modification and interpretation of thinking itself. According to recent theorizing, metacognition is an important factor in the development and maintenance of psychological disorder.

Ruminations: Rumination is a maladaptive emotion regulation strategy that is characterized by the tendency to respond to a stressful event with repetitive, perseverative, and negative thinking.

Chapter 8
Characterising Attention Deficit Hyperactivity Disorder

Mishab A. K.
University of Calicut, India

ABSTRACT

ADHD is a neurodevelopmental disorder that affects children. ADHD can often persist in adulthood too. Children diagnosed with ADHD have significantly increased across the globe and range between 3-10% of the population. The cardinal features of ADHD are inattention, hyperactivity, and impulsivity. Clinically significant impairment affects bio-psychosocial functioning. Theoretical understanding reveals the central role of genetics, environmental factors, and cognition in ADHD symptoms. The gold standard for ADHD diagnosis relies on clinical history, mental status examination, and diagnostic tools. Pharmacological intervention is the first-line evidence-based treatment for ADHD. However, studies also report that children don't respond to or can't tolerate medications and suffered from adverse side effects. There are also evidence-based treatments such as neurofeedback training that uses technology to regulate brain activity through modifying brain waves. Hence, developing devices for assessment and intervention using technology that targets the cognitive deficits is the need of the hour.

DOI: 10.4018/978-1-7998-9534-3.ch008

"Phil, stop acting like a worm,

The table's not a place to squirm"

Thus speaks the father to the son,

Severely says, not in fun.

Mother frowns and looks around,

But Philip will not take advice,

He'll have his way at any price.

He turns,

And churns,

He wiggles

And giggles

Here and there on the chair;

"Phil, these twists I cannot bear."

"Fidgety Phil, translated from a German book illustrating childhood misbehavior "(1845)

NEURODEVELOPMENTAL DISORDER

Neurodevelopmental disorder is group of disorder broadly defined as a disorder that evident in the developmental period of the children primarily associated with the functioning of nervous system and brain. These disorders are characterized by impairment that can impact bio-psychosocial functioning of the individual. Neurodevelopmental Disorders includes intellectual disability, communication disorders, Autism Spectrum disorder, Attention-deficit/Hyperactivity disorder, specific learning disorder, motor disorders and other developmental disorder. Table 1 shows the classification of Neurodevelopmental disorder (American Psychiatric Association, 2013).

Table 1.

Neurodevelopmental Disorder
Intellectual Disabilities
Intellectual Disability (Intellectual Developmental Disorder)
Global Developmental Delay
Unspecified Intellectual Disability (Intellectual Developmental Disorder)
Communication Disorder
Language Disorder
Speech Sound Disorder (previously Phonological Disorder)
Childhood-Onset Fluency Disorder (Stuttering)
Social (Pragmatic) Communication Disorder
Unspecified Communication Disorder
Autism Spectrum Disorder
Autism Spectrum Disorder
Attention-Deficit/Hyperactivity Disorder
Attention-Deficit/Hyperactivity Disorder
Other Specified Attention-Deficit/Hyperactivity Disorder
Unspecified Attention-Deficit/Hyperactivity Disorder
Specific Learning Disorder
Specific Learning Disorder
Motor Disorders
Developmental Coordination Disorder
Stereotypic Movement Disorder
Tic Disorders
Tourette's Disorder
Persistent (Chronic) Motor or Vocal Tic Disorder
Provisional Tic Disorder
Other Specified Tic Disorder
Unspecified Tic Disorder
Other Neurodevelopmental Disorders
Other Specified Neurodevelopmental Disorder
Unspecified Neurodevelopmental Disorder

ATTENTION DEFICIT HYPERACTIVITY DISORDER (ADHD)

History

The literature suggests that children with ADHD symptoms have been described by several authors at the beginning of the 18th Century. However, the manifestations, characterizations, underlying concepts, etiology have changed over time.

Sir Alexander Crichton, a Scottish physician, was the first person who has described a similar case of ADHD in his book on attention and its diseases. According to Crichton (1978) attention is the ability to focus on one particular stimulus and ignoring the other stimuli stimulus. He also emphasizes that attention can vary from person to person and within a person at different times. The distraction of attention is not necessarily qualifying for pathological every time. Crichton distinguishes inattention as the result of increased or decreased ''sensibility of the nerves'' (Crichton 1798). All the symptoms depicted by Crichton are associated with attention deficit disorder. Crichton has failed to recognize the symptom of hyperactivity or correlation of hyperactivity with inattention. Thus, his description meets the criteria of the ADHD subtype but could not meet the criteria of ADHD clinical diagnosis. Still, it is not sure that Crichton was referring to ADHD.

Another important figure was the German physician Heinrich Hoffmann who has created some illustrated children's stories including ''Fidgety Phil'' (''Zappelphilipp''). In the story of Fidgety Phil, Hoffmann illustrates an event which was happened in a family during dinner. The scene illustrates a child who was falling with the food on the table due to his fidgeting behavior. This can be viewed as a case of ADHD. At the beginning of the story, the father requesting the child to remain seated. The presumptive statement suggests that the father had anticipated some misbehavior of his son at a table, indicating that this was not an occasional event (Thome & Jacobs, 2004). This wans another example of an early ADHD case.

Another Story relevant to the ADHD has been added in the 5th edition of "Johnny look- in the air" (Bader et al., 2018). In this story Hoffman describes a boy showing the symptoms of inattention. Johnny was always ''looking at the sky and the clouds that floated by'' (Hoffmann, 1846) and were, therefore often easily distracted by extraneous stimuli. Johnny's inattentiveness resulted in the collision with an approaching dog and climaxed in an accident as ''Johnny watched the swallows'' (Hoffmann, 1846). He finally fell into a river.

Immediately after the great encephalitis epidemics of 1917–1918, attention towards the ADHD diagnosis increases in North America. It was observed that children surviving this encephalitis had many behavioural issues that are in line with ADHD symptoms (Ebaugh 1923; Hohmann, 1922; Stryker, 1925). Moreover, the other brain infection arose from birth trauma, head injury, toxin exposure, and infections also associated with behavioral problems. This observation led to research that can identify the etiology of ADHD.

By the late 1950s, attention shifted away from etiology and towards the more specific characterization of these children such as hyperactivity and poor impulse control which eventually labeled the children as "hyperkinetic impulse disorder" or "hyperactive child syndrome" (Burks, 1960; Chess, 1960). The disorder was believed to be poor thalamic filtering of the stimuli entering in the brain which results from cortical over stimulation (Knobel et al.,1959; Laufer et al.,1957). The clinicians and researchers of this era strongly believed that the condition had some sort of neurological origin. However, when the second edition of the Diagnostic and Statistical Manual of Mental Disorders (DSM-II) appeared, all childhood disorders were described as "reactions," and the hyperactive child syndrome became "Hyperkinetic reaction of childhood".

By the 1970s, research also emphasized inattention and impulsivity in addition to hyperactivity (Douglas, 1972). Douglas (1980, 1983) theorized that the disorder involved major deficits in (1) attentional factors 2) inhibitory deficit (3) the diminished regulation of arousal-activation levels to meet situational demands 4) abnormal reward response and increased behavioral variability. This has eventually led to the renaming of the disorder "attention deficit disorder" (ADD) in 1980 (DSM-III; American Psychiatric Association, 1980). DSM III has come up with the distinction of two types of ADD; ADD with hyperactivity and without it. Later the concern arose within a few years regarding the label of ADD that the important features of hyperactivity and impulse control were being not emphasized. In 1987, the disorder was renamed "attention-deficit hyperactivity disorder" in DSM-III-R and incorporated the three core symptoms of ADHD.

During the 1980s the research was focused on the motivation factors in ADHD. The research was demonstrating conditions that are not reinforcing, the children with ADHD showed significant declines in their performance (Douglas & Parry, 1983, 1994; Parry & Douglas, 1983). The deficits in the control of behaviour by rules are governed by external factors rather than the internal.

Later DSM IV once again permitted the diagnosis of a subtype of ADHD that consisted primarily of problems with attention (ADHD predominantly inattentive type). It also permitted, for the first time, the distinction of a subtype of ADHD that consisted of hyperactivity and impulsivity without intention (ADHD, predominantly hyperactive-impulsive type). Children having significant problems from both inattention and hyperactivity were described as having ADHD, combined type.

The debate still continues over the major deficits in ADHD, with increasing focus given to issues with behavioral inhibition, self-regulation, and the related domain of executive functioning (Barkley, 1997a, 1997b, 2001c; Douglas, 1999; Nigg, 2001; Quay, 1997). The characterization of ADHD has been evolved over time.

Prevalence of ADHD

According to the Centers for Disease Control and Prevention National Parents survey revealed that children diagnosed with ADHD have significantly increased across the globe. The worldwide estimated prevalence of ADHD ranges between 3-10%. ADHD is more frequent in boys than in girls with a ratio of approximately 2:1 in children and 1.6:1 in adults. Girls are more likely than girls to be diagnosed with predominantly inattentive subtype. The official prevalence of ADHD in the United States was 3-7% (APA, 2000). The prevalence of ADHD in India ranges from 1.6 to 17.9% (Pingali S, 2014). A similar study carried out in children revealed that 6% of children who are diagnosed with ADHD are between 10- 15 years of age. Various studies conducted among parents/ teachers yielded a double-digit prevalence of ADHD. However, such studies cannot be fully reliable due to a single informant which doesn't meet the diagnostic criteria.

ADHD can occur as a comorbidity of other conditions. The most prevalent comorbidity reported in children with ADHD is oppositional defiant disorder. Other comorbidities can be associated with ADHD are conduct disorder, Specific learning disorder, bipolar affective disorder, substance use disorder, major depressive disorder, obsessive-compulsive disorder, tic disorder, elimination disorder, social phobia, and separation anxiety disorder (Palaniappan P, 2013).

Diagnostic Features and Criteria of ADHD

Attention Deficit Hyperactivity Disorder (ADHD) is a neurodevelopmental disorder that affects children. However, ADHD can often persist in adulthood too. The cardinal features of ADHD are inattention, hyperactivity, and impulsivity. ADHD has a differential brain development in which inattention can manifest in children as short attention span, increased distractibility, inability to complete tasks, careless mistakes, and difficulties of organizing tasks. Hyperactivity and impulsivity can manifest trouble in waiting their turn, sitting, fidgets, and interrupts others. Many of these symptoms are present in all children and adults to some degree at some point in their life. Consequently, the parents reading this chapter will conclude that all their children have attention deficit hyperactivity disorder. What characterizes children with ADHD is the intensity, the persistence, and the patterning of these symptoms.

Diagnostic Criteria (DSM 5,2020)

A persistent pattern of inattention, hyperactivity, and impulsivity that interferes with the development level or functioning of the child.

1. **Inattention**: Six or more of the following symptoms that persist for at least 6 months to a degree that is inappropriate with the age level and that impact his/her social, academic, psychological, and occupational life.
    ◦ Careless mistakes in activities or miss important details
    ◦ Difficulty to sustain attention in task/ activities at hand
    ◦ Lack of patience to listen when spoken to directly
    ◦ Often difficult to follow through on instructions or absent-minded
    ◦ Difficulty in organizing tasks/ activities
    ◦ Avoids tasks that are needed sustained mental effort
    ◦ Often loses track of their things/task/activities
    ◦ Easily distractible
    ◦ Easily forgetful
2. **II. Hyperactivity & Impulsivity**: Six or more of the following symptoms that persist for at least 6 months to a degree that is inappropriate with the age level and that impact his/her social, academic, psychological, and occupational life.
    ◦ Often fidgeting hand and feet
    ◦ Difficulty to remain seated when seating is expected
    ◦ Often runs or climb in situations where it is inappropriate
    ◦ Often difficulty stay quiet when needed
    ◦ Always "on the go" acting as if "driven by a motor" (often restless)
    ◦ Often talks excessively
    ◦ Often utter out the answer before question finishes
    ◦ Inability to wait for his/her turn
    ◦ Often interrupt others

The above symptoms should begin in childhood and present before the age of 12 years. Manifestation of the symptoms should be present in two or more settings such as at home, school, work, or with friends/relatives. Moreover, there should be clear evidence that symptoms are interfering in his/her psychological, social, academic, and occupational functioning. Parents may observe hyperactivity when the child is a toddler, but symptoms are difficult to distinguish before the age of 4 years. It's also the normal phenomenon of a toddler being restless, excessive motor activity, and distracted. Often these behaviors have not met the criteria of ADHD.

Attention deficit hyperactivity disorder is divided into three subtypes according to the criteria set by the DSM 5.

- **Predominantly inattentive:** If criteria 1 is met but criteria 2 fit not met for at least 6 months
- **Predominantly hyperactive and impulsive:** If criteria 1 is met but criteria 2 fit not met for at least 6 months
- **Combined Subtype:** If both criteria 1 and criteria 2 are met for at least 6 months

Adult ADHD

The manifestation/presentation of ADHD in adults is slightly different from children with ADHD. Hyperactivity is one of the common manifestations in children. However, hyperactivity is likely to be less in adults and may replace or with other symptoms such as restlessness. The Utah criteria for Adult ADHD are as follows;

1. Childhood history consistent with ADHD &
2. Adult symptoms
    a. Hyperactivity and poor concentration and two of the following
        - Hot temper
        - Inability to complete tasks and disorganization
        - Stress intolerance
        - Impulsivity
        - Affective inability

Theoretical Understanding of ADHD

ADHD, like other common psychiatric disorders, is not known what causes ADHD. There is no one particular cause of ADHD and exposure to a risk factor does result in disorder. However, researchers believe that a combination of multiple genes, brain, non-inherited factors, environment, and their interplay contributes to the development of the disorder. Also, risk factors that contribute to the development of ADHD might not always be the same as those that contribute to its course and outcomes. To be clear, genetic factors can exert indirect risk effects through interaction with environmental factors. Genes can alter through the interaction with the environmental risks. Inherited factors can also influence the possibility of exposure to certain environmental risks. This means that environmental and genetic risk effects cannot be separable.

GENETICS

Inherited Contribution to ADHD

The wide range of study designs of ADHD genetics has confirmed the importance of genes in etiology. Findings from family studies found that ADHD is twofold to eightfold increased risk in parents and siblings of affected probands compared with relatives of unaffected controls. Twin studies have estimated that monozygotic twin pairs have higher concordance rates for ADHD than dizygotic twin pairs. Similar way, adoption studies have also found higher rates of ADHD in the biological parents of ADHD adoptees (Sprich et al., 2020). Mean heritability estimates are around 79%, suggesting non-inherited factors also contribute to ADHD.

ADHD is also found to have an inherited answerability with other neurodevelopmental disorders and psychiatric issues such as autism spectrum disorder, learning problems, intellectual disability, conduct, and mood problems. These comorbidities in many cases suggestive of the same inherited and familial risks can contribute to the manifestation of different clinical phenotypes.

ADHD Susceptibility Genes

There has been a lot of efforts to identify susceptibility genes in ADHD. There is an enormous literature on candidate genes that are reported to be associated with ADHD, but very few are meta-analyses and studies that are consistently replicated. The Dopamine D4 receptor gene (DRD4) variant has been shown for the strongest association with ADHD. There have been extensive studies findings that the Dopamine D4 receptor gene binds with both dopamine and norepinephrine and there is a functional polymorphism (variable number tandem repeat—VNTR) in exon III of the gene. Meta-analysis studies show that the seven-repeat allele of this polymorphism has been found to be strongly associated with ADHD.DRD5 is another dopamine receptor gene, which is consistently implicated in multiple studies.

The dopamine transporter gene (DAT1) responsible for the reuptake of dopamine in the presynaptic cleft was primarily considered the most likely ADHD candidate gene. The gene encoding catechol O methyltransferase (COMT) has a modifying effect on the ADHD phenotype rather than increase the risk of the disorder itself. COMT helps in catalyzes the degradation of dopamine.

Literature suggests that high rates of ADHD are associated with different chromosomal anomalies such as abnormalities in the structure and number of chromosomes (e.g., sex chromosome aneuploidies). More commonly, It is also found that inattentive subtype of ADHD as a comorbidity with fragile X syndrome, tuberous sclerosis, and several microdeletion syndromes.

ENVIRONMENTAL RISK FACTORS

Maternal Smoking, Alcohol, Drug Use, and Stress/Anxiety in Pregnancy

Maternal stress during pregnancy has one of the important roles in all neurodevelopment disorders. Among them, maternal stress has a significant association with offspring ADHD symptoms. There are several studies that reported a significant correlation with offspring ADHD symptoms. One of the other environmental risk factors is maternal smoking and drug use. Clinical and epidemiological studies reveal a consistent association between dose-response relationship and prenatal exposure to maternal cigarette smoking (maternal reports and urinary cotinine levels) and offspring ADHD symptoms. Alcohol use during pregnancy can result in fetal alcohol syndrome. The behavioral aspects of fetal alcohol syndrome include symptoms of inattention and hyperactivity. However, associations between less extreme alcohol use in pregnancy and offspring ADHD/ADHD symptoms are inconclusive due to inconsistent findings across the studies. In summary, it plays a significant role with ADHD symptoms and maternal smoking, drug use, stress during pregnancy but there is no one-to-one casual relationship.

Low Birth Weight and Prematurity

Meta-analyses study findings provide evidence of a relatively high risk of ADHD symptoms/attention problems in premature and/or low birth weight children. Out of that, high-risk low birth weight child appears to have the strongest association with inattention symptoms.

Toxins and Diet

Specific environmental exposures have an important role to play in ADHD phenotype include organic pollutants (e.g., pesticides, polychlorinated biphenyl (PCBs)) and lead. These may affect or damage cognitive and neural systems known to be implicated in ADHD. Research study on neurobehavioral outcomes of polychlorinated biphenyl exposure suggests impairment in working memory, response inhibition, and cognitive flexibility. Similarly, lead exposure has similar impairments on executive functions and attention, with cognitive flexibility, vigilance, and alertness being most affected.

Dietary constituents such as sugar, artificial food colorings, zinc, iron, magnesium, and omega-3 fatty acids have been studied in relation to ADHD symptoms. However, there is no convincing evidence yet that diet plays a major causal role in ADHD. But there are several research findings that reveal the use of dietary change to modify ADHD symptoms. A recent randomized controlled trial of a restricted elimination diet based on high or low IgG foods findings reveal a reduction of ADHD symptoms as an effect of a restricted elimination diet on children with ADHD.

Psychosocial Adversity

Psychosocial adversity such as low parental education, social class, poverty, bullying/peer victimization, parenting, maltreatment, and family discord play significant association with ADHD. None of the study designs used so far have cannot conclude these are definite causes of ADHD. However, psychosocial factors might increase the vulnerability of ADHD presentation in children especially in those who are genetically susceptible.

BARKLEY'S THEORY OF ADHD

Barkley proposed a theory of ADHD that emphasizes the role of cognition in ADHD. The theory postulate's role of executive functions such as inhibitory control, working memory and attentional regulation in the manifestation of ADHD symptoms. According to him, Inhibitory control is the primary deficit that disrupts other executive function process.

Figure 1 illustrates the hybrid model of executive functions and the relationship of these four functions to the behavioural inhibitions and motor control systems. Non verbal working memory is the capacity to hold and maintain an information temporarily to guide a later motor response. As this theory predicts, deficits in behavioural inhibition will result in deficit in non verbal working memory that manifest as deficit in hindsight, poor anticipatory set, diminished sense of time, impaired imitation of complex sequences, limited self awareness and impaired non verbal rule governed behaviour.

Figure 1. Berkeley theory of ADHD

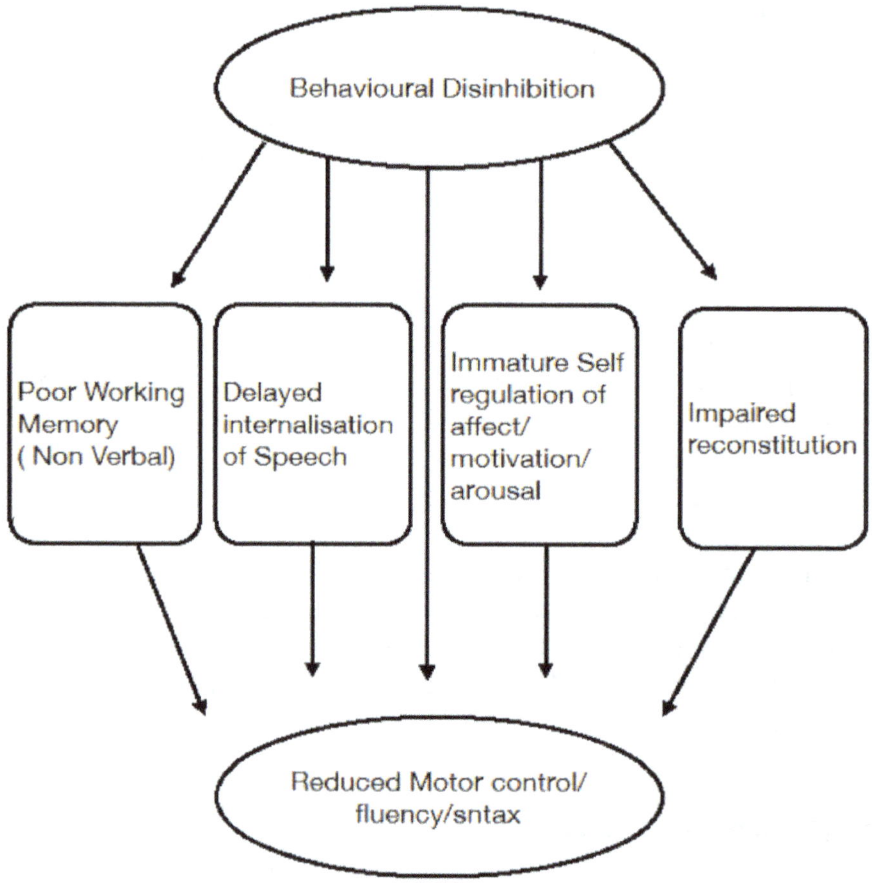

Children with ADHD has significant difficulty in internalization of speech. Inability to internalize the speech will lead to excessive talking, acts without thinking, less organized, difficulty in following the rules and instructions of others. Research Evidence suggests that delayed internalization of speech is the result of deficits in verbal working memory. The model portrays how internalization and self regulation plays role in ADHD. Those with ADHD shows immediate emotional expression in their reactions to stimulus, less objectivity in the choosing of a response to stimulus, reduced social perspective taking and diminished ability to persist in goal-directed behavior. Children with ADHD remain more dependent upon the immediate environmenttal reinforcement to sustain the motivation in the task at hand (Barkley, 1997). The model also explains the inability to mentally visualize, manipulate, and then generate multiple plans of action in the service of goal-directed behavior in ADHD children. This impairment in reconstitution will be evident in everyday functioning of ADHD children such as deficits in verbal and nonverbal fluency, planning, problem solving, and strategy development.

BRAIN REGIONS IMPLICATED IN ADHD

Neuroimaging studies implicate brain regions in ADHD: (1) the prefrontal cortices (2) the basal ganglia (3) the cerebellum (Swanson & Castellanos, 2002).

The major area associated with ADHD is the dorsolateral prefrontal cortex (mostly associated with working memory), orbital prefrontal cortex (response inhibition), and anterior cingulate cortex (connection with emotional control and to cognitive control). These areas are highly interconnected both with other cortical regions and with major subcortical structures in a series of neural circuits. Through these circuits, prefrontal structures are involved in emotion regulation, executive functioning (working memory, controlling interference, response inhibition), temporal organization of behavior, motivational responding (identifying potential reward), social judgment, and motor control (Fuster, 1997). Thus, ADHD is also interconnected with these circuits and brain areas. It's also a known fact that developmentally, the prefrontal cortices are among the last areas of the brain to mature fully. They continue to undergo changes in adolescence and even into early adulthood (Benes, 2006).

The most consistent and replicated findings suggest the involvement of the right inferior prefrontal cortex in children with ADHD. Both structure and activity in this region lead to impairment in response inhibition and the ability to organize complex response sequences in children with ADHD (Casey et al., 1999 Rubia et al., 1999).

The other key area relevant to ADHD is the caudate and the putamen. These structures are closely interconnected with prefrontal regions that form bidirectional "loops" of circuitry which work in coordinates to control unwanted response and to monitor whether the current response is matching toward the targeted/expected goal. As part of these circuits, these structures thus help with motor control, with motivation and emotion (e.g., response to reward, possible consequences), and with executive and cognitive functions (including attention and suppression of a motor response). Several studies ' findings also indicate abnormalities of the caudate.

The cerebellum, a differentiated subcortical structure located in the back of the brain is involved in a wide array of timing and temporal information processing abilities, including detecting when expected consequences should occur (Ivry, 1997). The cerebellum may be involved in other cognitive control operations as well, perhaps by detecting and coordinating the timing of their activation (Diamond, 2000). Research findings indicate that the cerebellar vermis is to be smaller in children with ADHD compared to the control group (Swanson & Castellanos, 2002). A consistent finding from several studies suggests that the exact regions involved in ADHD are lobules VIII–X. Castellanos (2001) has revealed that the vermis modulates catecholamine functions. Therefore, these cerebellar regions have a possible role to modulate the operations of the prefrontal subcortical circuits.

EEG STUDIES IN ADHD

QEEG Spectrum analysis shows that Children with ADHD have commonly shown high levels of slow waves (predominantly theta) and low levels of beta activity compared to the normal group (Barry et al., 2003). It is also found that these abnormalities seem to be more evident in children with the combined type of ADHD than the inattentive ADHD (Barry et al., 2003; Chabot & Serfontein, 1996). These findings were replicated in a large-scale multicenter study (Monastra et al., 1999) as well as a meta-analysis conducted by Boutros et al (2005). They concluded that higher levels of theta waves are biomarkers of

ADHD. However, the literature is less consistent regarding the low level of beta in ADHD (Callaway et al., 1983; Dykman et al., 1989).

TOOLS TO ASSESS ADHD

The diagnosis is based on the evaluation of the child's symptoms by the clinician. Rating scales, which can be completed by parents, teachers, and/or patients, are used to evaluate the presence of symptoms as well as the degree of interference in a child's social, psychological, academic, and occupational functioning. Rating scale combined with neuropsychological evaluation and a clinical interview is needed to determine the onset, course, duration, and impairment associated with symptoms. A particular challenge of the clinician is to distinguish ADHD from other conditions that may appear similar (e.g., anxiety, conduct disorders, speech or language delay, other developmental disorders) and to ADHD symptoms or is present as a comorbid diagnosis.

Table 2.

Widely Used Performa & Rating Scales
Interview • Standard Clinical interview • K-SADS (kiddie SADS) • Diagnostic Interview schedule for children (DISC/DISC IV) Rating Scales in ADHD • National Institute for children's Health Quality (NICHQ) • Vanderbilt Assessment Scale • Conners Rating Scales • Swanson, Nolan and Pelham Revision (SNAP-IV) • Disruptive Behavior Disorder Rating Scale (DBDRS) • ADHD Rating Scale (ADHD- RS) • Strengths and Difficulties Questionnaire (SDQ) • Behavior Rating Inventory of Executive Function (BRIEF) • Childhood Executive Functioning Inventory (CHEXI) • Attention and Executive Function Rating Inventory (ATTEX)

Table 3.

Test of Cognitive function in ADHD
Attention
• Continuous Performance Test (Conners CPT)
• Integrated Visual and Auditory Continuous Performance Test (IVA CPT)
• Tests of Variables of Attention (TOVA)
• Letter cancellation test
• Digit vigilance test
• Digit span forward task
• Spatial span forward task
Working memory
• N-back Task
• Digit span backward task
• Spatial span backward task
• Paced Serial addition test (PASAT)
Set Shifting
• Trail Making Test
• Wisconsin Card Sorting Test
Response Inhibition
• Go No Go Task
Planning
• Porteous mazes test
• Tower of London

COMPUTATIONALLY SUPPORTED DIAGNOSIS AND ASSESSMENT

As we already discussed, the diagnosis is relying on series of behavioral observations and reports (parents & teachers) combined with neuropsychological assessments and self-report. Technological tools have been developed to obtain diagnostic information that is useful to clinicians. Computerized assessment owes unique advantages, particularly beneficial for cognitive testing due to the potential for greater recording accuracy and precision of timed tasks, easy scoring, and standardized administration without biases. There is n number of assessments that are widely used to test cognitive function. One of the frequently used technological tools to assess attention is Conner's Continuous Performance Test (CPT-3) and Test of Variables of Attention (TOVA). This task-oriented test is used to assess sustained attention.

There are many approaches that have been explored to develop non-biased computerized diagnostic tests for ADHD. However, there are too many limitations for these tests to advocate as diagnostic tools. Some of the computational diagnostic and assessment approaches are:

1. Computer and smartphone-based assessments
2. Virtual and augmented reality to assess cognitive function
3. Diagnostic and assessment games
4. Visual observational methods
5. Multimodal and Physical Interfaces
6. Biofeedback -Wearable and physiological sensors

These approaches are the need of the hour and are attempts to make diagnosis and assessment easier, more measurable, and more reliable through technological means. Computerized tests are promising, interactive, and applicable in the everyday lives of children and adults with ADHD. These tests can be used to evaluate, monitor, and as an intervention for children and adults with ADHD.

MANAGEMENT OF ADHD

The treatment of ADHD consists of pharmacological, psychosocial intervention, cognitive retraining. In this chapter, we discuss the technology-based intervention in ADHD.

ADHD can cause significant impairment in multiple domains considering the chronic course of ADHD, intervening early in the trajectory of illness during childhood may lessen the extent of negative impact during adulthood. Interventions in children with ADHD were largely based on medication management. However, studies report that a substantial number of children do not respond to, or cannot tolerate, medications and suffered from their adverse side effects and that there is a lack of clear positive long-term effects. This suggests that there is a strong need for alternative treatment modalities for ADHD.

Pharmacological intervention is the first-line evidence-based treatment for ADHD. However, studies also report that children do not respond to or cannot tolerate medications and suffered from adverse side effects. Psychotherapeutic interventions are also widely used and evidence-based treatment for ADHD. Another widely used evidence-based treatment is cognitive retraining

COGNITIVE RETRAINING

Cognitive Training or Retraining has been defined as an intervention aimed at providing guided practice on a set of standardized tasks which are designed to target specific cognitive function(s) such as attention, executive functions, and memory (Gates & Valenzuela, 2011). The underlying assumption is that cognitive functioning in a specific domain can be improved by practice and that effects of practice have the potential to get generalized beyond the context of training (Buschert et al., 2010). The strategies used in cognitive retraining include restorative strategies and internal compensatory strategies.

Cognitive Rehabilitation has been broadly defined as the use of any strategy or technique which intends to facilitate patients and their families, to manage or sidestep patient's cognitive deficits (Buschert et al., 2010). It involves the identification of needs and goals which are personally relevant to the client and strategies are devised to address these goals. The prominence is given to developing ways for compensating for cognitive impairments and thereby improving the daily functioning of the patient (Clare & Woods, 2003). Cognitive rehabilitation relies greatly on internal compensatory strategies as well as external aids (Buschert et al., 2010).

EEG NEUROFEEDBACK TRAINING IN ADHD

Electroencephalogram (EEG) neurofeedback training is an advanced technology-based rehabilitation. Neurofeedback is a method that helps subjects to self-regulate their brain waves. During the neurofeedback treatment Electroencephalography (EEG) is recorded. Then, its several components are extracted and real-time feedback in the form of audio, video or their combination will be provided to the subject during the Neurofeedback. This procedure provides insight to the subject regarding the changes that occur during the training and will help to assess his/her performance based on the feedback. There are several protocols that are widely used in treatment for multiple conditions. Neurofeedback treatment protocols target the pattern of brain waves such as alpha, beta, delta, theta, and gamma or a combination of those brain waves such as alpha-theta (Dempster, 2012; Vernon, 2005).

Delta (1–4 or 1–3.5 Hz) activity is seen predominantly in infants and it is associated with sleep. Its also commonly seen during problem-solving in the awake EEG. Research findings suggest abnormal activation of delta and theta bands in children with attention deficit hyperactivity disorder (ADHD). Down training the delta band with the theta band may be helpful in these conditions. Theta (4–7, 4–7.5, or 4–8 Hz) is known to be related to creativity and spontaneity. Otherwise, it is also associated with distractibility and other deficits of attention, daydreaming, depression, and anxiety. Alpha waves (associated with meditation and a state of relaxation) are commonly seen in the occipital, parietal, and posterior temporal lobes regions of the brain. Alpha amplitudes are normally higher in posterior regions and lower in anterior regions of the brain. Beta (13–21 Hz), increased beta activity in the left frontal cortex is a marker for depression, and decreased activity in the right frontal cortex is a marker for anxiety. Sensorimotor rhythm (12–15 or 12–16 Hz) sometimes referred to as low beta, is primarily found in the sensorimotor cortex. Barry Sterman and his colleagues are pioneers in SMR training. Uptraining of SMR at Cz or C4 sites is a well-established protocol in treatment for ADHD children.

In 1976, Lubar and Shouse were the first to publish on the use of neurofeedback interventions in children with ADHD. During the initial phase, they have used sensory motor rhythm training (SMR) training to help children with ADHD. In their initial study, they tested the idea that neurofeedback training (Sensorimotor Rhythm training [SMR] frequency of 12–14 Hz), over the sensorimotor strip of the brain, could be used to help children with hyperkinesis. During the neurofeedback training, the child was rewarded whenever the child inhibits theta activity (4–7 Hz) and produce SMR activity. It was found that the child up-regulated the SMR by threefold the amount of the initial recording along with fewer behavioural issues in the classroom. These studies were again replicated in hyperkinetic children. An experimental ABA design study design was conducted with the addition of the gradual withdrawal of Ritalin (Lubar & Shouse, 1976). Children were able to regulate their SMR by two times the amount of the initial recording along with fewer behavioural problems. These two initial studies pay the way to multiple studies which investigated neurofeedback as a treatment for ADHD.

Randomized controlled trials on neurofeedback in ADHD were published by Gevensleben showed that the neurofeedback trained group but not the control group showed reduced EEG theta power (Gevensleben, Holl, Albrecht, Vogel, et al., 2009), thereby establishing the specificity of this intervention. Another recently published meta-analysis on neurofeedback in ADHD by Arns et al. (2012) concluded that neurofeedback had large effect sizes on the domains of impulsivity and inattention and medium effect size on hyperactivity. Neurofeedback efficacy is level 5 (efficacious and specific).

CONCLUSION

There is no doubt that ADHD has a significant impact on the individual. ADHD is not only affecting the psychological, social, academic, and occupational life of the person but it also affects the family members too. There are many management programs available for ADHD children such as pharmacological, psychosocial management and cognitive retraining that are efficacious. Research findings also suggest that computerized cognitive retraining can often improve performance in cognitive functions such as attention, working memory, and other executive functions. However, there is a scarcity of evidence-based computer-based interventions that can help people with ADHD. Clinician monitored computerized assessment, follow up and intervention is the need of the hour for the long-term management of ADHD. Developers, researchers, and clinicians should work together to develop computerized cognitive programs to enhance the well-being of the patient. Treatment such as neurofeedback is one of the well-established examples of how computerized intervention can help in these specific conditions. Thus, the future direction should target how technology can be designed in a way that helps clinicians to readily and consistently deliver evidence-based services that are generalizable in client's real life and thereby improve the quality of life.

REFERENCES

American Psychiatric Association. (1980). Diagnostic and statistical manual of mental disorders (Vol. 3). Washington, DC: American Psychiatric Association.

American Psychiatric Association & American Psychiatric Association. (2013). *Diagnostic and statistical manual of mental disorders: DSM-5*. Author.

Arns, M. (2012). EEG-based personalized medicine in ADHD: Individual alpha peak frequency as an endophenotype associated with nonresponse. *Journal of Neurotherapy, 16*(2), 123–141. doi:10.1080/10874208.2012.677664

Bader, M., Tannock, R., & Hadjikhani, N. (2018). The Zappel-Philipp a historical example of ADHD Clinics. *Attention Deficit and Hyperactivity Disorders, 10*(2), 119–127. doi:10.100712402-017-0239-4 PMID:28905267

Barkley, R. A. (1997). *ADHD and the nature of self-control*. Guilford press.

Barkley, R. A. (1997). Behavioral inhibition, sustained attention, and executive functions: Constructing a unifying theory of ADHD. *Psychological Bulletin, 121*(1), 65–94. doi:10.1037/0033-2909.121.1.65 PMID:9000892

Barkley, R. A. (2001). The executive functions and self-regulation: An evolutionary neuropsychological perspective. *Neuropsychology Review, 11*(1), 1–29. doi:10.1023/A:1009085417776 PMID:11392560

Barkley, R. A., & Edwards, G. H. (2006). *Attention-deficit*. Academic Press.

Barry, R. J., Clarke, A. R., & Johnstone, S. J. (2003). A review of electrophysiology in attention-deficit/hyperactivity disorder: I. Qualitative and quantitative electroencephalography. *Clinical Neurophysiology, 114*(2), 171–183. doi:10.1016/S1388-2457(02)00362-0 PMID:12559224

Benes, F. M. (2006). *The development of the prefrontal cortex: The maturation of neurotransmitter systems and their interactions*. Academic Press.

Boutros, N., Fraenkel, L., & Feingold, A. (2005). A four-step approach for developing diagnostic tests in psychiatry: EEG in ADHD as a test case. *The Journal of Neuropsychiatry and Clinical Neurosciences, 17*(4), 455–464. doi:10.1176/jnp.17.4.455 PMID:16387983

Burks, H. F. (1960). The hyperkinetic child. *Exceptional Children*, *27*(1), 18–26. doi:10.1177/001440296002700105

Buschert, V., Bokde, A. L., & Hampel, H. (2010). Cognitive intervention in Alzheimer disease. *Nature Reviews. Neurology*, *6*(9), 508–517. doi:10.1038/nrneurol.2010.113 PMID:20717104

Callaway, E., Halliday, R., & Naylor, H. (1983). Hyperactive children's event-related potentials fail to support underarousal and maturational-lag theories. *Archives of General Psychiatry*, *40*(11), 1243–1248. doi:10.1001/archpsyc.1983.01790100089012 PMID:6639294

Casey, B. J., Castellanos, F. X., Giedd, J. N., Marsh, W. L., Hamburger, S. D., Schubert, A. B., Vauss, Y. C., Vaituzis, A. C., Dickstein, D. P., Sarfatti, S., & Rapoport, J. L. (1997). Implication of right frontostriatal circuitry in response inhibition and attention-deficit/hyperactivity disorder. *Journal of the American Academy of Child and Adolescent Psychiatry*, *36*(3), 374–383. doi:10.1097/00004583-199703000-00016 PMID:9055518

Castellanos, F. X. (2001). Neuroimaging studies of ADHD. *Stimulant drugs and ADHD, Basic and Clinical Neuroscience*, 243–258.

Chabot, R. J., & Serfontein, G. (1996). Quantitative electroencephalographic profiles of children with attention deficit disorder. *Biological Psychiatry*, *40*(10), 951–963. doi:10.1016/0006-3223(95)00576-5 PMID:8915554

Chess, S. (1960). Diagnosis and treatment of the hyperactive child. *New York State Journal of Medicine*, *60*, 2379–2385. PMID:13809736

Crichton, A. (1798). *An inquiry into the nature and origin of mental derangement: comprehending a concise system of the physiology and pathology of the human mind. and a history of the passions and their effects* (Vol. 2). Academic Press.

Dempster, T. (2012). *An investigation into the optimum training paradigm for alpha electroencephalographic biofeedback*. Canterbury Christ Church University.

Diamond, A. (2000). Close interrelation of motor development and cognitive development and of the cerebellum and prefrontal cortex. *Child Development*, *71*(1), 44–56. doi:10.1111/1467-8624.00117 PMID:10836557

Douglas, V. I. (1983). Attention and cognitive problems. *Developmental Neuropsychiatry*, 280-329.

Douglas, V. I. (1999). Cognitive control processes in attention deficit/hyperactivity disorder. In *Handbook of disruptive behavior disorders* (pp. 105–138). Springer. doi:10.1007/978-1-4615-4881-2_5

Douglas, V. I., & Parry, P. A. (1983). Effects of reward on delayed reaction time task performance of hyperactive children. *Journal of Abnormal Child Psychology*, *11*(2), 313–326. doi:10.1007/BF00912094 PMID:6619440

Dykman, R. A., Holcomb, P. J., Oglesby, D. M., & Ackerman, P. T. (1982). Electrocortical frequencies in hyperactive, learning-disabled, mixed, and normal children. *Biological Psychiatry*. PMID:7104419

Ebaugh, F. G. (1923). Neuropsychiatric sequelae of acute epidemic encephalitis in children. *American Journal of Diseases of Children*, *25*(2), 89–97.

Fuster, J. M. (1997). Network memory. *Trends in Neurosciences*, *20*(10), 451–459. doi:10.1016/S0166-2236(97)01128-4 PMID:9347612

Gates, N. J., Valenzuela, M., Sachdev, P. S., Singh, N. A., Baune, B. T., Brodaty, H., ... Singh, M. A. F. (2011). Study of Mental Activity and Regular Training (SMART) in at risk individuals: A randomised double blind, sham controlled, longitudinal trial. *BMC Geriatrics*, *11*(1), 1–15. doi:10.1186/1471-2318-11-19 PMID:21510896

Gevensleben, H., Holl, B., Albrecht, B., Vogel, C., Schlamp, D., Kratz, O., Studer, P., Rothenberger, A., Moll, G. H., & Heinrich, H. (2009). Is neurofeedback an efficacious treatment for ADHD? A randomised controlled clinical trial. *Journal of Child Psychology and Psychiatry, and Allied Disciplines*, *50*(7), 780–789. doi:10.1111/j.1469-7610.2008.02033.x PMID:19207632

Ivry, R. (1997). Cerebellar timing systems. *International Review of Neurobiology*, *41*, 555–573. doi:10.1016/S0074-7742(08)60370-0 PMID:9378608

Knobel, M., Wolman, M. B., & Mason, E. (1959). Hyperkinesis and organicity in children. *A.M.A. Archives of General Psychiatry*, *1*(3), 310–321. doi:10.1001/archpsyc.1959.03590030094011 PMID:14410146

Laufer, M. W., Denhoff, E., & Solomons, G. (2011). Hyperkinetic impulse disorder in children's behavior problems. *Journal of Attention Disorders*, *15*(8), 620–625. doi:10.1177/1087054711413043 PMID:22131306

Lubar, J. F., & Shouse, M. N. (1976). EEG and behavioral changes in a hyperkinetic child concurrent with training of the sensorimotor rhythm (SMR). *Biofeedback and Self-Regulation*, *1*(3), 293–306. doi:10.1007/BF01001170 PMID:990355

Marzbani, H., Marateb, H. R., & Mansourian, M. (2016). Neurofeedback: A comprehensive review on system design, methodology and clinical applications. *Basic and Clinical Neuroscience*, *7*(2), 143. doi:10.15412/J.BCN.03070208 PMID:27303609

Monastra, V. J., Lubar, J. F., Linden, M., VanDeusen, P., Green, G., Wing, W., Phillips, A., & Fenger, T. N. (1999). Assessing attention deficit hyperactivity disorder via quantitative electroencephalography: An initial validation study. *Neuropsychology*, *13*(3), 424–433. doi:10.1037/0894-4105.13.3.424 PMID:10447303

Nigg, J. T., & Casey, B. J. (2005). An integrative theory of attention-deficit/hyperactivity disorder based on the cognitive and affective neurosciences. *Development and Psychopathology*, *17*(3), 785–806. doi:10.1017/S0954579405050376 PMID:16262992

Palaniappan, P., Seshadri, S., Girimaji, S. C., & Srinath, S. (2013). Pattern of comorbidities in Indian children and adolescents with attention deficit hyperactivity disorder. *European Psychiatry*, *28*, 1. doi:10.1016/S0924-9338(13)77398-X

Pingali, S. (2014). Sunderajan J. A study of comorbidities in attention deficit hyperactivity disorder: A retrospective analysis of case records. *AP J Psychol Med*, *15*(2), 206–210.

Quay, H. C. (1997). Inhibition and attention deficit hyperactivity disorder. *Journal of Abnormal Child Psychology*, *25*(1), 7–13. doi:10.1023/A:1025799122529 PMID:9093895

Rubia, K., Overmeyer, S., Taylor, E., Brammer, M., Williams, S. C., Simmons, A., & Bullmore, E. T. (1999). Hypofrontality in attention deficit hyperactivity disorder during higher-order motor control: A study with functional MRI. *The American Journal of Psychiatry*, *156*(6), 891–896. doi:10.1176/ajp.156.6.891 PMID:10360128

Sprich, S., Biederman, J., Crawford, M. H., Mundy, E., & Faraone, S. V. (2000). Adoptive and biological families of children and adolescents with ADHD. *Journal of the American Academy of Child and Adolescent Psychiatry*, *39*(11), 1432–1437. doi:10.1097/00004583-200011000-00018 PMID:11068899

Stryker, S. (1925). Encephalitis lethargica: The behavior residuals. *The Training School Bulletin*, *22*, 152–157.

Swanson, J. M., & Castellanos, F. X. (2002). *Biological bases of ADHD--Neuroanatomy, genetics, and pathophysiology*. Academic Press.

Thome, J., & Jacobs, K. A. (2004). Attention deficit hyperactivity disorder (ADHD) in a 19th century children's book. *European Psychiatry*, *19*(5), 303–306. doi:10.1016/j.eurpsy.2004.05.004 PMID:15276664

Vernon, D. J. (2005). Can neurofeedback training enhance performance? An evaluation of the evidence with implications for future research. *Applied Psychophysiology and Biofeedback*, *30*(4), 347–364. doi:10.100710484-005-8421-4 PMID:16385423

Chapter 9
Artificial Intelligence in the Detection of Alzheimer's Disease

Mohammad Gouse Galety
https://orcid.org/0000-0003-1666-2001
Catholic University in Erbil, Iraq

Shweta Gupta
Jain University, India

ABSTRACT

Dementia is a neurological illness that causes diversion from a variety of important cognitive activities. Common examples include memory, reasoning, orientation, understanding, computation, verbal communication, and decision making. Alzheimer's disease (AD) is one of the most common dementias affecting the elderly. It was projected that more than 47 million people globally will be affected by dementia in 2015; these predictions were verified, and forecasts for 2050 are much more concerning, with 131 million people living with dementia. The basic objective of AI is to improve human decision-making and automate operations that are too time-consuming or resource-intensive for people to accomplish. AI can operate as a fast, accurate, and in the long run, cost-effective method to assist human experience and intuition through predictive analytics. AI is an effective technique for AD detection as these methods are employed as a computer-aided diagnosis (CAD) system in clinical practices and play a crucial role in identifying variations in the brain images to detect AD.

INTRODUCTION

Memory suffers from poor function at times because of distraction, information overload, or mild melancholy. Unless anything goes wrong, we maintain a vast store of general knowledge, the capacity to organise and control our affairs, and our orientation in time and location. Attention, memory, executive cognitive function, language, and visuospatial ability are examples of the distinct cognitive domains that

DOI: 10.4018/978-1-7998-9534-3.ch009

define cognitive talents. The brain's ability to retain and retrieve memories across decades is one of its many notable abilities. Forgetting happens just as regularly as learning in our daily lives. The amnesia condition occurs after a severe traumatic brain injury or illness, with brain damage having severe memory problems and the inability to learn.

Dementia has its roots in Latin *de* and *men's* (translated, respectively, as *out of* and *mind*). Ageing brings a lot of ills, and dementia tops the list of greatest fears. We have yet to decipher the complexities of the brain. Major Neurocognitive Disorder is a new term for dementia.

Dementia is a degenerative condition in which the patient's mental capacity consistently deteriorates progressively or chronically and worsens with time. It is a challenging condition that impairs many functions, including memory, concentration, understanding, computation, learning ability, language, and judgment. Being aware, or being conscious, is not altered. Because of emotional Control, social behaviour, and decreased motivation, most people who have a cognitive disability also experience behavioural problems.

Dementia happens when the brain is affected by Alzheimer's disease or stroke and other diseases and traumas. Of all dementia cases, 70% are linked to Alzheimer's. Being diagnosed with a mental illness is difficult for the patient and on the patient's family members and friends.

A degenerative brain illness was seen in humans; Alzheimer's disease (AD) is the most prevalent cause of dementia and has several possible triggers that might result in dementia. A person's capacity to do everyday tasks can be hindered by memory, language, and other cognitive skills. Cognitive capabilities can be compromised by decreased memory, speech, and different cognitive abilities. In general, the five A's of Alzheimer's disease are amnesia, aphasia, apraxia, agnosia and abnormal executive function. It's because nerve cells (neurons) in the brain's cognitive-function areas have been destroyed and are no longer operating as they should.

In 2015, the Alzheimer's Association study (Association, 2015) found that 5.3 million Americans had Alzheimer's. Even though almost 5.1 million people over 65 have Alzheimer's, about 200,000 people under 65 also have the condition. As people age, the rate of AD goes up dramatically. More than 40% of the elderly have AD by the time they reach 85 years of age, but the disease affects fewer than 5% of the general population when they become 65. The 2014 Alzheimer's Disease International Report (Alz.co.uk) gives the estimated number of individuals in the Asia Pacific regions who have dementia. For instance, it is projected that there will be 40.3 million people in India in 2015, but by 2030, that number will be much higher, at 67.4 million. Those with dementia in the Asia Pacific area are expected to swell from 13.7 million in 2005 to 64.6 million by 2050 (PACIFIC, 2006) In approximately 50 - 60 years, the US population has grown by 34 million, and life expectancy has increased by nine years. Over 6 million Americans now have Alzheimer's disease, and without early diagnosis or a cure, this figure might rise to nearly 14 million by 2050.

BACKGROUND

The aberrant accumulation of proteins within and around brain cells is suspected to be the origin of Alzheimer's disease. A protein known as amyloid, which forms plaques around brain cells, is significant. Brain cells are tangled with the presence of a protein called tau. Scientists have discovered that this process begins years before symptoms ever arise. However, they do not know the specific mechanism that triggers it. Neurons become weakened, causing chemical messengers neurotransmitters, which are used to carry messages between brain cells, to drop as well. People with Alzheimer's disease have notably reduced levels of acetylcholine, a neurotransmitter, in their brains. The brain atrophies, shrinking with time. The first afflicted regions are generally associated with memories.

Generally, three major phases of the disease are classified, including early-stage (lasting 2–3 years), middle, and terminal stage, where the patient becomes bedridden and incontinent in addition to suffering a multitude of other ailments. The early stages are frequently ignored. Patients at the beginning of dementia, some of whom exhibit symptoms including memory loss that particularly affects events that just transpired, have trouble speaking because they struggle to find the right words and are confused even in familiar environments. As the illness advances, the restrictions become more obvious and more restrictive. People lose track of time, date, location, and events; become disoriented at home and in the community; struggle with communication (speech and understanding), and require assistance with personal care. Finally, the last stage is characterised by near-complete reliance and immobility. The disease's effect on memory is critical, and the disease's impact on physical health are now plainly visible. People sometimes cannot perceive time and location, comprehend what is happening around them, recognise family members or familiar items.

To have quality dementia care, it is important to make a correct and accurate diagnosis. The large number of persons with dementia who go without diagnosis is quite concerning. People generally find out they have received a diagnosis when too late to make important life decisions or get support. Knowing about a disease as early as possible might help a person be treated so that their cognition and mental symptoms can be mitigated or prevented to avoid setbacks. According to the Alzheimer's World Report, the following are the advantages of early diagnosis: Increasing the efficiency of existing medical management, achieving more decisional autonomy, enhancing patient access to treatments, risk reduction, preparing for the future, improving clinical outcomes, avoiding or lowering future expenditures are all important goals. Diagnosis is a fundamental human right.

Alzheimer's disease begins with an asymptomatic stage and only later show obvious symptoms. Biomarkers can assist identify high-risk persons who have chronic illnesses so that these people can receive treatment as soon as feasible. There are several kinds of biomarkers, including imaging biomarkers (such as CT, MRI, and PET) and molecular biomarkers, divided into three subtypes: volatile biomarkers, such as breath; bodily fluid biomarkers, such as CSF; and biopsy biomarkers.

Artificial intelligence (AI) in healthcare and medicine is simply the application of machine learning algorithms to provide favourable patient outcomes through effective data utilisation. Artificial intelligence's primary goal is to help humans make better decisions and do things that individuals cannot do quickly or need an excessive amount of resources. This goal is accomplished by implementing several processes such as data collection, analysis, and utilisation to answer important challenges with an objective, data-driven approach. An AI may work well for predictive analytics in helping humans learn to work with intuition and experience via serving as a rapid, accurate, and in the long run, cost-effective tool. Using artificial intelligence, CAD systems may collaborate with neuroradiologists, speeding up the diagnosis of patients while still helping the doctor perform their duties. The CAD system delivers a neuropsychological evaluation to reduce the consequences of AD, an enormous public health concern. This assessment, which occurs early on, helps detect the illness.

IMAGING BIOMARKERS

During the previous decade, many breakthroughs have been achieved in identifying AD biomarkers utilising neuroimaging. The Food and Drug Administration (FDA) considers an ideal biomarker specific, sensitive, predictive, robust, simple, accurate, and affordable. An AD biomarker with more than 80% sensitivity and specificity is regarded as In detecting Alzheimer's disease (AD) and other types of dementia, the ability to identify and validate biomarkers is becoming critical.

The techniques under consideration are particularly well-suited to examining both structural, functional, and white matter changes that may occur in the brain (Márquez & Yassa, 2019). These methods are highly diverse in their capability to identify and understand disease mechanisms, such as structure decay, like a decrease in volume, cortical thinning, and functional decay, such as the emergence of hyperactive regions via fMRI, changes in network connectivity, white matter decay, such as a reduction in diffusion anisotropy, white matter pathology, and pathology aggregation, such as amyloid and tau PET.

STRUCTURAL IMAGING

Structural magnetic resonance imaging (MRI), the most often used sequence being T1-weighted, provides excellent contrast between grey and white matter, making it one of the easiest, cheapest, and most extensively used methods for diagnosing AD (Kehoe, McNulty, Mullins, & Bokde, 2014).

Figure 1. MRI images [Magnetic resonance imaging - Wikipedia]

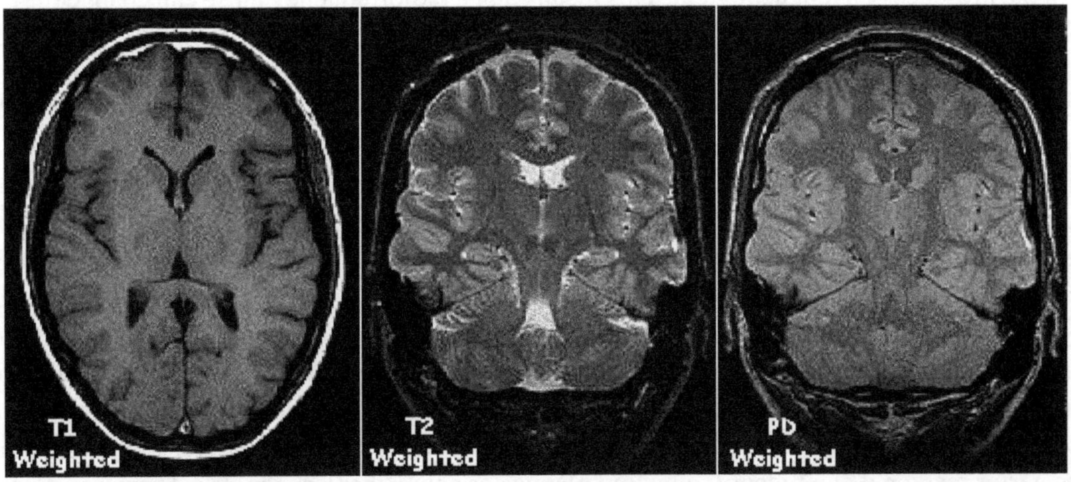

Figure 2. fMRI image [Functional magnetic resonance imaging - Wikipedia]

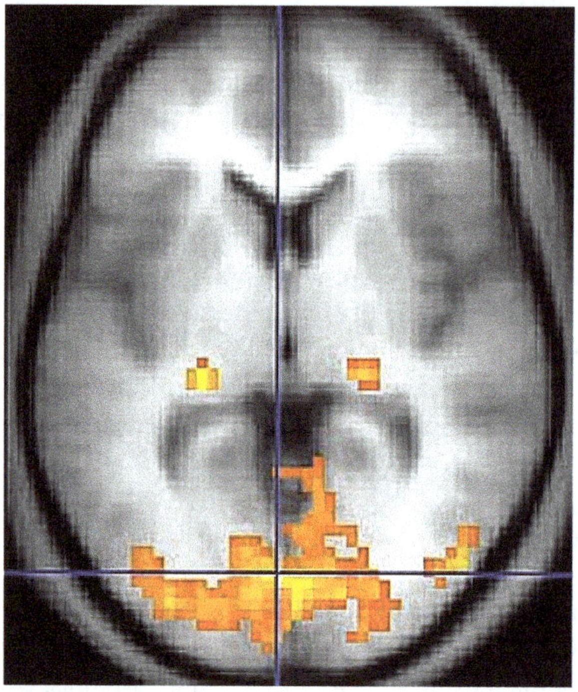

The imaging process employs the fact that protons have inherent angular momentum and their polarisation in the presence of a magnetic field. This means that a radiofrequency pulse can change the energy state of protons and, after the pulse stops, the protons will release a radiofrequency signal after reverting to their previous energy level. A technique is known as sequences, which uses a mix of various gradients and pulses to create something responsive to tissue features. On the whole, structural MRI in AD may be split between finding quantities of atrophy (or shrinkage) and examining how tissue features, such as white matter hyperintensity on T2-weighted MRI, originate from vascular injury. The MRI image of the brain is as shown in Figure 1.

An MRI's clear advantage is its availability. European and American recommendations, respectively, advocate structural imaging (MRI or CT) on patients with cognitive loss, and it is a requirement of proposed AD diagnostic criteria and similar dementia standards. MRI is harmless and doesn't include ionising radiation, so patients may be scanned repeatedly without worrying about getting cancer. In one examination, MRIs can yield several distinct tissue-image types that provide different kinds of information for diagnosis and study. MRI's lack of molecular specificity affects structural imaging. Although it's a posterior marker, it can't identify amyloid plaques or neurofibrillary tangles. Therefore it's farther back than the molecular pathology (Johnson, Fox, Sperling, & Klunk, 2012).

FUNCTIONAL IMAGING

By detecting the movement of blood flow, the results of a functional magnetic resonance imaging scan can reveal which region of the brain is active (or functioning) in response to the patient doing a certain activity. Magnetic resonance is present in all atoms and molecules and may be detected as the presence of radio waves. The protons are caused by these structures (Wright, 2010).

Functional magnetic resonance imaging (fMRI) is becoming increasingly popular for investigating the functional integrity of brain networks supporting memory and other cognitive domains in ageing and early Alzheimer's disease. Neuronal activity may be measured indirectly using functional magnetic resonance imaging (fMRI), which measures variations in the blood oxygen level-dependent (BOLD) MR signal. fMRI image of the brain is as shown in Figure 2.

Longitudinal fMRI investigations in individuals with progressive dementias provide several difficulties. Because these methods are sensitive to head motion, fMRI is likely to be difficult to evaluate individuals with more severe cognitive impairment. One of the main benefits of task fMRI activation investigations is lost if the patients cannot properly execute the cognitive task.

POSITRON EMISSION TOMOGRAPHY

Figure 3. PET

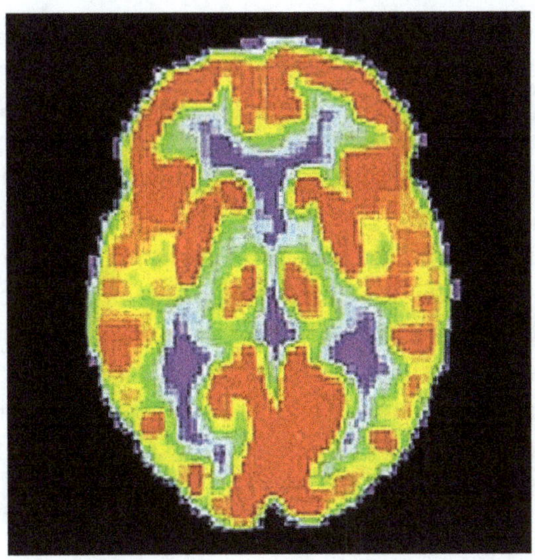

A further measure of neurological damage is through F-fluorodeoxyglucose-positron emission tomography (FDG-PET) imaging (Biscetti, et al., 2019). It indicates cerebral activity by monitoring the brain's glucose metabolic rate, often compromised before structural anatomic brain abnormalities become visible. Additionally, it notes vascular issues and blood-brain barrier problems, which AD patients frequently have. PET scan image is as shown in Figure 3.

Functional activities in the brain may be seen in a full 3D image with positron emission tomography scanning. PET is a nuclear medicine imaging method that uses a radioactive tracer (FDG) in sugar. The tracer is administered into the circulation through a tiny injection. Radioactive materials produce gamma-rays, a kind of high-energy electromagnetic radiation. Radioactive substance gets delivered to the brain via the body. Aing of detectors outside the skull detects pairs of Gamma rays produced by the positron-emitting radionuclide (tracer) (Young, et al., 1999).

FDG PET, like all PET techniques, is expensive and limited in availability. It is complex, requiring intravenous access and exposure to low levels of radioactivity, even though that is far below any harmful levels (Ou, et al., 2019). Brain FDG retention is a nonspecific metabolic biomarker that can be disrupted by ischemia or inflammation and may be irrelevant or only indirectly associated with AD in certain people.

DETECTING AMYLOID IN VIVO USING PET

Because early detection of amyloid disease in the brain is essential in AD research, PET scans using Aβ -specific radiolabeled tracers are becoming more prevalent. PET scans use the notion that positron-emitting radioligands cluster in a particular location. In the event of electron-positron annihilation, gamma photons are released and received by scintillation detectors (Evans, et al., 2018). By radiolabeled tracers that are administered through an injection followed by a delay to allow for absorption by brain tissue, it is possible to visualise Aβ.

The in-vivo imaging of amyloid is a unique use of PET imaging. One of the pathological indicators of AD is the presence of neurotic plaques, which are composed of the protein amyloid β (Frisoni, et al., 2013). A few amyloid-imaging tracers have been released in the last few years after years of preclinical work.

Two major reasons why many people don't use amyloid PET scanning are its expense and limited availability. Initially, amyloid burden imaging was investigated using carbon-based tracers [11C] such as Pittsburgh Compound B (PiB). However, the introduction of fluorine-based tracers [18F] has allowed greater availability of these longer-lasting tracers, allowing for more general usage. The introduction of F-18-labeled drugs which can be used in PET scanners outside of cyclotrons has increased availability. Even while Aβ42 quantification offers equivalent information to determine the presence or absence of amyloid plaque, the cost of this method is a problem because it provides only redundant information. Amyloid PET is not a useful predictive induction measure during the clinical stage for detecting AD. Images for amyloid provide a considerably clearer two-state diagnostic output than MRI and FDG PET methods.

SINGLE-PHOTON EMISSION TOMOGRAPHY

Figure 4. SPECT image of brain (Sin, Kim, Park, Joo, & Kim, 2018)

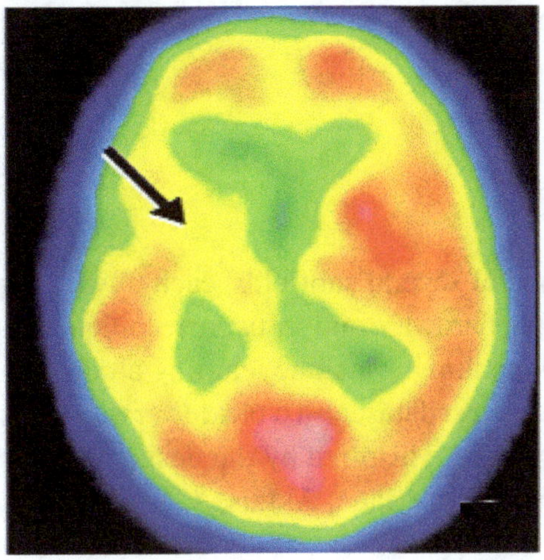

Single-photon emission tomography (SPECT) captures gamma-ray signals using two or more synchronised gamma cameras, and the numerous 2-D images are processed, tomographically rebuilt, to 3-D. SPECT image is as shown in Figure 4. One portion may be viewed from many perspectives but is blurry compared to a PET image. SPECT scanner is more affordable than a PET scanner, and it employs long-lived isotopes that are relatively commonly found. Identification of the regions of metabolism inside the brain is possible by tracing blood flow, which provides information on brain activities (Frankle, Slifstein, Talbot, & Laruelle, 2005). A false-positive result and a lack of additional value relative to MRI have slowed the use of SPECT in clinical practice.

DIFFUSION TENSOR IMAGING (DTI)

Diffusion tensor imaging is an MRI procedure used to examine brain activities as they take place (in vivo). Measurement is taken of how water spreads out in the brain tissue being studied. It is very useful for imaging white matter. For each pixel, a tensor, describing the diffusion anisotropy, is derived using MRI's magnetic field changes, which may be applied in up to six distinct directions (Lazar, et al., 2003).

FLUID BIOMARKERS

Some research teams have identified the following biomarkers, although they haven't proven accurate: AD biomarkers found in biofluids such as Cerebrospinal fluid (CSF) biomarkers. Patients with AD exhibited higher neurofilament light concentrations (NFL) than healthy controls. This finding is also present in other neurodegenerative diseases, thus preventing the diagnostic accuracy of the marker from being accurate enough to add as a specific biomarker for AD (Zetterberg, et al., 2016) β amyloid (1–42)

[Aβ (1–42)] is one of three biomarkers. It is well-established and globally proven to diagnose AD in CSF. Furthermore, the subjects in the test were shown to have total tau and phospho-tau-181.

In clinical studies, unlike with amyloid imaging, CSF measurement of amyloid or tau pathology has not yet been approved as a diagnostic tool. Despite strong results in classifying AD patients from healthy individuals based on CSF biomarkers, these markers couldn't correctly identify the dementia type (AD vs other types) (Simonsen, et al., 2017).

ARTIFICIAL INTELLIGENCE

AI is extensive research comprised of several subfields, each of which tackles the entire job differently, with the ultimate goal of developing hardware and software techniques capable of performing cognitively difficult tasks, including decision making. Machine learning algorithms are trained to execute specific functions by learning patterns from vast datasets. To tackle very complicated issues, the artificial neural networks employed by deep learning are inspired by the design of the human brain and often combine with huge amounts of data (Erickson, Korfiatis, Akkus, & Kline, 2017) (McCollough & Leng, 2020).

MRI TECHNOLOGY-BASED CAD SYSTEMS FOR BRAIN DISORDERS

Figure 5. Basic principle of computer-aided detection system

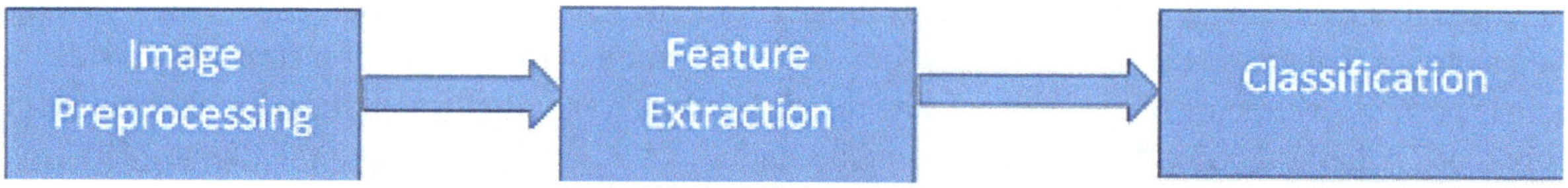

Figure 5 shows the many procedures carried out in a CAD system related to a brain image. The first step in the method is for the CAD programme to use MRI images as a source for its training data by determining which samples to use based on the image. Then comes preprocessing and defining the region of interest (ROI). Then the voxel's distinctive features are extracted. Finally, the last step is to segment and classify. Segmentation will organise the voxels into different areas by following the image properties. The classification permits the images to be classified as normal or abnormal.

FEATURES DERIVED FROM STRUCTURAL MAGNETIC RESONANCE IMAGING (MRI)

Patients with Alzheimer's disease have substantial brain shrinkage as the disease develops. Different parts of the brain have various roles: the grey matter is crucial for thinking, white matter organises communication between brain areas, and the hippocampus is critical for creating new memories.

When AD affects brain regions, MRI brain imaging might show variations in the size of these brain regions. The hippocampus's size, cortical thickness, and the likelihood of distinct tissues, namely grey matter (GM), white matter (WM), and cerebrospinal fluid (CSF), being present in a particular voxel, where voxel represents a single value in a three-dimensional grid, are retrieved from structural MRI. These characteristics can be used to distinguish people with Alzheimer's disease who have progressed to the advanced stage.

The Features Derived from PET and Functional MRI Scans

Some areas of the brain of AD patients have less activity in their brain cells. Patients' brain cell activity is examined using PET and fMRI imaging. Compared to inactive neurons, blood puts out more oxygen to the active neurons in the brain. This variation in the blood oxygen levels manifests as a shift in several locations. Functional MRI scanners can detect the differences in magnetic characteristics between oxygenated and deoxygenated blood. During a brain test, magnetic changes in blood can be utilised to determine active brain regions. Resting-state fMRI (rs-fMRI or R-fMRI) is now being used to assess brain activity in patients at rest. It employs BOLD, a measure of changes in blood flow from fMRI imaging, to assess functional connectivity between active brain areas. If the activity of two brain areas exhibits a high degree of correlation in their time series, they are functionally linked.

The Cerebral Metabolic Rate for glucose (CMRgl) is the term used to describe the rate of glucose metabolism in the brain. The cortical areas of AD patients have lower CMRgl than non-AD individuals. Fluorodeoxyglucose Positron Emission Tomography (FDG-PET) measures CMRgl by injecting fluorodeoxyglucose (FDG-glucose with positron-emitting radioactive isotope Florine-18). The absorption of FDG by tissues implies glucose intake, which is seen using a PET scanner.

Tau proteins are abundant in neurons. Microtubules are tube-like components of cells that maintain cell shape and transfer nutrients. Tau proteins connect and stabilise microtubules. AD patients' brains have tau proteins that cannot link to microtubules, rendering them destabilised. The microtubules begin to deteriorate, leading to cell shape degradation and nutrition distribution problems. Eventually, the cell will perish. Unbound tau proteins cluster together to form neurofibrillary tangles (NFT) (Lee, et al., 2005). In the beginning, NFTs could only be detected via biopsy. Several tau PET tracers, including T807, THK-5117, and PBB3, have been created recently, allowing PET imaging of p-tau tangles (Okamura, et al., 2014).

Synapses contain a large number of proteins known as amyloid precursor proteins. These amyloid proteins are broken down by beta and gamma secretases to produce beta-amyloid (amyloid β). In healthy people, alpha-secretase functions to cut apart the amyloid proteins instead of beta-secretase, and as a result, amyloid-β is not produced. Plaques formed by sticky beta-amyloid protein clusters are harmful to brain cells. Aside from that, they also interfere with the transmission of information between neurons at synapses. With the radioactive Pittsburgh compound B (PiB) or Florbetaben, positron emission tomography (PET) scans neurons for beta-amyloid. Apolipoprotein E (APOE) is a protein involved in transferring cholesterol to the brain (Feero, Guttmacher, & Collins, 2010). Everyone gets two copies of ApoE in one of three variant forms: ApoE2, ApoE3, or ApoE4. ApoE3 is the most prevalent type seen in the majority of the population. In late-onset sporadic Alzheimer's disease, the ApoE4 allele is revealed to represent a genetic risk factor for late-onset dementia. An individual who has inherited two copies of ApoE4 has a massive eight times the chance of AD. A blood test can identify different variations of ApoE in an individual. Researchers have not determined why ApoE4 puts individuals at risk for AD.

According to a recent study, the ApoE4 genotype is less effective than ApoE2 and ApoE3 at clearing beta amyloid plaques in the brain.

SUPERVISED MACHINE LEARNING CLASSIFICATION

Some studies in the literature describe computer-aided Alzheimer's disease diagnoses using MRI scans. Classification methods were employed in CAD systems, which relied on supervised or unsupervised training for their implementation. The system's performance was assessed by looking at the following performance measures: Sensitivity (SE) reflects the real positive rate, specificity (SP) estimates the true negative rate and accuracy (AC) denotes the proportion of correct findings in the database.

Support vector machine (SVM), artificial neural network (ANN), and deep learning are extremely popular classification methods. One of the main distinctions between SVM and ANN is the optimisation problem each solves. ANN and SVM yield a locally or globally optimum solution, respectively (Bisgin, et al., 2018). Extraction of features is crucial in both SVM and ANN. According to (Shi, He, Suzuki, Nakamura, & Itoh, 2009), neural networks and intelligent agents can be used to analyse medical images. While deep learning does not require a separate feature extraction phase, it is part of the learning model. Deep learning is particularly effective for huge datasets. The use of ensemble techniques to enhance the accuracy of Alzheimer's disease categorisation has also been reported (Liu, Zhang, Shen, Initiative, & others, 2012) (Plant, et al., 2010).

SVM Classifier

Fan et al. (Fan, Resnick, Wu, & Davatzikos, 2008) proposed that PET scans offer additional information to sMRI scans, increasing the classification accuracy of Control normal (CN) versus mild cognitive impairment (MCI) using SVM. Studies such as those conducted by Dukart et al. (Dukart, et al., 2013) corroborate the notion that FDG-PET is more useful in discriminating CN vs AD than MRI. T scans appear to be 100% accurate at differentiating CN from AD (Álvarez, et al., 2008), but SPECT pictures are only 97.5% accurate. The same conclusion is reached in a later study (Segovia, et al., 2010) regarding CN versus AD with greater PET image accuracy 96.67% than SPECT image correctness 94.5%. Kamathe et al. (Kamathe & Joshi, 2018) utilised T1, T2 and PD scans to classify CN versus AD. Both Hojjati et al. (Hojjati, et al., 2017) and Sheng et al. (Sheng, et al., 2019) employed connection information from fMRI data to classify MCIc vs MCInc.

SVM is widely employed for classifying Alzheimer's, and many kernel types have been utilised for the task. For multiclass classification of CN, MCI, and AD, Lahmiri et al. (Lahmiri & Boukadoum, 2014) employed a polynomial kernel. Zhang et al. discovered that polynomial kernel helps classify PCA features for CN versus AD (Zhang, et al., 2015). Certain researchers have also utilised ensemble kernels. Alam et al. (Alam, Kwon, & Initiative, 2017) use multiple kernel SVM (MK-SVM) to categorise CN, MCI, and AD. Kamathe et al. (Kamathe & Joshi, 2018) utilised linear, polynomial, and RBF kernel methods to classify AD and CN.

Artificial Neural Network (ANN)

The most significant drawback of the prior research is that it only evaluated basic low-level characteristics such as grey matter tissue volumes from MRI, mean signal intensities from PET, and biological measures from CSF. An artificial neural network (ANN) is utilised as a classification approach in numerous studies connected to neuroimaging (Islam & Zhang, 2017) (Joshi, Rana, & Misra, 2010) (Latif, Butt, Khan, Butt, & Al-Asad, 2017). and has been widely used as a classifier to discriminate in the validation dataset. They are adaptable nonlinear models for simulating complicated real-world situations. They self-adapt to data without explicit functional or distributional form definition in the underlying model. They can estimate probabilities needed to create classification rules and statistical analyses. In contrast, the learning period for large ANNs tends to belong, and adjusting the parameters to be as little as possible necessitates a great deal of calculation.

Deep Learning

In one of the first studies to use deep learning in Alzheimer's disease and mild cognitive impairment, Gupta et al. (Gupta, Ayhan, & Maida, 2013) argued that because low-level features in natural images and brain imaging are similar, and therefore interchangeable, and realistic images, in contrast to neuroimaging, are abundant, natural images could be used to learn low-level features, which could then be used to identify lesions along the surface and ventricles of the brain. Transfer learning is a term used to describe a process in which the characteristics learnt in one data set are utilised to solve a problem in another data set. The authors developed a sparse autoencoder, which learned features from natural pictures, applied to structural MRI data through a CNN to get a 94.7% classification accuracy for AD, 86.4% for MCI, and 88.1% for AD vs MCI. Payan and Montana (Payan & Montana, 2015) discovered equivalent classification accuracies utilising features learnt from structural MRI data. This might be explained by the fact that Payan and Montana (2015) used a considerably bigger sample size and the fact that the author's used 3D brain images rather than 2D, which could include more valuable patterns for categorisation. the 3D model was reported by (Payan & Montana, 2015) to outperform the 2D model in almost all of the comparisons (AD vs HC (2D/3D) = 95.4%/95.4%; AD vs MCI (2D/3D) = 82.2%/86.8%; MCI vs HC (2D/3D) = 90.1%/92.1%). In terms of accuracy, Hosseini-Asl et al. (Hosseini-Asl, Gimel'farb, & El-Baz, 2016) delivered the highest results with 97.6 per cent. This was done with the help of transfer learning. Rather than using two datasets (raw image and AD dataset) to train and test an algorithm, (Hosseini-Asl, Gimel'farb, & El-Baz, 2016) utilised only one Alzheimer's dataset for pre-training another independent Alzheimer's dataset to fine-tune the model.

According to Suk et al. (Suk & Shen, Deep learning-based feature representation for AD/MCI classification, 2013), stacked autoencoders (SAEs) may be better than linear autoencoders in improving the accuracy of Alzheimer's disease (AD), mild cognitive impairment (MCI), and MCIc diagnoses. Based on MRI and PET scans, Suk et al. (Suk, Lee, Shen, Initiative, & others, 2014) utilised patch-based characteristics to classify AD and MCI patients from CN through deep Boltzmann machine learning (DBM). Most accurate classifications were obtained by using a combination of low-level features (LLF), and SAE learnt elements (SAEF) with multi-kernel SVM (MK-SVM). By collecting high-level characteristics and a soft-max logistic regressor, Liu et al. (Liu, et al., Multimodal neuroimaging feature learning for multiclass diagnosis of Alzheimer's disease, 2014) employed SAE-based DL architecture for the diagnosis of Alzheimer's disease in four phases.

MULTIMODAL IMAGE LEARNING

Magnetic resonance imaging (MRI) is a non-invasive method to diagnose disorders since it does not require ionising radiation, making it safe. However, magnetic resonance imaging (MRI) is sensitive to movement, which restricts its usefulness in some situations, such as the diagnosis of mobile organs. Multiple researchers have sought to merge MRI with other modalities through multimodal fusion to overcome this issue and improve the performance of the computer-aided design system. Using this method, one might forecast and recreate missing information that was not present in the MRI. It can also extract additional features that were not evident in the MRI scans.

Regarding multimodal research, Liu et al. (Liu, et al., Early diagnosis of Alzheimer's disease with deep learning, 2014) used a stacked autoencoder (SAE) to structural and PET data. They effectively differentiated Alzheimer's disease (AD) and mild cognitive impairment (MCI) from controls with an accuracy of 87.8 per cent and 76.9 per cent, respectively. The correlation between the two imaging modalities, sMRI and PET, was better captured, which resulted in higher performance (Liu, et al., Multimodal neuroimaging feature learning for multiclass diagnosis of Alzheimer's disease, 2014) . This was done by allowing the hidden layers of the model to learn correlations between the two modalities (sMRI and PET). It distinguished between those with AD and MCI from controls, with an accuracy of 91.4% and 82.1%, respectively. The same model was used for structural data alone, and while the results weren't quite as exciting, the application nevertheless yielded an AD accuracy of 82.6% and an MCI accuracy of 72%. This disagreement between the two models suggests better classifier accuracy if we combine the structural and functional data.

(Song, et al., 2021) propose an image fusion approach to help AD diagnosis strengthen the multimodal fusion process. A novel fusion modality dubbed "GM-PET" is created by registering and mask coding the grey matter (GM) tissue region of MRI and FDG-PET images. The single composite image highlights the GM region while maintaining the shape and metabolic properties of the subject's brain tissue to diagnose AD. 3D Simple CNN and 3D Multi-Scale CNN are used to assess the image fusion method's performance in binary and multiclass classification tasks.

Finally, several recent studies have attempted to strengthen classifications by integrating clinical data with neuroimaging information. A stacked auto-encoder model with deep learning-based feature representation is employed (Suk & Shen, Deep learning-based feature representation for AD/MCI classification, 2013) . Low-level features include underlying complex patterns, such as nonlinear correlations. Combining latent and low-level features helps create a robust AD/MCI classification model with good diagnostic accuracy. Along with the brain imaging data, two types of clinical ratings are supplied for each subject: Minimum Mental State Examination (MMSE) and Alzheimer's Disease Assessment Scale-Cognitive subscale (ADAS-Cog) to the model.

VBM-BASED ALZHEIMER'S DISEASE DETECTION

With the use of magnetic resonance imaging (MRI) scans, voxel-based morphometry (VBM) may be used to examine the anatomic morphology of the brain and its connected parts by measuring the intensity value of each voxel contained in the image. It is commonly used in conjunction with other statistical parametric mapping techniques to compare tissue contents between two or more groups of patients subjected to various hypothesis tests. Features of the three tissue distributions in each voxel (grey matter, white matter, and cerebrospinal fluid) are extracted by VBM. An advanced methodology is known as Voxel-based Morphometry (VBM) effectively studies structural brain alterations in dementia. An image processing and statistical approach permits automated voxelwise studies of GM volume (GMV) anomalies in the brain as measured by MRI and utilising Statistical Parametric Mapping (SPM) software. VBM consists of three preprocessing steps: tissue categorisation, spatial normalisation, and spatial smoothing, followed by statistical analysis (Kurth, Gaser, & Luders, 2015).

Bijen Khagi et al. (Khagi, et al., 2021) studied the VBM technique for MRI classification using SPM 12. The standard VBM pipeline is coupled with a feature extraction technique to assist the categorisation of the normalised feature vectors. Following the VBM execution process, an at-map picture indicating the locations where two groups (CN and AD/MCI) can be distinguished is utilised in the t-test. The t-map is used to locate ROIs and produce classification features. A Gaussian smoothing process has weighted average feature vectors without any feature reduction. The smoothed components are then input into a neural network with their labels and trained using Bayesian optimisation techniques.

Yubraj Gupta (Gupta, Lama, Lee, & Kwon, 2020) presented a unique feature fusion approach to enhance AD, aAD, mAD, and HC classification accuracy. First, sMR images were preprocessed and utilised the SPM12 software's integrated with CAT12 to extract particular ROIs. Using Freesurfer, extracted CSC and HV characteristics from 326 samples. Finally, linearly combined, these three characteristics are used to detect AD early. The combination of morphometric, cortical, and HV characteristics outperformed any single feature.

LINKING S-MRI AND PET FOR AD DIAGNOSIS

The use of multi-modality data to diagnose brain diseases such as Alzheimer's disease (AD) has been shown to result in better performance than the use of a single modality in many cases. However, training a multi-modality model remains a tough task since it is rare in clinical practice to acquire robust data that contains data from all modality sources simultaneously. Obtaining both magnetic resonance imaging (MRI) and positron emission tomography (PET) images of a single subject is, on the whole, a challenging task. ET imaging is expensive and requires the injection of radioactive tracer into the patient's body. In contrast, magnetic resonance imaging (MR imaging) is less expensive, safer, and more commonly utilised in clinical practice. Samples lacking PET data were routinely discarded in earlier research. However, the drop in sample numbers will result in a loss in the model's ability to predict the outcome. To resolve these issues, Reconstructing missing data using the Reversible Generative Adversarial Network (RevGAN) model developed by Wanyun Lin (Lin, et al., 2021). A 3D convolutional neural network (CNN) classification model with multi-modality input was developed for use in Alzheimer's disease diagnosis and classification.

CONCLUSION

Structured brain abnormalities on magnetic resonance imaging (MRI), molecular neuroimaging changes on positron emission tomography (PET), and changes in cerebrospinal fluid (CSF) biomarkers are now recognised as distinct indicators of the disease. Brain imaging methods benefit from having a greater level of spatiotemporal sensitivity than fluid biomarkers, making it possible to track illness development.

Imaging biomarkers such as MRI or PET scans give critical information on the disease stage. Imaging biomarkers have an advantage over fluid biomarkers because they can accurately discriminate between the different phases of the illness and its various anatomical locations. There is no proof of a biomarker that outperforms another (CSF versus imaging) in AD diagnosis. Availability and affordability are what influence biomarker selection the most. Although several biomarkers are known to have varying degrees of success in properly diagnosing AD, it is clear that no one biomarker is sufficient to do so. The diagnostic potential of distinguishing between Alzheimer's disease and cognitively healthy controls is maximised when many biomarkers are used in a set.

There are several challenges to overcome in imaging biomarkers, including the reliability of test results over time, histological validation, specificity for disease process and sensitivity to detect subtle abnormalities, practical feasibility in research settings, and correlation with cognitive and clinical outcomes. Additionally, radiation exposure is an unavoidable outcome of PET imaging and is related to the injected ligand's radioactivity, half-life, and the number of injections. Although MRI does not carry the risk of radiation exposure, it cannot be used in several situations, such as on individuals with cardiac stents or pacemakers (Levine, et al., 2007). Future research should also focus on the relationship between neuroimaging biomarkers (particularly amyloid) and cognition (Márquez & Yassa, 2019). An amyloid PET scan can identify dementia but not discriminate between stages/severity.

ANN, Bayesian networks, k-NN, GMM, HMM, decision tree induction, rule-based classification, PCA, and SVM have been used to classify brain images in the literature. Noise and artefacts in real-world applications restrict single-modality MRI-based CAD systems' efficacy and classification algorithms. Binary classification is easier to verify than multi-classification of AD, MCI and normal controls, but it is still important to determine the various phases of dementia.

The different imaging contexts and modalities provide important information when combined. This enhances the diagnostic system's performance over a single modality system. It also helps to establish appropriate standards for each modality to retain its informative richness and avoid overpowering the features of each image type. It is hard to assess the significance of each modality and its impact on the classifier.

Encouragingly, VBM can be used to research neurological disorders. It can help to understand disease processes better, both scientifically and anatomically, which can aid in disease differential diagnosis. Other imaging modalities, including fMRI and PET, can use similar voxel-level statistical methods. However, due to the statistical nature of the approach, VBM's value resides in group analyses.

REFERENCES

Alam, S., Kwon, G.-R., & Initiative, A. D. (2017). Alzheimer disease classification using KPCA, LDA, and multi-kernel learning SVM. *International Journal of Imaging Systems and Technology*, *27*(2), 133–143. doi:10.1002/ima.22217

Álvarez, I., López, M., Górriz, J. M., Ramírez, J., Salas-Gonzalez, D., Puntonet, C. G., & Segovia, F. (2008). Automatic classification system for the diagnosis of alzheimer disease using Component-Based SVM aggregations. *International Conference on Neural Information Processing*, 402–409.

Arul Kumar, M. G. (2019). WCBAODV: An Efficacious approach to detect Wormhole attack in VANET using CBAODV Algorithm. *International Journal of Advanced Trends in Computer Science and Engineering*, 20-25.

Arulkumar, N. G. M. (2020). CPAODV: Classifying and Assigning 3 Level Preference to the Nodes in VANET Using AODV Based CBAODV Algorithm. In Intelligent Computing Paradigm and Cutting-edge Technologies. ICICCT 2019. Learning and Analytics in Intelligent Systems (pp. 432-445). Springer. doi:10.1007/978-3-030-38501-9_42

Association, A. (2015). 2015 Alzheimer's disease facts and figures. *Alzheimer's & Dementia*, *11*(3), 332–384. doi:10.1016/j.jalz.2015.02.003 PMID:25984581

Sahu, B., Gouse, M., Ranjan Pattnaik, C., & Nandan Mohanty, S. (2021, February). MMFA-SVM: New bio-marker gene discovery algorithms for cancer gene expression. *Materials Today: Proceedings*. Advance online publication. doi:10.1016/j.matpr.2020.11.617

Biscetti, L., Salvadori, N., Farotti, L., Cataldi, S., Eusebi, P., Paciotti, S., & Parnetti, L. (2019). The added value of Aβ42/Aβ40 in the CSF signature for routine diagnostics of Alzheimer's disease. *Clinica Chimica Acta*, *494*, 71–73. doi:10.1016/j.cca.2019.03.001 PMID:30844364

Bisgin, H., Bera, T., Ding, H., Semey, H. G., Wu, L., Liu, Z., Barnes, A. E., Langley, D. A., Pava-Ripoll, M., Vyas, H. J., Tong, W., & Xu, J. (2018). Comparing SVM and ANN-based machine learning methods for species identification of food contaminating beetles. *Scientific Reports*, *8*(1), 1–12. doi:10.103841598-018-24926-7 PMID:29695741

Dukart, J., Mueller, K., Barthel, H., Villringer, A., Sabri, O., & Schroeter, M. L. (2013). Meta-analysis based SVM classification enables accurate detection of Alzheimer's disease across different clinical centers using FDG-PET and MRI. *Psychiatry Research: Neuroimaging*, *212*(3), 230–236. doi:10.1016/j.pscychresns.2012.04.007 PMID:23149027

Erickson, B. J., Korfiatis, P., Akkus, Z., & Kline, T. L. (2017). Machine learning for medical imaging. *Radiographics*, *37*(2), 505–515. doi:10.1148/rg.2017160130 PMID:28212054

Evans, N. R., Tarkin, J. M., Buscombe, J. R., Markus, H. S., Rudd, J. H., & Warburton, E. A. (2018). Erratum: PET imaging of the neurovascular interface in cerebrovascular disease. *Nature Reviews. Neurology*, *14*(5), 313–313. doi:10.1038/nrneurol.2018.42 PMID:29611539

Fan, Y., Resnick, S. M., Wu, X., & Davatzikos, C. (2008). Structural and functional biomarkers of prodromal Alzheimer's disease: A high-dimensional pattern classification study. *NeuroImage*, *41*(2), 277–285. doi:10.1016/j.neuroimage.2008.02.043 PMID:18400519

Fareed & Al-Atroshi. (2021). *Australia Patent No. 2020103911*. Australian Government.

Feero, W. G., Guttmacher, A. E., & Collins, F. S. (2010). Genomic medicine—An updated primer. *The New England Journal of Medicine*, *362*(21), 2001–2011. doi:10.1056/NEJMra0907175 PMID:20505179

Frankle, W. G., Slifstein, M., Talbot, P. S., & Laruelle, M. (2005). Neuroreceptor imaging in psychiatry: Theory and applications. *International Review of Neurobiology*, *67*, 385–440. doi:10.1016/S0074-7742(05)67011-0 PMID:16291028

Frisoni, G. B., Bocchetta, M., Chételat, G., Rabinovici, G. D., De Leon, M. J., Kaye, J., Reiman, E. M., Scheltens, P., Barkhof, F., Black, S. E., Brooks, D. J., Carrillo, M. C., Fox, N. C., Herholz, K., Nordberg, A., Jack, C. R., Jagust, W. J., Johnson, K. A., Rowe, C. C., ... DeCarli, C. (2013). Imaging markers for Alzheimer disease: Which vs how. *Neurology*, *81*(5), 487–500. doi:10.1212/WNL.0b013e31829d86e8 PMID:23897875

Md, G., & Gouse, D. K. (2009). Web Mining: A Review of Present Research Techniques, and Its Software. *Journal of Computer Information Systems*, 75–83.

Galety, M. G. A. A. (2020). Improved Crypto Algorithm for High-Speed Internet of Things (IoT) Applications. Springer. doi:10.1007/978-3-030-38501-9_28

Galety, M. G. (2019). OSSR-P: Ontological service searching and ranking system for PaaS services. *Int. J. Adv. Trends Comput. Sci. Eng*, 271-276.

Gouse, D. G. (2018). Improved Reconfigurable based Lightweight Crypto Algorithms for IoT based Applications. *Journal of Advanced Research in Dynamical & Control Systems*, 186-193.

Gupta, A., Ayhan, M., & Maida, A. (2013). Natural image bases to represent neuroimaging data. *International conference on machine learning*, 987–994.

Gupta, Y., Lama, R. K., Lee, S.-W., & Kwon, G.-R. (2020). An MRI brain disease classification system using PDFB-CT and GLCM with kernel-SVM for medical decision support. *Multimedia Tools and Applications*, *79*(43-44), 32195–32224. doi:10.100711042-020-09676-x

Hojjati, S. H., Ebrahimzadeh, A., Khazaee, A., Babajani-Feremi, A., & Initiative, A. D. (2017). Predicting conversion from MCI to AD using resting-state fMRI, graph theoretical approach and SVM. *Journal of Neuroscience Methods*, *282*, 69–80. doi:10.1016/j.jneumeth.2017.03.006 PMID:28286064

Hosseini-Asl, E., Gimel'farb, G., & El-Baz, A. (2016). *Alzheimer's disease diagnostics by a deeply supervised adaptable 3D convolutional network.* arXiv preprint arXiv:1607.00556.

Islam, J., & Zhang, Y. (2017). A novel deep learning based multiclass classification method for Alzheimer's disease detection using brain MRI data. *International conference on brain informatics*, 213–222. 10.1007/978-3-319-70772-3_20

Johnson, K. A., Fox, N. C., Sperling, R. A., & Klunk, W. E. (2012). Brain imaging in Alzheimer disease. *Cold Spring Harbor Perspectives in Medicine*, *2*(4), a006213. doi:10.1101/cshperspect.a006213 PMID:22474610

Joshi, D. M., Rana, N. K., & Misra, V. (2010). Classification of brain cancer using artificial neural network. *2010 2nd international conference on electronic computer technology*, 112–116.

Kamathe, R. S., & Joshi, K. R. (2018). A novel method based on independent component analysis for brain MR image tissue classification into CSF, WM and GM for atrophy detection in Alzheimer's disease. *Biomedical Signal Processing and Control*, *40*, 41–48. doi:10.1016/j.bspc.2017.09.005

Kehoe, E. G., McNulty, J. P., Mullins, P. G., & Bokde, A. L. (2014). Advances in MRI biomarkers for the diagnosis of Alzheimer's disease. *Biomarkers in Medicine*, *8*(9), 1151–1169. doi:10.2217/bmm.14.42 PMID:25402585

Khagi, B., Lee, K. H., Choi, K. Y., Lee, J. J., Kwon, G.-R., & Yang, H.-D. (2021). VBM-Based Alzheimer's Disease Detection from the Region of Interest of T1 MRI with Supportive Gaussian Smoothing and a Bayesian Regularized Neural Network. *Applied Sciences (Basel, Switzerland)*, *11*(13), 6175. doi:10.3390/app11136175

Kurth, F., Gaser, C., & Luders, E. (2015). A 12-step user guide for analysing voxel-wise gray matter asymmetries in statistical parametric mapping (SPM). *Nature Protocols*, *10*(2), 293–304. doi:10.1038/nprot.2015.014 PMID:25591011

Lahmiri, S., & Boukadoum, M. (2014). New approach for automatic classification of Alzheimer's disease, mild cognitive impairment and healthy brain magnetic resonance images. *Healthcare Technology Letters*, *1*(1), 32–36. doi:10.1049/htl.2013.0022 PMID:26609373

Latif, G., Butt, M. M., Khan, A. H., Butt, M. O., & Al-Asad, J. F. (2017). Automatic multimodal brain image classification using MLP and 3D glioma tumor reconstruction. *2017 9th IEEE-GCC Conference and Exhibition (GCCCE)*, 1–9.

Lazar, M., Weinstein, D. M., Tsuruda, J. S., Hasan, K. M., Arfanakis, K., Meyerand, M. E., Badie, B., Rowley, H. A., Haughton, V., Field, A., & Alexander, A. L. (2003). White matter tractography using diffusion tensor deflection. *Human Brain Mapping*, *18*(4), 306–321. doi:10.1002/hbm.10102 PMID:12632468

Lee, H., Perry, G., Moreira, P. I., Garrett, M. R., Liu, Q., Zhu, X., Takeda, A., Nunomura, A., & Smith, M. A. (2005). Tau phosphorylation in Alzheimer's disease: Pathogen or protector? *Trends in Molecular Medicine*, *11*(4), 164–169. doi:10.1016/j.molmed.2005.02.008 PMID:15823754

Levine, G. N., Gomes, A. S., Arai, A. E., Bluemke, D. A., Flamm, S. D., Kanal, E., Manning, W. J., Martin, E. T., Smith, J. M., Wilke, N., & Shellock, F. S. (2007). Safety of magnetic resonance imaging in patients with cardiovascular devices: an American Heart Association scientific statement from the Committee on Diagnostic and Interventional Cardiac Catheterization, Council on Clinical Cardiology, and the Council on Cardiovascular Radiology and Intervention: endorsed by the American College of Cardiology Foundation, the North American Society for Cardiac Imaging, and the Society for Cardiovascular Magnetic Resonance. *Circulation*, *116*(24), 2878–2891. doi:10.1161/CIRCULATIONAHA.107.187256 PMID:18025533

Lin, W., Lin, W., Chen, G., Zhang, H., Gao, Q., Huang, Y., Tong, T., & Du, M. (2021). Bidirectional Mapping of Brain MRI and PET With 3D Reversible GAN for the Diagnosis of Alzheimer's Disease. *Frontiers in Neuroscience*, *15*, 357. doi:10.3389/fnins.2021.646013 PMID:33935634

Liu, M., Zhang, D., Shen, D., & Initiative, A. D. (2012). Ensemble sparse classification of Alzheimer's disease. *NeuroImage*, *60*(2), 1106–1116. doi:10.1016/j.neuroimage.2012.01.055 PMID:22270352

Liu, S., Liu, S., Cai, W., Che, H., Pujol, S., Kikinis, R., Feng, D., Fulham, M. J., & Adni. (2014). Multimodal neuroimaging feature learning for multiclass diagnosis of Alzheimer's disease. *IEEE Transactions on Biomedical Engineering*, *62*(4), 1132–1140. doi:10.1109/TBME.2014.2372011 PMID:25423647

Liu, S., Liu, S., Cai, W., Pujol, S., Kikinis, R., & Feng, D. (2014). Early diagnosis of Alzheimer's disease with deep learning. *2014 IEEE 11th international symposium on biomedical imaging (ISBI)*, 1015–1018.

Márquez, F., & Yassa, M. A. (2019). Neuroimaging biomarkers for Alzheimer's disease. *Molecular Neurodegeneration*, *14*(1), 1–14. doi:10.118613024-019-0325-5 PMID:31174557

McCollough, C. H., & Leng, S. (2020). Use of artificial intelligence in computed tomography dose optimisation. *Annals of the ICRP*, *49*(1_suppl), 113–125. doi:10.1177/0146645320940827 PMID:32870019

Mohammad Galety, F. H. (2021). Deep Neural Network Concepts for Classification using Convolutional Neural Network: A Systematic Review and Evaluation. *Technium: Romanian Journal of Applied Sciences and Technology*, 58-70. doi:10.47577/technium.v3i8.4554

Okamura, N., Harada, R., Furumoto, S., Arai, H., Yanai, K., & Kudo, Y. (2014). Tau PET imaging in Alzheimer's disease. *Current Neurology and Neuroscience Reports*, *14*(11), 500. doi:10.100711910-014-0500-6 PMID:25239654

Ou, Y.-N., Xu, W., Li, J.-Q., Guo, Y., Cui, M., Chen, K.-L., Huang, Y.-Y., Dong, Q., Tan, L., & Yu, J.-T. (2019). FDG-PET as an independent biomarker for Alzheimer's biological diagnosis: A longitudinal study. *Alzheimer's Research & Therapy*, *11*(1), 1–11. doi:10.118613195-019-0512-1 PMID:31253185

Pacific, A. S. (2006). *Dementia in the Asia Pacific Region: The Epidemic Is Here*. Academic Press.

Payan, A., & Montana, G. (2015). *Predicting Alzheimer's disease: a neuroimaging study with 3D convolutional neural networks.* arXiv preprint arXiv:1502.02506.

Plant, C., Teipel, S. J., Oswald, A., Böhm, C., Meindl, T., Mourao-Miranda, J., Bokde, A. W., Hampel, H., & Ewers, M. (2010). Automated detection of brain atrophy patterns based on MRI for the prediction of Alzheimer's disease. *NeuroImage*, *50*(1), 162–174. doi:10.1016/j.neuroimage.2009.11.046 PMID:19961938

Ronald, T. (1998). Consensus report of the working group on: "Molecular and biochemical markers of Alzheimer's disease. *Neurobiology of Aging*, *19*, 109–116. PMID:9558143

Samanta, D. D. S. (2021). *A Novel Approach for Web Mining Taxonomy for High-Performance Computing. Kolkata, India.* Springer., doi:10.1007/978-981-16-4284-5_37

Segovia, F., Górriz, J. M., Ramírez, J., Salas-González, D., Álvarez, I., López, M., Chaves, R., & Padilla, P. (2010). Classification of functional brain images using a GMM-based multi-variate approach. *Neuroscience Letters*, *474*(1), 58–62. doi:10.1016/j.neulet.2010.03.010 PMID:20227464

Sheng, J., Wang, B., Zhang, Q., Liu, Q., Ma, Y., Liu, W., Shao, M., & Chen, B. (2019). A novel joint HCPMMP method for automatically classifying Alzheimer's and different stage MCI patients. *Behavioural Brain Research*, *365*, 210–221. doi:10.1016/j.bbr.2019.03.004 PMID:30836158

Shi, Z., He, L., Suzuki, K., Nakamura, T., & Itoh, H. (2009). Survey on neural networks used for medical image processing. *International Journal of Computational Science*, *3*, 86. PMID:26740861

Simonsen, A. H., Herukka, S.-K., Andreasen, N., Baldeiras, I., Bjerke, M., Blennow, K., Engelborghs, S., Frisoni, G. B., Gabryelewicz, T., Galluzzi, S., Handels, R., Kramberger, M. G., Kulczyńska, A., Molinuevo, J. L., Mroczko, B., Nordberg, A., Oliveira, C. R., Otto, M., Rinne, J. O., ... Waldemar, G. (2017). Recommendations for CSF AD biomarkers in the diagnostic evaluation of dementia. *Alzheimer's & Dementia*, *13*(3), 274–284. doi:10.1016/j.jalz.2016.09.008 PMID:28341065

Sin, D. S., Kim, M. H., Park, S.-A., Joo, M. C., & Kim, M. S. (2018). Crossed cerebellar diaschisis: Risk factors and correlation to functional recovery in intracerebral hemorrhage. *Annals of Rehabilitation Medicine*, *42*(1), 8. doi:10.5535/arm.2018.42.1.8 PMID:29560319

Song, J., Zheng, J., Li, P., Lu, X., Zhu, G., & Shen, P. (2021). An Effective Multimodal Image Fusion Method Using MRI and PET for Alzheimer's Disease Diagnosis. *Frontiers in Digital Health*, *3*, 19. doi:10.3389/fdgth.2021.637386 PMID:34713109

Suk, H.-I., & Shen, D. (2013). Deep learning-based feature representation for AD/MCI classification. *International Conference on Medical Image Computing and Computer-Assisted Intervention*, 583–590. 10.1007/978-3-642-40763-5_72

Suk, H.-I., Lee, S.-W., Shen, D., & Initiative, A. D. (2014). Hierarchical feature representation and multimodal fusion with deep learning for AD/MCI diagnosis. *NeuroImage*, *101*, 569–582. doi:10.1016/j.neuroimage.2014.06.077 PMID:25042445

Wright, A. (2010). Brain scanning techniques (ct, mri, fmri, pet, spect, dti, dot). *Cerebra: Positively Different*, 1–14.

Young, H., Baum, R., Cremerius, U., Herholz, K., Hoekstra, O., Lammertsma, A. A., Pruim, J., & Price, P. (1999). Measurement of clinical and subclinical tumour response using [18F]-fluorodeoxyglucose and positron emission tomography: Review and 1999 EORTC recommendations. *European Journal of Cancer*, *35*(13), 1773–1782. doi:10.1016/S0959-8049(99)00229-4 PMID:10673991

Zetterberg, H., Skillbäck, T., Mattsson, N., Trojanowski, J. Q., Portelius, E., Shaw, L. M., Weiner, M. W., & Blennow, K. (2016). Association of cerebrospinal fluid neurofilament light concentration with Alzheimer disease progression. *JAMA Neurology*, *73*(1), 60–67. doi:10.1001/jamaneurol.2015.3037 PMID:26524180

Zhang, Y., Dong, Z., Phillips, P., Wang, S., Ji, G., Yang, J., & Yuan, T.-F. (2015). Detection of subjects and brain regions related to Alzheimer's disease using 3D MRI scans based on eigenbrain and machine learning. *Frontiers in Computational Neuroscience*, *9*, 66. doi:10.3389/fncom.2015.00066 PMID:26082713

KEY TERMS AND DEFINITIONS

Agnosia: The failure to correctly interpret a sensory input, or *agnosia*, is common in AD.

Aphasia: The earliest changes are word finding difficulties and at this stage syntax may appear superficially intact, but close analyses may reveal unfinished sentences, inappropriate usage of tense and other minor errors.

Apraxia: Difficulties with complex motor tasks not due to primary motor deficits resulting in increasingly poor self-care and risk of harm.

Cognition: Is defined as the mental processes used to obtain knowledge or to become aware of and interact with the environment. These processes include perception, imagination, judgement, memory, and language.

Chapter 10
The Influence of Artificial Intelligence on People With Autism Spectrum Disorder:
A Methodical Literature Review

Shushma G. B.
GITAM University, India

I. Jeena Jacob
GITAM University, India

ABSTRACT

This literature review examines the past and recent relevant research on autism disorder. As undergoing many changes in the whole world, especially after the deadly effect of the COVID-19 widespread in the year 2020, has led to drastic adoption of more intelligent devices for quicker detection of certain human diseases and delivering the results quicker via electronic media, the research will focus on the autism disorder intelligent device detection and feed these data to machine learning models to predict the issues without human intervention. Based on the outcome of the results, the diseases can be treated accordingly in an appropriate manner. The individual suffering from autism disorder can be detected early using AI or machine learning, and this domain can be integrated with the IoT sensors. Such sensors can be combined with the human body, and this sensor will extract the data and send it to the centralized healthcare system. Such data will be removed from the data storage and processed using the AI algorithm to get the desirable results to give an appropriate treatment at the correct stages.

INTRODUCTION

ASD is a neurological syndrome that starts initial in the infant and continues during a human begin life. It disturbs how an individual acts, reacts, cooperates with other people, learns, and communicates (Gamaethige, 2017). The ASD is also known as "Asperger" syndrome and "pervasive" evolving disor-

DOI: 10.4018/978-1-7998-9534-3.ch010

ders. Pervasive developmental disorders fall into two categories: social skills communication and normal communication problems, and second confined and monotonous patterns of actions, interests, or activities. They are analyzing ASD can be challenging as there is no medical test to diagnose the disorders, like a blood test. Physicians look at the kid's activities and growth to make an identification. ASD can occasionally be spotted at 18 months or younger kids. By age 2, a diagnosis by a skilled person can be measured actual trustworthy. As even a few times there are human errors, to overcome these human errors, we propose in our research an intelligent device as well as analyses the machine-generated data using AI models the results values can detect the ASD at an early stage of childhood (Liu, 2013).

ASD will affect the intellectual functioning of the brain throughout the lifetime, and such disorder makes an individual with social and language communication issues or social interaction skills, memory summarizing, focus skills. These can be identified at the earlier stage of childhood and usually lead to deficiencies in effect growth of the child. Furthermore, these discrepancies have remained exposed to undesirably influence adaptive social behavior and operative. Consequently, initial analysis and interference are key elements so that in the future, these issues will not occur in the world population (Wedyan, 2016).

ASD is an extraordinarily predominant and harmful neuro-developmental syndrome that affects one out of twenty-four individual human beings over the world. In the recent several years, the analyses result from the frequency of ASD in the developing and non-developing nations has increased hypothetically, with the proper awareness of the ASD and initial treatment can reduce the ASD in most of the countries.

The ASD does not follow any ethnic, cultural, and regional groups, as similar to the COVID-19 outbreak, but in the case of the ASD, it can be earlier stages it can be detected (Orlandi, 2012), and doctors can take appropriate actions to treat the ASD disorder by giving proper medications for the ASD affected children, as figure 1, mentions the stages or levels of ADS severity as it has 3 phases, each phase will play a very critical role as sooner it's treated at level 1 stage then it's better and significantly more straightforward to cure the ASD disorder among the younger or early-born children's.

Figure 1. Levels of the ASD disorder in the children's

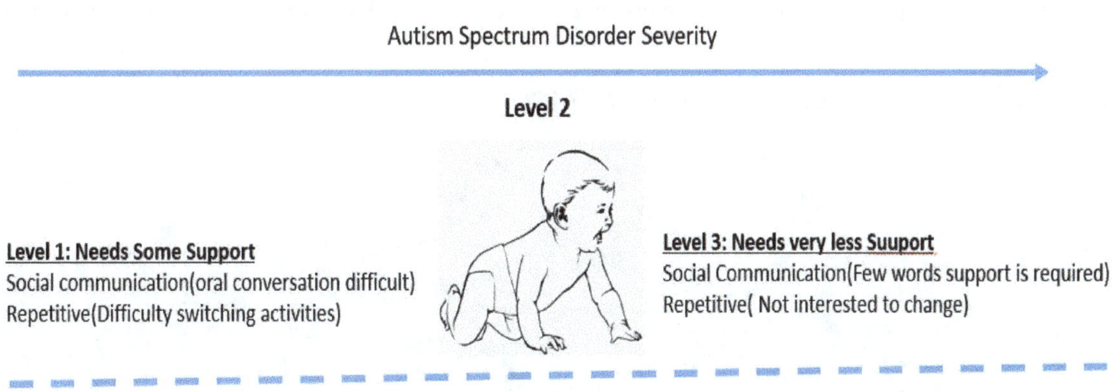

The ASD in males specifically at the age of 22 to 23 in the recent analysis's has been found, as the investigations are done not only the children but all the mid-age individual are also subjected to the ASD, from the female individual point of view it's closer to 3 is to 1 ratio, previously reported results are four is to 1 ratio. Usually, the studies have shown that the girls have a higher risk of ASD as well as not receiving appropriate treatment or clinical diagnosis. Female autism phenotype might lead a role in girl's child being misdiagnosed, diagnosed late (Dris, 2019), or ignored. As the regional factors also will play an improvement role in the case of females getting treated for the ASD disorder. If the earlier interpretation at the earlier stage needs to be identified for male or female, if it's ignored, then it will turn into significant disorder issues as well as it will be life treating issues.

In the current scenario of COVID-19 or for parents who stay in a remote location, it's challenging the tracing of the ASD in their children without any support from the health care system as parents lack the correct knowledge (Wu, 2019), knowledge, or help in dealing with the ASD disorder. Many parents in the remote village sense the guilt or question why we lack such information in the identification of the ASD, and they always think their kids are in the regular stage of their growth, as it's complicated to identify the ASD. If the child is spotted with ASD, the parents never aspect such a child into their lives. In the case of a financially weaker section of the parents, they lack to take appropriate action by not giving the proper medical treatment. This impacts the kids as well as it will create a burden for the family members as the child requires more timer or attention to take care of such ASD disorder impacted kids. In the next section, we will analyze the earlier signs of the ASD disorder (Taha Ahmed, 2020).

AUTISM EARLY SIGNS

The early signs of ASD can be tracked, or it may give an impression, when a child is as early as a few months old from the birth (Muty, 2016), in few cease it is not traceable until of the age range between 3 to 4 children's.

The appropriate developmental and behaviors screening tests can help to spot the ASD in the kids as the initial signs. Such a task is classically achieved by a clinician through a repetitive check-up to measure a child's social behavior (Taffoni, 2014), speech test, book learning capability, and body movement. Significant how mutual ASD is in your family member's past may also give a hint to the doctor to take a call on the child is affected with ASD as well as day-to-day close observing of the kids is very critical.

Figure 2. Five types of Autism Spectrum Disorder (ASD)

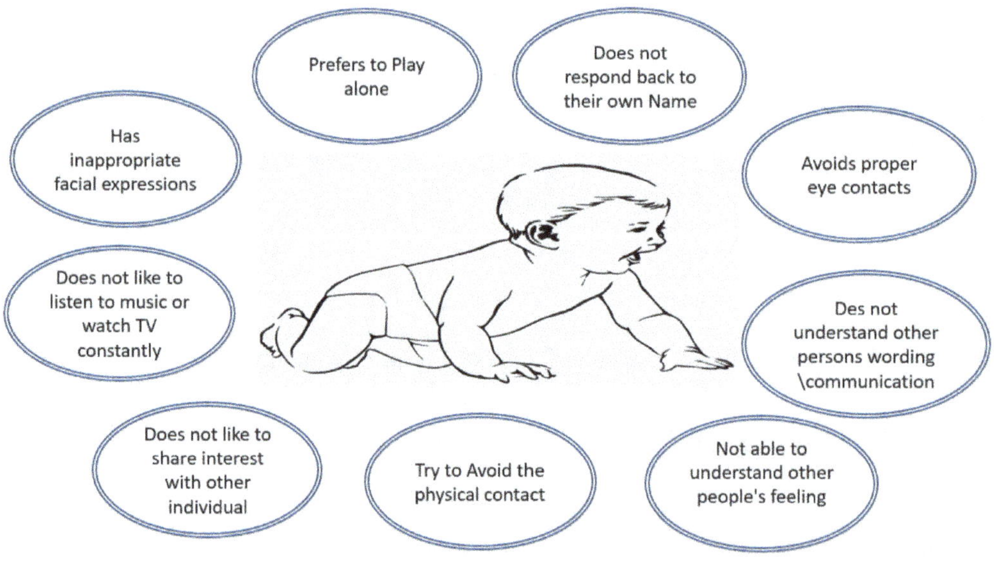

Parents can watch for primary signs by one-to-one care of their child's social behavior. By monitoring each day, they can know what are the different kinds of ASD disorder by looking at figure 2, and there are few parameters which will help the parents to monitor their child; if a few of the parameters matches, then it's the root of the concerns issues, where parents should get in touch with the nearby health center. Social deficiencies such as the lack of social skills may become an early sign of ASD (Ramirez-Duque, 2018). Nearly of these ASD early signs may surface, such as evading eye contact as well as the physical contact, not answering when the kid's name is called or on the repeated time, likes to be unaccompanied, or an incapability to understand the emotional state of another individual (Sadato,2012).

In addition, that parents can become an observer for talkative impairments, such as difficult while in the speaking (or) absence of facial expressions (Ahmadi, 2014) or mental impairments such as not showing curiosity in preferred dolls or indifference to surfaces and room lights. The monotonous actions can also be revealing primary signs of ASD. For example, kids might consist of retelling the words or performances, shaking their body such as hand or head regularly, or flustering their hands (Gamaethige, 2019).

STUDIES TOWARDS DIFFERENT TYPES OF AUTISM SPECTRUM DISORDER (ASD) DISORDER CAUSES

The person with ASD naturally has major social and communication issues and uncommon actions and interests. Most individual with ASD also have knowledgeable frailty (Mohd, 2020). The person with "Asperger syndrome" typically has slighter signs of ASD. They might have public challenges and uncommon interests and behaviors. Moreover, they naturally do not have complications with intellectual disability or language (Chrisman, 2018). PDD-NOS is occasionally termed "atypical autism." (Zhang,2019) The person who meets some of the principles for ASD, nevertheless not everyone, might not be diagnosed with "atypical autism" (Anurekha,2018). These individual typically have fewer and milder symptoms than those with "Autistic disorder." The indications might affect only communication challenges and social interaction issues. There are five syndrome categories of ASD (Qidwai,2018), as shown in Figure 1. The Rett syndrome, one of the foremost causes of mental hindrance and developmental worsening in girls, and rare X-linked prevailing genetic disorder affecting only girls. The disorder is generally regarded as a neurodevelopmental condition rather than a neurodegenerative disorder. With Rett syndrome girls, had abnormal movements of the upper limbs and hypotonic, ataxic (Cheng,2016). Youthful disintegrative syndrome, an occasional, insistently progressive neurologic disorder, first defined by "Heller" in 1908, remains a disorder of great interest. It has extended remained discussed whether it is a distinct disorder or simply a late-onset variant of childhood autism, and also known as Heller syndrome (or) as disintegrative mental illness, is a moderately infrequent illness that has variably been encompassed in official diagnostic systems (SARANYA,2021).

Table 1 shows the various symptoms of ASD associated to social interaction and communication difficulties, as well as other Symptoms.

Figure 3. Signs of autism or autism spectrum disorder (ASD) typically appear during early childhood but can often go undetected until young adulthood

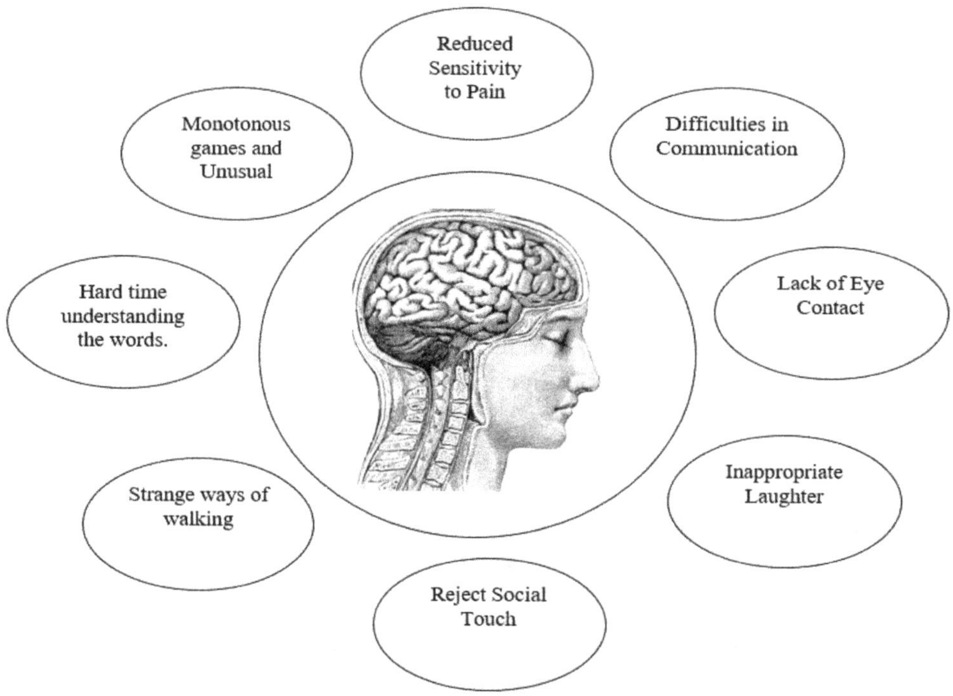

Table 1. Summary of Study towards signs and symptoms of ASD

Everyday social interaction and communication problems like as:	Unusual Interests and Behaviors	Other Symptoms
No sensitivity or pain and Want to live alone.	Rocks body, or spins self in circles, Flaps hands.	Causing self-injury, Temper tantrums
Not able to make eye contact correctly and No interaction with others	Follow certain routines	Unusual sleeping and eating habits, Short attention span.
No proper response to sound and Inappropriate laughing and to giggle	Obsessive interests and Gets upset by minor changes	Unusual mood or emotional reactions
May not have a wish for cuddling, Using echo words, etc	Lines up toys or other entities	Absence of agitation or further fear than expected
Not able to express their gestures	Has to follow certain routines	Abnormal reactions to the way things sound, look or feeling, smell.
Inappropriate objects attachment	He plays with toys the identical way each time	Hyperactivity (active)

FIVE TYPES OF AUTISM SPECTRUM DISORDER (ASD) DISORDER

Figure 4. Five types of Autism Spectrum Disorder (ASD)

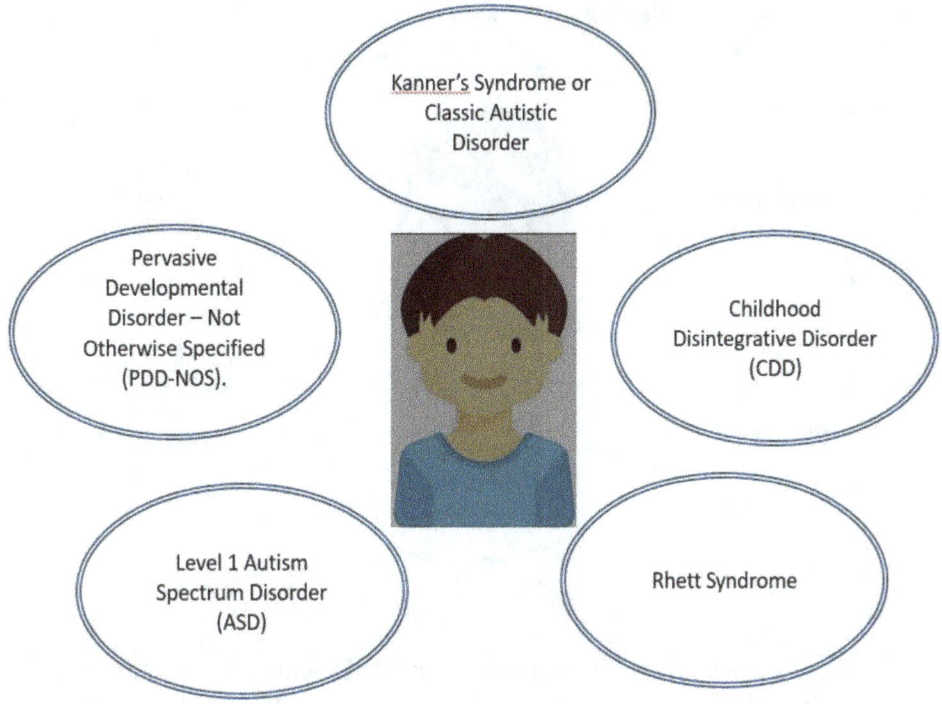

Type 1: Autism or Asperger's Spectrum Disorder

Asperger's Syndrome currently it's not measured as a formal diagnosis, but still, it's been the common term used in the autism spectrum disorders community discussion. The correct way to quote is that it's a type 1 ASD. Usually, people or the individual affected with such type of level 1 ASD of above-average or average intellect and processes more vital verbal communication skills, but in the case of the social communication is a significant challenge (Sariya,2016). Figure 5 showcases the level 1 signs usually found among the children.

Figure 5. Asperger's Syndrome sings in the children's

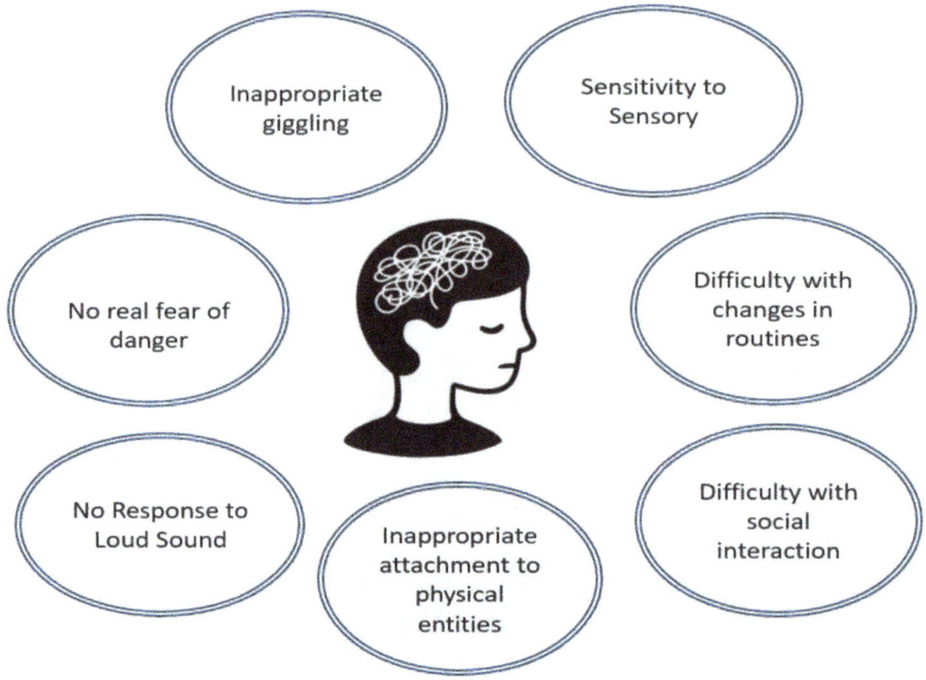

The Level 1 Asperger's can be categorized as part of the ASD, and in the current years, the doctors do not consider it as a significant issue; usually, such type of individual will struggle to properly communicate with another individual, as well as such people tend to grow interested into the multiple subjects areas. As such, an individual has a delay in their speech in a few of the individual or children or in other few cases few of the children possess advanced vocabulary skills at their age. The level 1 severity is lesser compare to different types of ASD types, the level 1 people can recover from these from giving an appropriate treatment which generally involves one or many social, educational, or behavioral interventions.

Type 2: Rett Syndrome

As similar to the Level 1 type, the type 2 "Rett's" Syndrome was excluded as a part of the ASD in current years (Hu,2021). Nevertheless, it principally affects girl's children, and the symptoms can be seen around six months old. The symptoms related to "Rett's" Syndrome contain public communication skills and an impaired capability to use one's hands or other things monotonous hand and arms flapping; it's a common sign of the "Rett's" Syndrome. Type 2 is scarce, as mentioned; it's usually found in female children, as it's a neurological disorder. These can be identified in the first two years of the girl's child (Jaganathan,2017). Such a children's diagnosis with such Syndrome can feel overwhelming. Usually, such types of Syndrome are treated as genetically based, where the child's parents derive from their grand family members. As shown in figure 6, the different hand position of the child, which occurs at the age of 10 to 18-year-old children's.

The symptoms of type 2 may vary amongst the individual children, but most of the babies with the type 2 "Rett" syndrome seem to grow as usual for the first six months before any signs can be identified.

The type 2 disorder is evident. The most obvious thing or changes usually show up which the child is between 10 and 17 months old, and type 2 can be sudden or slow progress.

Usually, it's been identified that or as per the research, the growth of the brain is prolonged or doesn't correctly grow as per the age progress, and the head of the child is usually smaller than compare to an average growth children babies. The growth can be analyzed only when the child grows older (Wang,2018).

Figure 6. Rare neurological disorder sings in the children's

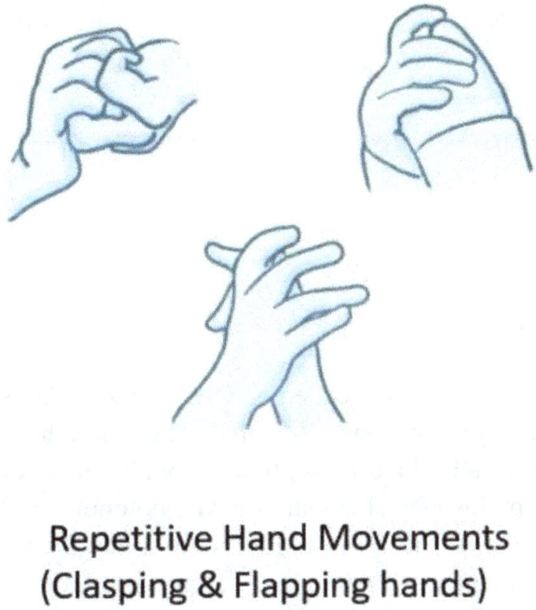

Type 3: Childhood Disintegrative Disorder (CDD)

The CDD is an illness in which kids generally progress through the age of three or four. After a few months, they will start losing social skills or language and other skills they have already learned. Type 3 CDD can seem to hurt parents as it will create confusion and fear among parents. In such a case, they required appropriate suggestions from the health care expert. As per the figure, as type 3 CDD is gauged as significant severe mental retardation, if such classes are not diagnosed early then, it will become a substantial issue (Aslam,2021).

Type 3 is also called HS (heller syndrome) or dementia infantilize. This Syndrome was first traced in 1908, as it's an infrequent neuro-biological illness categorized by the worsening of verbal skills and public skills and by damage of logical functioning and normal development throughout life. Nevertheless, since the disorder is uncommon, happening in one in all or around 50,000 to 100,000 persons, it was not formally predictable as a growing illness until the 1990s.

The source of CDD is not identified yet, but as in recent years, the health care organization has grown at a faster phase, it can be traceable at the initial stage by the health care experts. Though, it is suspected that an irregularity in a gene involved in the expansion of the essential nervous system contributes to such a type 3 CDD disorder. Even though CDD has been related to other illnesses, similar to abnormalities in lipid storage and an immune reaction, none of these circumstances look as if to be an original reason for type 3 CDD.

Figure 7. The CCD is considered as major severity

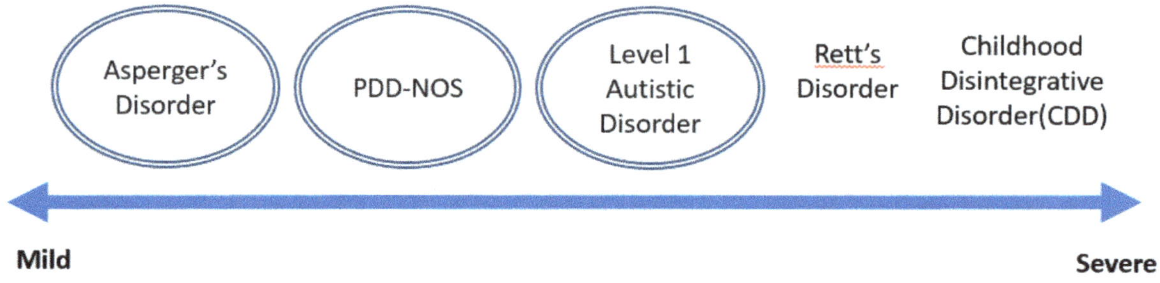

Type 4: Kanner's Syndrome

Type 4 is "Kanner's" Syndrome, or it's also called as CAD (classic Autistic Disorder), such type of symptoms usually include challenges interactive (or) understanding others individual, no eye contact, as well as an allergic reaction to light, loud noise, touch, not able to smell. The kids diagnosed with "Kanner's" Syndrome show a philosophical essential for monotonous or dull and frequently offer no notice in the individual around them. This type of kid usually shows their responsiveness innermost. It demonstrates a little wish to cooperate with others or socialize with others as shown that "Kanner's" Syndrome usually tends to have lower IQ knowledge, as compared to other normal children.

Figure 8. The "Kanner's" Syndrome children usually have lower IQ knowledge

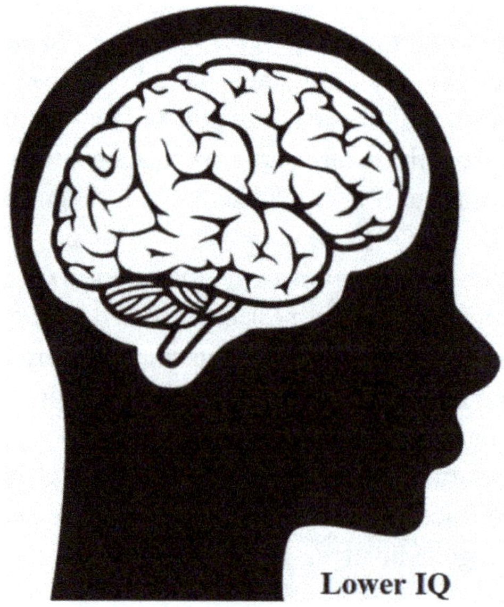

Type 5: Pervasive Developmental Disorder – Not Otherwise Specified (PDD-NOS)

These "PDD-NOS" usually have lesser severity than compared to other types of Autistic Disorder. In such variety of the kids typically have experienced delays in standards like talking to other (or) walking, and frequently lag behind other kids as compared to the other children's (Islam,2020). The kids with "PDD-NOS" symptom can succeed this milder form further effortlessly than those who have been detected with the more common forms of autism disorder. As shown in figure 9, the process of the "PDD-NOS" is given in detail.

Figure 9. The "PDD-NOS" Syndrome children usually effect the children below 2 to 4 years

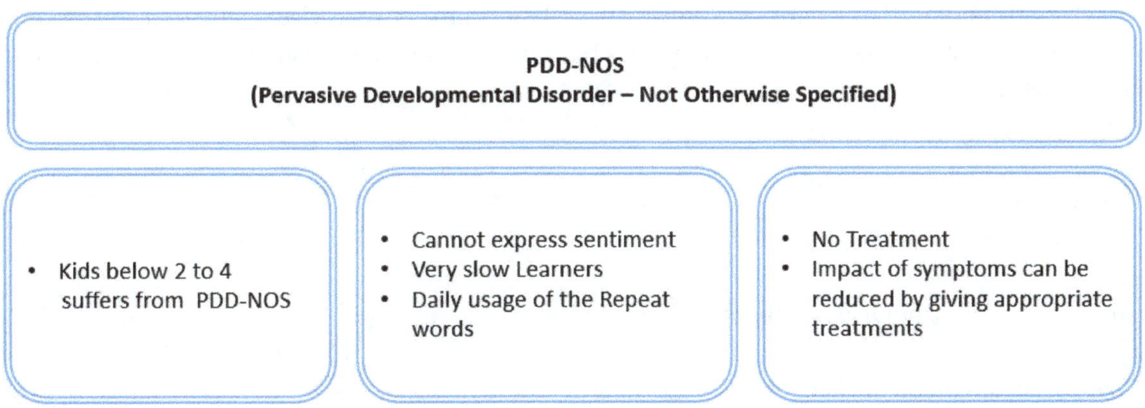

The Usage of the Data Sets

The commonly used tools for analyzing the dataset of autism are functional magnetic resonance imaging (fMRI), Electroencephalography (EEG), and more recently "eye-tracking". Eye-tracking is a system of monitoring of the gaze grouping together a set of techniques that make it possible to record the ocular movements and to measure several parameters such as the time of fixation of the image, the number of fixations of an area of the image, etc. The objective of the eye-tracking system is to examine perceptual characteristics of ASD and facilitate study into the abnormal behavior of visual attention and oculomotor patterns that contribute to clinical characteristics of ASD. The detailed and objective measures of pupil eye behavior, eye tracking system are used to identify disorder-specific characteristics, enhance early identification, and inform treatment. Particularly, examiners of ASD have benefited from integrating eye-tracking into their research paradigms.

The most frequently used technologies to detect early ASD were electroencephalogram, magnetic resonance imaging, and eye-tracking

Electroencephalography (EEG) is a technique used to record the electrical activity of the brain. For an EEG, multiple electrodes are placed on the patient's scalp. These electrodes measure features of the brain's spontaneous electrical activity and display these as waveforms on a computer screen. The advantages of the EEG can be used for real-time tracking of the neural activity of the brain in milliseconds and detecting subtle differences in neural oscillations more sensitively, thus quickly and accurately distinguishing children with ASD and typically developing (TD) children with EEG signals.

What is MRI?

Magnetic-resonance (MR) examination provides a powerful tool for investigating brain structural changes in children with Autism Spectrum Disorder (ASD) MRI uses a powerful magnetic field, radiofrequency pulses, and a computer to produce detailed pictures of internal body structures. MRI does not use radiation (x-rays). Detailed MR images allow doctors to examine the body and detect disease.

What is Eye Tracking?

Eye-tracking technology is a means of exploring the relationship between visual attention and consumer behavior. In the past, eye-tracking technology has been used to conduct research on consumer decision-making, marketing, and advertising
Eye tracking advantages:

1. Real visual data
2. Natural eye movements recorded

Eye-tracking equipment Disadvantages

1. Not all eyes can be tracked
2. Only track one individual at a time
3. Tracks only eye movement data

The most common and specific challenges associated with ASD are listed below:

1. Speech and language difficulties.
2. Intellectual disability.
3. Difficulties with fine and gross motor skills.
4. Sleep problems.
5. Attention problems.
6. Epilepsy.
7. Anxiety and depression.

The techniques required to overcome the challenges can be

Common autism treatments include **behavior therapy, speech-language therapy, play-based therapy, physical therapy, occupational therapy, and nutritional therapy**.

Studies towards Autism Spectrum Disorder (ASD) Diagnosis Treatment

The treatment considerations are well conventional that ASD cannot be treated; nonetheless, at the primary interference can fetch gratifying results. Furthermost of these recommendation based interferences necessitate of the expert health care system worker and extremely trained specialists available in only a one or two of government organizations (Matsumoto,2016). Private health care center established services deliver sessions on a day to day or substitute day basis. Still, the psychoanalyses are costly, and affordability turn out to be an important issue for children from lower income family member cannot afford such treatment. Also, furthermost of these health care centers emphasis on a specific characteristic of ASD-like speech, sensory problems, or researchers, and general management is barely considered. There is a more stress on professional therapy. Astonishingly, numerous professionals also emphasis more on social control, need-based communication, adaptive living, and functional academics rather than social communication skills, or play, practical language growth (Misman,2019).

Table 2. Summary of study towards early and later indicators for the (ASD) diagnosis

Primary signs that necessitate assessment by an expert include:	Later indicators include:
No particular terms by age 16 months or two word terms by age 2	Inflexible adherence to specific routines or rituals
No babbling or pointing by age one and poor eye contact	Preoccupation with particular objects or subjects
Loss of language or social skills previously knowledge	Repetitive or unusual use of language
Excessive lining up of toys or objects and abnormally intense or focused interest	Absence or impairment of imaginative and social play
No smiling or social responsiveness	Impaired ability to initiate or sustain a conversation with others
Inappropriate objects attachment and no response to name	Inadequate capacity to make friends with peers

The Influence of Artificial Intelligence for Autism Spectrum Disorder (ASD) Disorder

The applied AI domain to detecting ASD is the instrument to measure whether other social features might hypothetically be used as proof of identity of noticeable indications for the ASD diagnosis. In total, around 13 technical articles were studied. A mainstream of the studies used the supervised ML process, such as SVM, to differentiate between persons with and without ASD syndrome. As shown in figure 10, it's a classic example of how to assess ASD (Abhirami,2019). As the doctor does the observation of the children in the health care center, as well as taking the feedback of the parents about the day to day task or any strange behavior of the kids in the parent's observation, if any peculiar behavior such as social communication lacking skills, as well as the other parameter will be taken into consideration while performing the initial analyses, then the final result of the diagnosis details are shared across to parents to take an appropriate actions, as sooner or early-stage the ASD is detected its safer to give proper treatment (Huang,2019).

Figure 10. The traditional method of the identifying the ASD

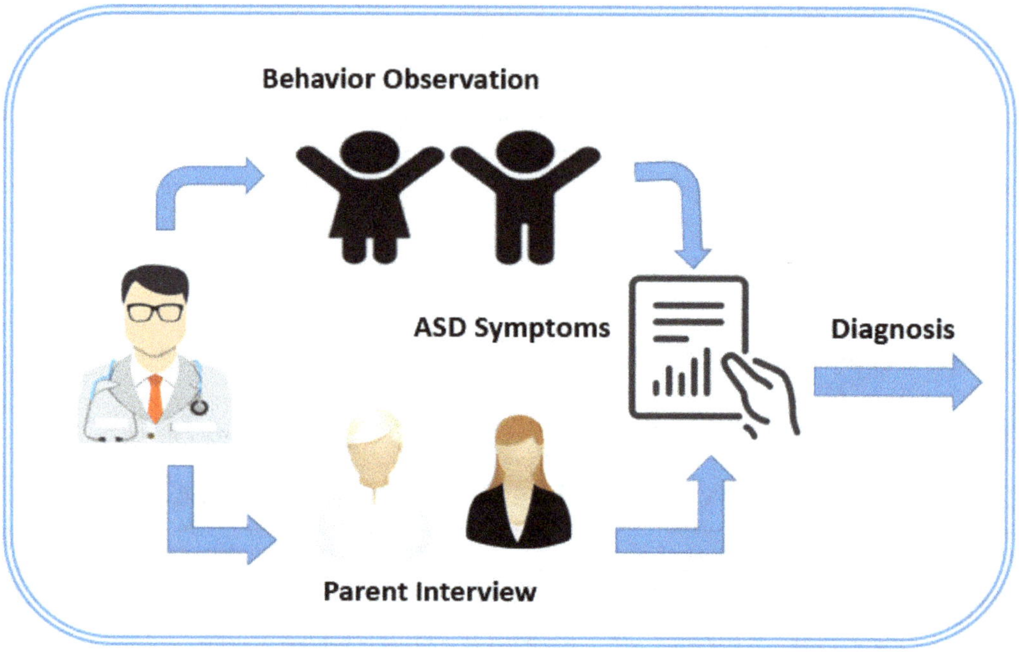

Figure 11. The AI method for classification of the healthy and non-healthy patient(ASD)

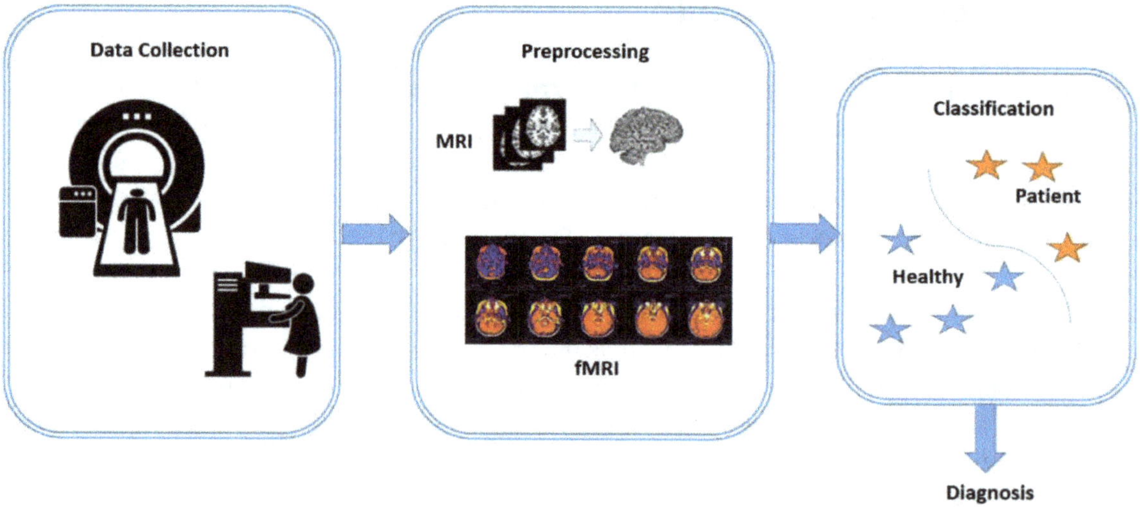

In the case of figure 11, all the systems are automated AI technology systems, where first the patient details or brain mapping images are scanned via MRI machine, the data are collected and transfer to the next level for pre-processing, and appropriate action or features are extracted, and then the is processed using the AI & machine learning algorithms, a helpful classification report is generated either the patient is healthy or unhealthy, and if the patient is sick then appropriate action is taken by the physician, and the patient will be monitored for few months with proper medication (Vittorias,2008).

In contrast to the field of AI and ML, it's a very quickly spreading health issue among the children in most of the developing and non-developing nations as the technology is getting progressive zones with AI and ML technology to perform the higher end analytical imaging, as well as for the genetics. As there is higher growth in medical image processing and analyses and pipelines that abstract very critical features are precious information to make a decision based (Othman,2010) on the supporting data, as the data processing of biomedical images are becoming much faster. Unfortunately, this inclination has been motivated in the fields of other critical cognitive diseases related to or anything related to the cardiovascular (or) nervous system. In the current medical industry, many issues or challenges need to be resolved as the traditional process is time-consuming and lengthy, as the evolution of the AI and ML methods can be applied in research and bio-clinical settings. AI and ML require big data for storage of the larger dataset. The bulk data stored in the big data are either used for the studies or research point of view in this examination used composing data from a data source. There are some limitations to executing AI and ML in the wide-ranging medical healthcare system as it faces frequent difficulties. AI the ML algorithm comprehensively be determined by on the training dataset values, there has not yet been in available research measuring in what way the superiority of the input dataset affects the accuracy of the data-set values outcome results, and on the other side the data-set collection and cleaning of the data is time-consuming, the data collected should be clean so that it can be feed into the ML or AI algorithm to extract the better results out of it (Cherdal,2016). On the next level requiring vast quantities of dataset values, the principled challenge around the customer or individual dataset privacy is also an additional topic that is under discussion. Moreover, while complicated illnesses like ASD impact both the social behavior and the brain mental health, there is an absence of intelligence reports on present AI and ML technology mixing numerous modalities for an additional inclusive understanding of an individual, the best way is to integrate the IoT with the AI and ML algorithm as well as integrating with blockchain to safeguard the dataset values of the patients or individual transferred over the insecure internet (Samad,2018).

Detection of the Autism Spectrum Disorder (ASD) using Smart Device and Influence of AI or Machine Learning.

There has been a noticeable increase in research literature evaluating the effectiveness of machine learning and AI for diagnosing ASD. Machine Learning has enormous potential to enhance diagnostic and intervention research in the behavioral sciences. The reliable machine learning-based diagnosis processes for ASD (Fadhil,2018) using structural magnetic resonance image (fMRI) (Gamaethige,2017)., functional magnetic resonance image (fMRI). ML can be a very less expensive (S. Gupta, 2020), easy technique to classify and categorize medical matters that achieve enhanced than utmost normally used standardized implements (S. Gupta, 2018).

Many machine learning techniques are used for classification (S. Gupta, 2018), such as k-NN, SVM, Naïve Bayes, Random Forest, Fuzzy Method, PCA, ANN, ICA, Decision Tree, LDA, Deep Learning, etcetera, giving the greatest results for feature extraction of ASD diagnostics (K. Nermand, 2018). There are multiple devices and toys which can be integrated with the IoT sensors, and as well as connected with the internet and their activities can be easily tracked, and more detailed analyses can be done. It can also be used in entertainment so that kids get entertained. The IoT can offer assistance with exterior features such as ambient room lighting and very relaxing music on request. As shown in figures 12, all the wearable devices, which can keep track of the day to day tasks, the integration of the IoT with AI or ML evolved over a couple of years, not only in the health care domain, in various fields such as financial services or more significant industrial center were IoT sensor devices are dominating with AI and ML when the kids are wearing the wearable watch their plus rate and other details can be tracked. Such information is sent directly to nearby health care centers to perform further analysis, as IoT also has vital help remote location areas for faster or quicker treatment, as patients can get treated over the telephone conversation or video conferencing. Table 3 contents are given an overview summary of studies towards ASD the influence of AI or Machine Learning. After performing the summary of reviews of the multiple research pepper over different journals or conference sessions, AI or ML, and IoT have played critical roles in diagnosing ASD (L. Cattaneo, 2007).

Figure 12. All the Wearable technology can be wearable to kids and their day to day activities can be tracked

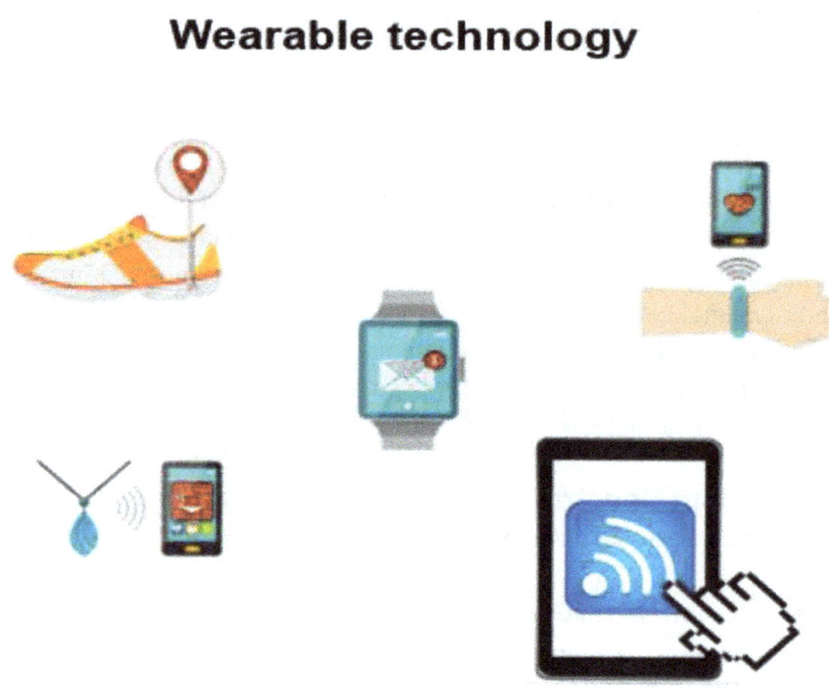

Table 3. Summary of study towards ASD the influence of AI or machine learning

Authors	Problems	Technique	Advantage	Limitation
(KS.Omar et al., 2019)	Sensing autism traits through screening tests is very costly and time consuming process.	CRF-CART and RF-Id3	With artificial intelligence and machine learning (ML), autism can be predicted at quite an early stage.	It was assessed with only the AQ-10 dataset.
(Matthew J. Maenner et al., 2016)	The number of assessments collected has intensely bigger since the year 2000, challenging the resources and appropriateness of the observation system.	RFC	The ML process predicted ASD case standings 86.5% concordant with the clinician-determined case statuses (84.0% sensitivity, 89.4% predictive value positive).	Restricted Amongst 8-year older kids in many US cities.
(Fadi Abdeljaberet al., 2018)	ASD diagnosis problem	ASD classification	To accelerate the screening time or to improve sensitivity	The consistency of these tools using the DSM-5 moderately than the DSM-5 manual

Use Case 1: Parent Feedback Analysis for ASD using BERT Machine Learning Process

The kids with ASD tend to show unique or different ways of voice patterns. At the same time, they speak as well as they make a weird voice that is the scared factor for the parents, to perform the analyses based on the inputs from the parents of the affected kids, the use case is about to interact with the parents and take a piece of information found on their conversation over a phone In the proposed method, as shown in figure 13, the parents are asked multiple questions day by day from different health care works, and the voice conversation is converted into the text values. These values are feed into the BERT model to forget any accurate results where the conversation is positive or negative. Such type of system will help the remote village people to have an easier conversation over the phone than using any internet connection, as in most developing nations, the internet connection is tough to connect, as the phone conversation is the best option to interact with the health care system workers.

Figure 13. Parents voice feedback analyses report generation

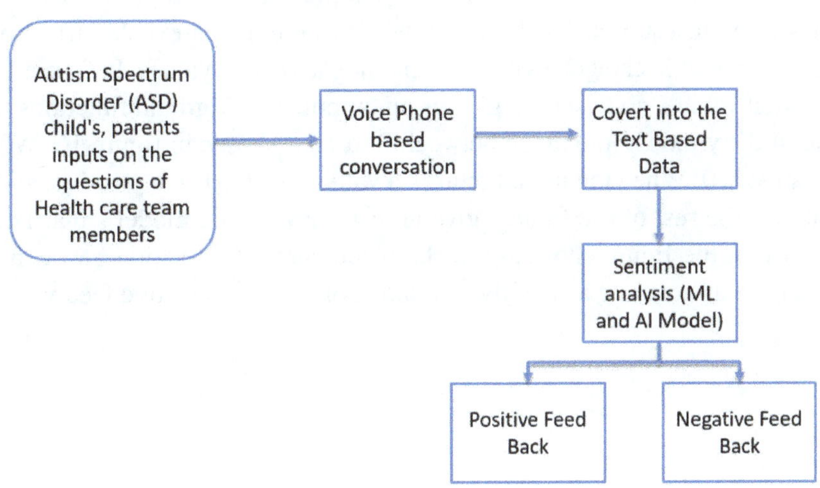

Natural language processing (NLP) is one of the most significant tasks in the current business that uses machine learning ideas. The NLP deals with whatever is associated with using the system to process and recognize human text or speech, the customary NLP prototypes that follow a procedure of the unidirectional process, that is, interpretation the data text one or the other from right to left or left to right, as in the case of the BERT reading the data values from the whole sequence of words at once. The BERT uses a modifier which is essentially a mechanism to build associations amongst the words in the dataset values. The BERT contains two handling models, one an encoder and the other one is a decoder. The encoder process read out the input data set text values and produces the predictions in the case of the decoder. But, since the primary objective of BERT is to create a pre-trained model, the encoder profits precedence in excess of the decoder. As shown in figure 14, the input data set values are ASD and their representation for BERT.

Figure 14. Text information classification using the BERT concepts

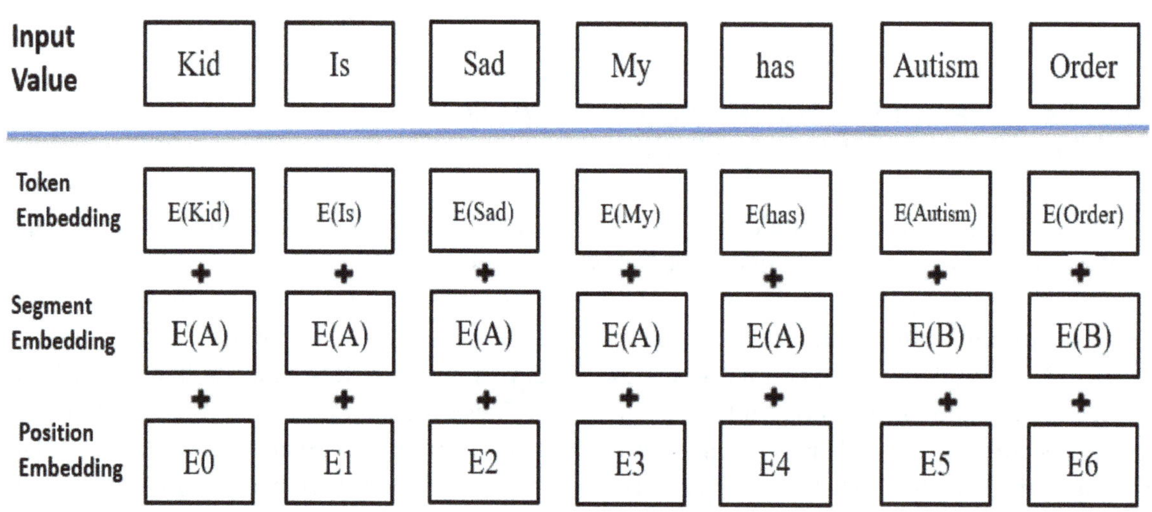

Implementation and Results

The data set values are divided into 80% of the dataset samples into a training subset, 10% into a validation subset, and 10% into a test subset. The Problem type is Single-label text classification since we want to classify text into two possible categories positive and negative data values. In figure 15, the activation process calculates what value a node should give as an output. The Sigmoid functions most often show a return data value of the y-axis in the range between 0 to 1, as shown in figure 16. Where the positive is one, and the negative is 0. When the model returns a value ≥ of 0.51, it's positive, and < 0.51 implies the image is negative—the rest of the figures give an overview of the model's matrix and ROC curve details. As in the case of the figure showcase of the healthcare conversation between the parents, the dialogue is either tagged as accurate as positive feedback or false as negative feedback.

Figure 15. The outcome of the result either true or false values based on the text classification

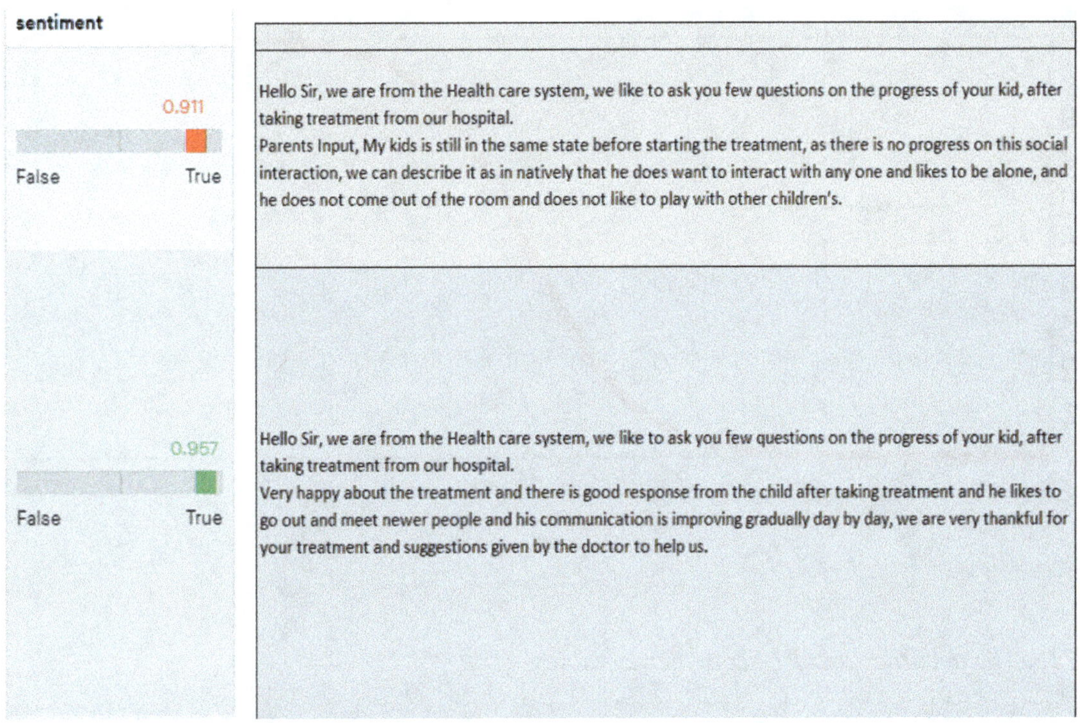

Figure 16. The flow diagram of the BERT model

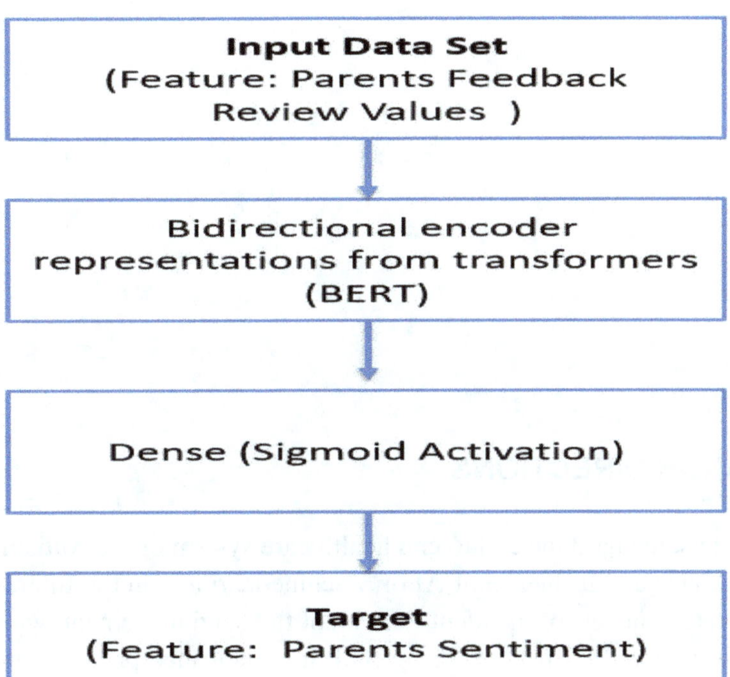

Figure 17. Y-axis value of the sigmoid function

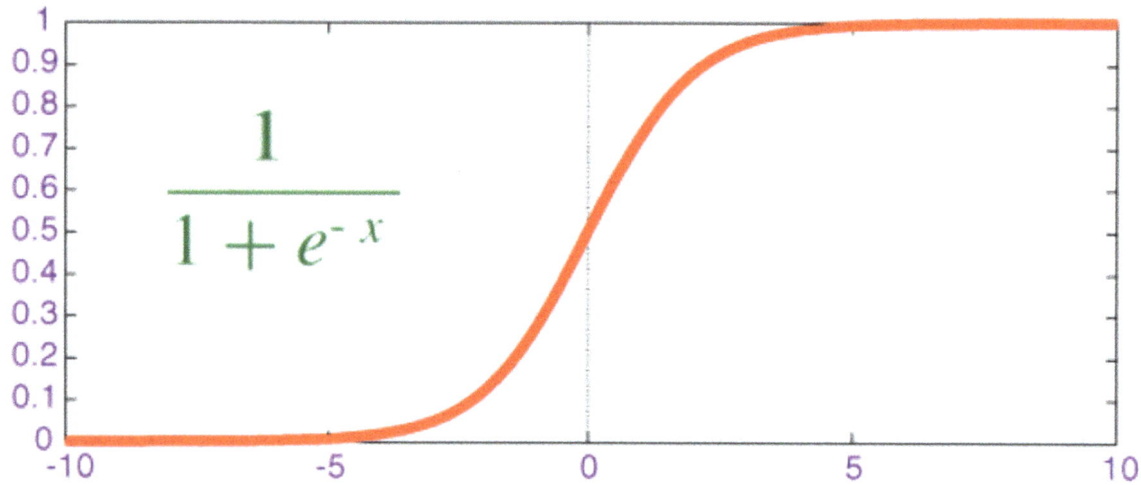

Figure 18. The accuracy and F1-score metrix values

Metric (y axis)	Validation	Training
Binary crossentropy (loss)	0.338	0.491
Accuracy	0.847	0.740
Recall	0.870	0.723
Precision	0.834	0.747
F1-score	0.852	0.735
PR AUC	0.929	0.838
ROC AUC	0.931	0.836
Error	0.153	0.260

FUTURE RESEARCH DIRECTIONS

The core objective is to safe guard the end to end health care system of the Autism Spectrum Disorder (ASD) using Smart Device and Influence of AI or Machine learning, in the future work to use the 2D or 3D computer vision techniques for the identification of the hand movement, with eye tracking of the Autism Spectrum Disorder (ASD) patient, along with more advance process can be integrated with

Quantum Artificial Intelligence sensors. As these process allow more detail information gather at faster phase, and these information can be shared across to the health care physician for detail analyses of the patient data accordingly recommend appropriate medication with in stipulated time limit.

CONCLUSION

From the above summary review survey, it is observed that social aspects play a significant role in primary diagnosis, management and identification of ASD, as well as the smart devices, play the vital roles in quicker identification of the autism spectrum disorder, the data collected out of these devices can effectively be analyzed using a machine learning algorithm. Its significance is that AI plays a vital role in predicting the correct issues in the autism spectrum disorder. Based on the above summary review, we will focus our research more on improving the machine learning model and bringing a novel approach to analyze autism spectrum disorder data set values. The system also needs to be enhanced using advanced technologies such as the use of the blockchain to provide the security of the individual customer data or protect the data, where the data can be encapsulated into the block chain and sent across to multiple health care centers without leakage of the customer data.

REFERENCES

Abhirami, A., & Sudheesh, P. (2019). Detection and Tracking of Anxiety Related Diseases for Autism Spectrum Disorder Using ECG. *2019 International Conference on Communication and Electronics Systems (ICCES)*, 1044-1052. 10.1109/ICCES45898.2019.9002160

Ahmadi, S. M. M., Mohajeri, N., & Soltanian-Zadeh, H. (2014). Connectivity abnormalities in autism spectrum disorder patients: A resting state fMRI study. *2014 22nd Iranian Conference on Electrical Engineering (ICEE),* 1878-1882. 10.1109/IranianCEE.2014.6999846

Anurekha, G., & Geetha, P. (2018). Evidence Based Adaptive Neuro-Fuzzy Inference System for ASD Detection. *2018 3rd IEEE International Conference on Recent Trends in Electronics, Information & Communication Technology (RTEICT),* 2188-2192. 10.1109/RTEICT42901.2018.9012400

Aslam, A. R., Hafeez, N., Heidari, H., & Altaf, M. A. B. (2021). An 8.62 μ W Processor for Autism Spectrum Disorder Classification using Shallow Neural Network. *2021 IEEE 3rd International Conference on Artificial Intelligence Circuits and Systems (AICAS),* 1-4. 10.1109/AICAS51828.2021.9458412

Cheng, Y., Luo, S., & Lin, H. (2016). Investigating the Performance on Comprehending 3D Social Emotion through a Mobile Learning System for Individuals with Autistic Spectrum Disorder. *2016 5th IIAI International Congress on Advanced Applied Informatics (IIAI-AAI),* 414-417. 10.1109/IIAI-AAI.2016.138

Cherdal, S., & Mouline, S. (2016). A Petri Net model to simulate and analyse cerebral folate deficiency and hyperhomocysteinemia effects in Autism Spectrum Disorder. *2016 7th International Conference on Sciences of Electronics, Technologies of Information and Telecommunications (SETIT),* 279-284. 10.1109/SETIT.2016.7939880

Chrisman, B. (2018). Analysis of Sex and Recurrence Ratios in Simplex and Multiplex Autism Spectrum Disorder Implicates Sex-Specific Alleles as Inheritance Mechanism. *2018 IEEE International Conference on Bioinformatics and Biomedicine (BIBM)*, 1470-1477. 10.1109/BIBM.2018.8621554

Dris, A. B., Alsalman, A., Al-Wabil, A., & Aldosari, M. (2019). Intelligent Gaze-Based Screening System for Autism. *2nd International Conference on Computer Applications & Information Security (ICCAIS)*, 1-5. 10.1109/CAIS.2019.8769452

Fadhil, T. Z., & Mandeel, A. R. (2018). Live Monitoring System for Recognizing Varied Emotions of Autistic Children. *2018 International Conference on Advanced Science and Engineering (ICOASE)*, 151-155. 10.1109/ICOASE.2018.8548931

Fadi, A., Carette, R., Elbattah, M., Dequen, G., Guérin, J.-L., & Cilia, F. (2018). Visualization of Eye-Tracking Patterns in Autism Spectrum Disorder: Method and Dataset. *2018 Thirteenth International Conference on Digital Information Management (ICDIM)*, 248-253. 10.1109/ICDIM.2018.8846967

Gamaethige, C., Gunathilake, U., Jayasena, D., Manike, H., Samarasinghe, P., & Yatanwala, T. (2017). "SenseA"-Autism Early Signs and Pre-Aggressive Detector through Image Processing. *2017 Asia Modelling Symposium (AMS)*, 125-130. 10.1109/AMS.2017.28

Gupta, S. (2020). Smartphone based Early Detection of Epileptic Seizures Using Machine Learning. *Proceedings of the 2020 12th International Conference on Bioinformatics and Biomedical Technology*. 10.1145/3405758.3405763

Hu, Z., Wang, J., Zhang, C., Luo, Z., Luo, X., Xiao, L., & Shi, J. (2021). Uncertainty Modeling for Multi center Autism Spectrum Disorder Classification Using Takagi-Sugeno-Kang Fuzzy Systems. *IEEE Transactions on Cognitive and Developmental Systems*, 1. Advance online publication. doi:10.1109/TCDS.2021.3073368

Huang, F., Elazab, A., OuYang, L., Tan, J., Wang, T., & Lei, B. (2019). Sparse Low-rank Constrained Adaptive Structure Learning using Multi-template for Autism Spectrum Disorder Diagnosis. *2019 IEEE 16th International Symposium on Biomedical Imaging (ISBI 2019)*, 1555-1558. 10.1109/ISBI.2019.8759487

Islam, S., Akter, T., Zakir, S., Sabreen, S., & Hossain, M. I. (2020). Autism Spectrum Disorder Detection in Toddlers for Early Diagnosis Using Machine Learning. *2020 IEEE Asia-Pacific Conference on Computer Science and Data Engineering (CSDE)*, 1-6. 10.1109/CSDE50874.2020.9411531

K. & Jaganathan. (2021). Graph Convolutional Model to Diagnose Autism Spectrum Disorder Using Rs-Fmri Data. *2021 5th International Conference on Computer, Communication and Signal Processing (ICCCSP)*, 1-5. 10.1109/ICCCSP52374.2021.9465490

Liu, M., An, Y., Hu, X., Langer, D., Newschaffer, C., & Shea, L. (2013). An evaluation of identification of suspected autism spectrum disorder (ASD) cases in early intervention (EI) records. *2013 IEEE International Conference on Bioinformatics and Biomedicine*, 566-571. 10.1109/BIBM.2013.6732559

Matsumoto, S., Horiguchi, S., Shigeno, H., & Okada, K. (2016). Visual Effect on the Odor Identification Ability of Children with Autism Spectrum Disorder. *2016 IEEE International Conference on Healthcare Informatics (ICHI)*, 349-355. 10.1109/ICHI.2016.63

Matthew, Yang, Islam, & Khaled. (2019). Functional connectivity magnetic resonance imaging classification of autism spectrum disorder using the multisite ABIDE dataset. *2019 IEEE EMBS International Conference on Biomedical & Health Informatics (BHI)*, 1-4. 10.1109/BHI.2019.8834653

Misman, M. F. (2019). Classification of Adults with Autism Spectrum Disorder using Deep Neural Network. *2019 1st International Conference on Artificial Intelligence and Data Sciences (AiDAS)*, 29-34. 10.1109/AiDAS47888.2019.8970823

Mohd, M. S., Aimie-Salleh, N., Wahab, A. H. A., Sahalan, M., & Ashari, U. M. M. (2020). Heart Rate Variability Response on Autism Spectrum Disorder and Typical Development Children. *2020 4th International Symposium on Multidisciplinary Studies and Innovative Technologies (ISMSIT)*, 1-3. 10.1109/ISMSIT50672.2020.9255015

Muty, N., & Azizul, Z. (2016). Detecting arm flapping in children with Autism Spectrum Disorder using human pose estimation and skeletal representation algorithms. *2016 International Conference On Advanced Informatics: Concepts, Theory And Application (ICAICTA)*, 1-6. 10.1109/ICAICTA.2016.7803118

Omar, Mishra, & Bajpai. (2018). Machine Learning Techniques to Predict Autism Spectrum Disorder. *2018 IEEE Punecon*, 1-5. . doi:10.1109/PUNECON.2018.8745405

Orlandi, S., Manfredi, C., Bocchi, L., & Scattoni, M. L. (2012). Automatic newborn cry analysis: A Non-invasive tool to help autism early diagnosis. *Annual International Conference of the IEEE Engineering in Medicine and Biology Society*, 2953-2956. 10.1109/EMBC.2012.6346583

Othman, M., & Wahab, A. (2010). Affective face processing analysis in autism using electroencephalogram. *Proceeding of the 3rd International Conference on Information and Communication Technology for the Moslem World (ICT4M)*, E23-E27. 10.1109/ICT4M.2010.5971907

Qidwai, U., & Connor, O. (2018). A General Purpose Game Module for Children with Autism Spectrum Disorder. *2018 IEEE-EMBS Conference on Biomedical Engineering and Sciences (IECBES)*, 426-431. 10.1109/IECBES.2018.8626699

Ramirez-Duque, A. A., Frizera-Neto, A., & Bastos, T. F. (2018). Robot-Assisted Diagnosis for Children with Autism Spectrum Disorder Based on Automated Analysis of Nonverbal Cues. *2018 7th IEEE International Conference on Biomedical Robotics and Biomechatronics (Biorob)*, 456-461. 10.1109/BIOROB.2018.8487909

Roopa, B. S., & Manjunatha Prasad, R. (2019). Concatenating framework in ASD analysis towards research progress. *2019 1st International Conference on Advanced Technologies in Intelligent Control, Environment, Computing & Communication Engineering (ICATIECE)*, 269-271. 10.1109/ICATIECE45860.2019.9063816

Sadato, N., & Tanabe, H. C. (2012). Neural substrates and inter-individual functional connectivity during mutual gaze and joint attention using dual functional MRI. *2012 ICME International Conference on Complex Medical Engineering (CME)*, 527-530. 10.1109/ICCME.2012.6275596

Samad, M. D., Diawara, N., Bobzien, J. L., Harrington, J. W., Witherow, M. A., & Iftekharuddin, K. M. (2018, February). A Feasibility Study of Autism Behavioral Markers in Spontaneous Facial, Visual, and Hand Movement Response Data. *IEEE Transactions on Neural Systems and Rehabilitation Engineering*, *26*(2), 353–361. doi:10.1109/TNSRE.2017.2768482 PMID:29432106

Saranya & Anandan. (2021). Autism Spectrum Prognosis using Worm Optimized Extreme Learning Machine (WOEM) Technique. *2021 International Conference on Advance Computing and Innovative Technologies in Engineering (ICACITE)*, 636-641. 10.1109/ICACITE51222.2021.9404729

Taffoni, F., Focaroli, V., Keller, F., & Iverson, J. M. (2014). A technological approach to studying motor planning ability in children at high risk for ASD. *2014 36th Annual International Conference of the IEEE Engineering in Medicine and Biology Society*, 3638-3641. 10.1109/EMBC.2014.6944411

Taha Ahmed, Z. A., & Jadhav, M. E. (2020). A Review of Early Detection of Autism Based on Eye-Tracking and Sensing Technology. *International Conference on Inventive Computation Technologies (ICICT)*, 160-166. 10.1109/ICICT48043.2020.9112493

Vittorias, J., Petrantonakis, P., Bolis, D., Tsiligkyri, A., Kosmidou, V., & Hadjileontiadis, L. J. (2008). NOESIS: An Enhanced Educational Environment for Kids with Autism Spectrum Disorders. *2008 Eighth IEEE International Conference on Advanced Learning Technologies*, 1019-1020. 10.1109/ICALT.2008.44

Wang, J., Wang, Q., Zhang, H., Chen, J., Wang, S., & Shen, D. (2018). Sparse Multiview Task-Centralized Ensemble Learning for ASD Diagnosis Based on Age- and Sex-Related Functional Connectivity Patterns. IEEE Transactions on Cybernetics, 49(8), 3141-3154. doi:10.1109/TCYB.2018.2839693

Wedyan, M., & Al-Jumaily, A. (2016). Early diagnosis autism based on upper limb motor coordination in high risk subjects for autism. *IEEE International Symposium on Robotics and Intelligent Sensors (IRIS)*, 13-18. 10.1109/IRIS.2016.8066059

Wu, C., Liaqat, S., Cheung, S.-c., Chuah, C.-N., & Ozonoff, S. (2019). Predicting Autism Diagnosis using Image with Fixations and Synthetic Saccade Patterns. *2019 IEEE International Conference on Multimedia & Expo Workshops (ICMEW)*, 647-650. 10.1109/ICMEW.2019.00125

Zhang, M., Ma, Y., Zheng, L., Wang, Y., Liu, Z., & Ma, J. (2019). Comparison of Neural Networks' Performance in Early Screening of Autism Spectrum Disorders Under Two MRI Principles. *2019 International Conference on Networking and Network Applications (NaNA)*, 338-343. 10.1109/NaNA.2019.00065

KEY TERMS AND DEFINITIONS

AI: Artificial Intelligence.
ANN: Artificial Neural Network.
ASD: Autism Spectrum Disorder
BERT: Bidirectional Encoder Representations from Transformers.
CAD: Classic Autistic Disorder.
CDD: Childhood Disintegrative Disorder.
CRF-CART: Combining Random Forest-Classification and Regression Trees.

EEG: Electroencephalography.
FC: Random forest classifier.
fMRI: Functional Magnetic Resonance Image.
HS: Heller Syndrome.
IoT: Internet of Things.
IQ: Intelligence quotient.
LDA: Latent Dirichlet allocation.
ML: Machine Learning.
MRI: Magnetic Resonance Image.
PCA: Principal component analysis.
PDD-NOS: Pervasive Developmental Disorder – Not Otherwise Specified.
RF-Id3: Random Forest Iterative Dichotomiser.
ROC Curve: Receiver operating characteristic.
SVM: Support Vector Machine Algorithm.
US: Untied States.

Chapter 11
Artificial Intelligence, Machine Learning, and Internet of Drones in Medical Applications

Kavya J.
ICAR Sugarcane Breeding Institute, Coimbatore, India

Prasad G.
Dayananda Sagar University, Bangalore, India

Bharanidharan N.
Dayananda Sagar University, Bangalore, India

ABSTRACT

Internet of drones (IOD) plays an important role in the delivery of emergency medicine to remote locations. Furthermore, it is employed for blood transfer, disaster assistance, missing persons, discovering lost hikers in the hill station, and a variety of other emergency services. The use of drones for emergency response services, particularly in medical circumstances, offers new avenues for life-saving interventions. Using drones to have "eyes" on a risky scenario or to transport medical supplies to stranded patients may increase the capacity of emergency response physicians to provide care in dangerous conditions. IOD provides several emergency response services that have an influence on daily life. The Federal Aviation Administration (FAA) conducts completely autonomous missions beyond visual range and flights above people to provide critical medical supplies. Artificial intelligence and machine learning are the future of the unmanned aerial vehicle in multiple applications.

INTRODUCTION

As a result of rapid technological advancement, the aviation industry has undergone a paradigm shift. The introduction of unmanned aerial systems has aided in this. Advances in Unmanned Aerial Vehicle (UAV) technology have benefited military operations, civil applications, agricultural applications, and research and development. Unmanned aerial vehicles (UAVs) are attracting operators, manufacturers,

DOI: 10.4018/978-1-7998-9534-3.ch011

and industries from all over the world. Unmanned aerial vehicles (UAVs) are aircraft that do not have a human pilot on board. In recent years, unmanned aerial vehicles (UAVs) have grown in popularity in the field of research and development. The duration of flight (endurance) and the distance travelled are the two performance metrics that are examined (range). The two most significant limitations of UAVs are battery power and payload. To predict the performance characteristics of UAVs, the experimental work must be performed as a real-time problem. As a result, the range and endurance required for completing tasks with a UAV can be calculated (Balasingam et al., 2017; Sun, G et al., 2021).

Smaller aircraft, such as unmanned aerial vehicles (UAVs), are now being developed for a variety of applications. The main advantage is that, when compared to large planes, the cost and training requirements are significantly lower. These UAVs can also be controlled manually or programmed to fly autonomously. The functional capacity of the UAV varies greatly depending on the model (Bogle et al.,2019; Li, H. et al.,2021). Drones used for military purposes can reach speeds of up to 45 m/s, whereas small rotary wings can only reach speeds of 17–26 m/s. A UAV's flying time, endurance, and payload vary depending on its size. Small unmanned aerial vehicles (UAVs) have a payload capacity of 3–4 kg and a range of 20–40 minutes. Furthermore, depending on payload and fuel supply, small UAVs typically have a range of 32–96 kilometres. Military unmanned aerial vehicles, on the other hand, have a range of 1,500 kilometres (Amukele et al., 2016; Hua, M et al., 2021).

Drone technology for healthcare is still in its infancy in advanced countries. Much of the existing research in developed countries is theoretical and focuses on how to organise drone technology applications in healthcare (Braun et al., 2019). This article aims to map actual drone technology applications in industrial countries for healthcare and other health-related goals. The article's concept is to: (1) describe how drones are being used for healthcare in developed countries; (2) synthesise the knowledge base being generated in published descriptions of various applications; and (3) identify knowledge gaps within that foundation. This study provides an overview of the use of drones for healthcare and health-related purposes in developed countries and suggests future research objectives.

BACKGROUND

In this sample, various healthcare participants were extensively studied, including those involved in biomedical supply transport, emergency first responders, and telemedicine providers. While these are natural categories for academics seeking to have their drone applications implemented by healthcare policy and decision makers, little thought was given to how such applications might affect patient groups and communities. This begs the question of who is developing drone health applications and why. Eight of the studies had no authors with a background in health, medicine, or health-related fields. Working with target communities was advocated by less than one-third of the author groups (Claesson et al., 2017). Even fewer people actually follow through on their invitations to participate (Mulero et al., 2017). Taken together, these characteristics of drones for health indicate that some may be more interested in leveraging the health context to advance drone technology and markets than in designing drones to meet a specific health need. While this may not be a problem in some cases, it can be a problem when people with a good understanding of patient and healthcare system needs, such as system users, front-line workers, and administrators, are not given the opportunity to develop competence and autonomy in their own field. Engagement with a broader range of users may encourage the development of health-related drone apps that take a variety of health and digital literacies into account, facilitating their long-term integration into healthcare (Glauser et al., 2018).

Global Medical Corporation is constantly developing and implementing new technologies in order to improve efficiency and productivity. Industry 5.0 refers to smart machinery and modern technology such as the Internet of Things (IOT) and big data. This medical breakthrough adds a personal human touch to boost automation and efficiency (Prasad et al., 2018; S.G. Mohamed Jebran P, 2020).

Industry 5.0 technologies appear to be appropriate for dealing with medical emergencies. This new industrial revolution will be able to meet the precise and sophisticated needs for high-quality medical components. Telemedicine can help transform the health-care system in pandemic situations by allowing people to seek medical advice while remaining physically separated. Furthermore, following remote patient screening, this technology can assist in limiting patient input to hospitals by prioritising facilities for critical patients. The demand for medical devices made with 3D printing technology is increasing rapidly. Fabric production Advanced manufacturing technology allows for the rapid production of masks, face shields, respirators, and other critical medical items. These technologies have a high likelihood of meeting individualised healthcare needs during the COVID-19 pandemic. Industry 5.0 technologies create a new virtual working platform during the lockdown.

INTERNET OF THINGS IN INDUSTRY 5.0

Industry 5.0 technologies appear to be appropriate for dealing with medical emergencies. This new industrial revolution will be able to meet the precise and sophisticated needs for high-quality medical components.

The fifth industrial revolution is known as Industry 5.0. It consists of wirelessly connected novel technologies that can be used to improve manufacturing and healthcare automation. Industry 5.0 is a new technological innovation that improves the interaction between humans and machines. It introduced cutting-edge technology for the production of goods and services that are environmentally friendly, efficient, and safe. The concept of Industry 5.0 is gaining traction as smart and creative technologies emerge.

The Internet of Everything (IOE) is a technology that expands on the Internet of Things concept (IOT). In the context of IoT, it refers to a more complex domain that includes people and processes, as opposed to the machine-to-machine concept. In the event of a COVID-19 pandemic, this technology could be used to provide medical services and perform other daily tasks while maintaining social separation.

The Internet of Medical Things (IoMT) is a grouping of medical devices and software that can communicate with medical information technology systems and help manage multiple devices for multiple patients. During the COVID-19 epidemic, this technique could be useful in managing a limited number of ventilators for many patients.

Artificial intelligence (AI) is a tool that can help track the virus's spread and isolate high-risk patients. Furthermore, previous patient data can be used to estimate the risk of mortality (P. M. Jebran & S. Gupta, 2020; Bharanidharan N & Rajaguru H., 2020). Drones are unmanned flying machines that can be used for a variety of purposes, including surveillance to enforce social distancing norms, disinfectant spraying in affected areas without human intervention, delivery of essential commodities, medicines, and grocery items to affected areas, broadcast of critical information, and even temperature monitoring during COVID-19 scenarios (Rosser et al., 2018). Thanks to Industry 5.0 technologies, all machines and medical devices used in healthcare can now be connected. It is possible to improve machine-to-machine communication, which aids in the efficiency of the treatment process. Robots have been tasked with reducing the workload of healthcare workers, improving their safety, and lowering the risk of infection.

METHODOLOGY

Each flight controller has its own set of codes, which are kept up to date by software called Flight Control Software or Flight Controller Configurator. There is a diverse selection of flight controller software available. Each one is typically centred on a specific piece of hardware, technology, or goal. In this post, we've compiled a list of the top three flight controller firmware and software options, as well as some thoughts on each. This will give you a good idea of what is available and allow you to decide which you want to use or participate in. Instead of racing and freestyle software, Flight Controller Configurators are used in professional drones for industrial applications.

1. ArduPilot
2. PX4
3. FlightStack
4. iNAV

Unmanned aerial vehicles (UAVs), also known as drones, are emerging as a new medical tool capable of assisting in the alleviation of logistical issues and the improvement of health-care distribution. According to experts, drones could be used for everything from disaster relief to transferring transplant organs and blood samples. Drones can carry small payloads and deliver them quickly to their target. Figure. 1 shows Application use of medical drones.

Figure 1. Application use of medical drones

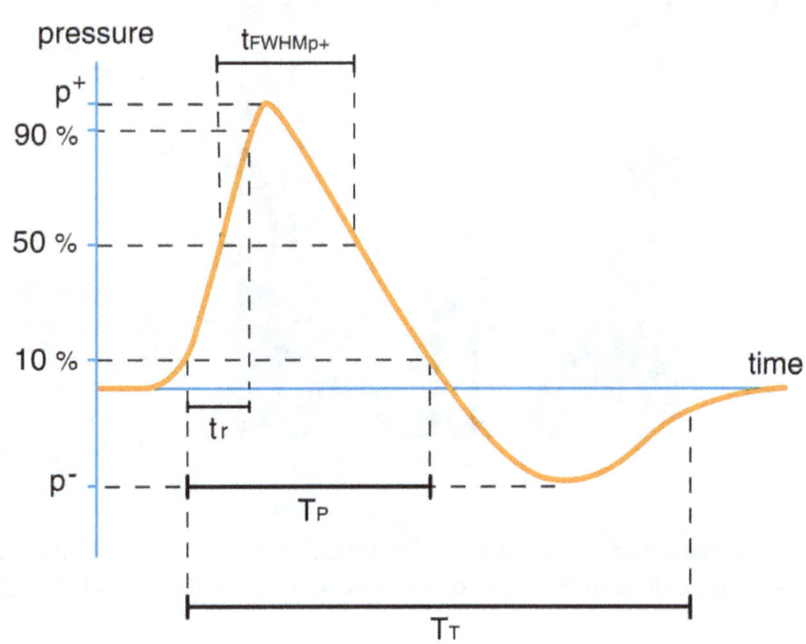

1) **Transportation of blood products and hazardous materials:** Hazardous materials must be transported safely and in accordance with hazmat laws. Because it's currently being done, this isn't necessarily a use case that fills an unmet need in the medical industry; however, it's quite expensive in many cases and time-sensitive in others.
2) **Vaccine and drug delivery:** Drones can improve access to and the speed with which life-saving pharmaceuticals and vaccines are delivered. Wingcopter, for example, provided immunizations for children in Vanuatu, a Pacific island nation, three years ago.
3) **Diagnostics:** One of the most common applications for drones is diagnostics. Because some diagnostic procedures are time and temperature sensitive, a patient sample must be submitted to the lab and the test must be completed within a specific timeframe, which could be as little as 2 hours. This is where unconnected communities come into play, and drones play a significant and growing role.
4) **Organ transfers:** Due to the short time frame for transferring organs from donor to patient, which can range from 4 to 36 hours depending on the organ type1, ultra-rapid transportation, such as a private jet charter or a helicopter, is required. The use of drones can make organ delivery faster, safer, and more cost-effective.

Figure 2. Revenue of Drones during the period of 2016 to 2025

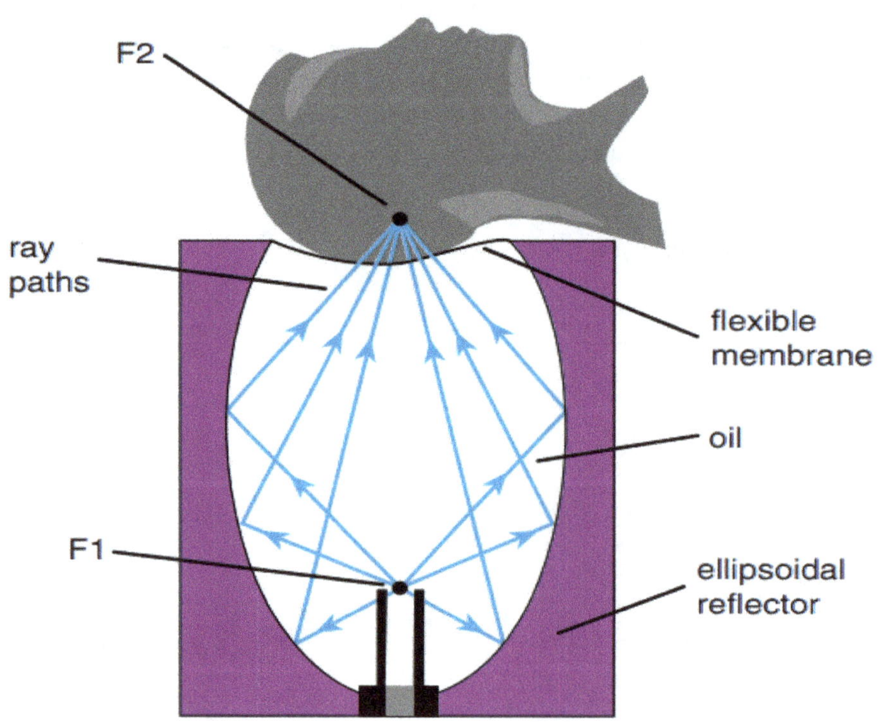

Figure 2 depicts the Revenue of Drones during the period of 2016 to 2025. Drones can also be used to transport small medical devices such as automated external defibrillators (AEDs). Some businesses have inquired as to whether our drone can transport AEDs or other minor medical devices from a hospital or emergency medical services to an accident or disaster site. The answer is yes; unfortunately, aviation officials will not allow this to happen right now, but it will undoubtedly happen in the future. Drone technology has several advantages over traditional modes of transportation, including the ability to avoid traffic in congested areas, bad road conditions when the terrain is difficult to manoeuvre, and safely reaching risky fly zones in war-torn countries. Despite the fact that drones are still underutilised in emergency situations and relief efforts, their contributions are being recognised more widely (Robakowska et al., 2019).

Although digital twins are used in engineering, health care, and urban planning, in most cases, each twin is a one-of-a-kind, proprietary solution that only works with a single application. The digital twin detects changes in the UAV's general state over time (due to processes such as mechanical wear and tear and logged flight time, among others) and updates its own state to match the physical UAV. This updated digital twin can then forecast how the UAV will evolve in the future, allowing the physical asset to be directed more effectively. The graphical model allows each digital twin "to be built on the same underlying computational model, but each physical asset must retain a distinct 'digital state,' resulting in a unique model configuration." The UAV was used for a variety of purposes, including calibration studies and a simulated "minor damage" scenario. Its digital twin was able to extract damage information from sensor data, predict how the structural health of the UAV would change in the future, and recommend manoeuvring changes to accommodate those changes (Zaman et al., 2017). In unmanned aerial vehicles (UAVs), augmented reality (AR) and virtual reality (VR) are popular technologies that can improve UAV operation by providing new ways to provide a digital context and feedback over a depiction of a real scenario. This section discusses how to build AR experiences and the technology required, as well as Web AR as a platform-independent alternative, and highlights the current state of augmented reality and examples of its application. The education, entertainment, tourism, fitness, and gaming industries are driving the growth of augmented reality (AR), virtual reality (VR), drones, and robots. Users of virtual reality equipment are immersed in a completely simulated environment through sight and sound, giving the impression that they are in a completely different location. In contrast, augmented reality (AR) augments the real world with intelligent data by digitally improving existing environments, such as 3D maps or scores and plays overlaid on sports telecasts, to make them more interactive and meaningful to the user. AR and VR devices are expected to grow rapidly, at rates comparable to smartphones. To achieve this level of growth, devices must become smaller, more compact, and more fashionable. For AR/VR applications, simultaneous location and mapping (SLAM) is a must-have feature. It entails mapping the room and extracting features from the environment around the user for positional tracking. Avoidance of Drone Collisions Consumer drones for aerial photography have grown in popularity as collision-avoidance technology has reduced crashes. Drones benefit from image sensors with ultra-high-resolution 4K video and global shutters. Pass-Through Viewing for Virtual Reality Headsets Pass-through viewing for virtual reality headsets allows users to move around the real world while playing in the virtual world without colliding with objects (Thiels et al., 2015; Feng, T et al., 2020). Fast frame rate imaging and global shutter technology with RGB sensors are two imaging methods that enable this. Human-Computer Interaction VR/IR applications with gesture-tracking capabilities enable human-computer interactions. Infrared (IR) light sources illuminate the area around the head-mounted display, while global shutter sensors with high near-IR (NIR) sensitivity record hand motions.

CONCLUSION

Drones for medical purposes have a number of benefits, including quick assistance, reduced travel time to the patient, reduced complications in the injured due to less time to wait for rescue, support and improvement of basic operations of medical emergency teams, and the ability to reach places inaccessible to basic medical transport (e.g., due to floods). Industry 5.0 improves smart manufacturing and a suitable information system in healthcare. It makes a significant contribution to the advancement of medical devices and instruments, ultimately improving the overall performance of the treatment process.

It is, however, critical to be aware of the current regulations. There are various safety awareness initiatives, but neither they nor the most perfect rules will protect against the dangers posed by the presence of a drone in an area where it was not intended. The appearance of an unmanned aircraft in controlled space has been identified as a global concern that poses a threat to aviation safety. Two examples are filming a large passenger plane from a close distance and disrupting the approach to an international airport due to the detection of a drone.

Although this sample demonstrates a wide range of healthcare and health-related drone applications in many developed countries, more research is required to fully comprehend the implications of their incorporation into healthcare services. More research should be conducted to see how involving patients, healthcare professionals, and cultural groups in drone development affects their digital and health literacy. This will ensure that as many end-user groups as possible are involved in their design and application; it will enable drone developers to design technologies that meet the current needs of their target populations; and it will gain acceptance and support from rural, remote, and Indigenous communities, which are often wary of outside interventions. Greater research into the costs of integrating various drone applications into existing healthcare services—including financial, human, and healthcare quality costs—is required to obtain a more holistic picture of how adopting various drone applications will influence a community. Such research could provide healthcare policymakers and decision-makers with the knowledge they need to integrate drones into the healthcare and health-related needs of their communities.

ACKNOWLEDGMENT

We acknowledge all the staff members of Aerospace Engineering, Dayananda Sagar University, Bangalore, India for the constant support and encouragement to carry out the research. I also thank Dr. K.N.B. Murthy (Vice Chancellor), Dr. A. Srinivas (Dean), Dr. BVN Ramakumar (Head of the Department), Dayananda Sagar University, Bangalore, India. I also thank my family members for the understanding and encouragement to preserve the research work. This research received fund from The Institution of Engineers (India) Ref No. R.4/2/UG/2017-18/RDUG2017026 and Tamilnadu State Council for Science and Technology Ref No. TNSCST/DIT/03/VR/2017-2018.

REFERENCES

Amukele, Ness, Tobian, Boyd, & Street. (2017). Drone transportation of blood products. *Transfusion*, *57*(3), 582–588.

Balasingam. (2017). Drones in medicine—the rise of the machines. *International Journal of Clinical Practice*, *71*(9). doi:10.1111/ijcp.12989

Bharanidharan, N., & Rajaguru, H. (2020). Performance enhancement of swarm intelligence techniques in dementia classification using dragonfly-based hybrid algorithms. *International Journal of Imaging Systems and Technology*, *30*, 57–74.

Braun, Gertz, & Furer. (2019). The promising future of drones in prehospital medical care and its application to battlefield medicine. *The Journal of Trauma and Acute Care Surgery*, *87*, S28–S34.

Bogle, Rosamond, Snyder, & Zègre-Hemsey. (2019). The case for droneassisted emergency response to cardiac arrest: An optimized statewide deployment approach. *North Carolina Medical Journal*, *80*(4), 204–212.

Claesson, Svensson, & Nordberg. (2017). Drones may be used to save lives in out of hospital cardiac arrest due to drowning. *Resuscitation*, *114*, 152–156.

Sachan, D. (2016). The age of drones: What might it mean for health? *Lancet*, *387*, 1803–1804.

Feng, T., Xie, L., Yao, J., & Xu, J. (in press). UAV-Enabled Data Collection for Wireless Sensor Networks with Distributed Beamforming. *IEEE Transactions on Wireless Communications*. Advance online publication. doi:10.1109/TWC.2021.3103739

Hua, M., Yang, L., Wu, Q., Li, C., & Swindlehurst, A. L. (2021). UAV-Assisted Intelligent Reflecting Surface Symbiotic Radio System. *IEEE Transactions on Wireless Communications*, *20*(9), 5769–5785.

Mulero-Pázmány, Jenni-Eiermann, & Strebel, Sattler, Negro, & Tablado. (2017). Unmanned aircraft systems as a new source of disturbance for wildlife: A systematic review. *PLoS One*, *12*(6).

Glauser. (2018). Blood-delivering drones saving lives in Africa and maybe soon in Canada. Canadian Medical Association Journal, 190(3), E88–E89.

Li, H., Li, J., Liu, M., Ding, Z., & Gong, F. (2021). Energy Harvesting and Resource Allocation for Cache-Enabled UAV Based IoT NOMA Networks. *IEEE Transactions on Vehicular Technology*, *70*(9), 9625–9630.

Prasad, G., Abhishek, P., & Karthick, R. (2018). Influence of Unmanned Aerial Vehicle in Medical Product Transport. *International Journal of Intelligent Unmanned Systems*, *7*(2), 88–94.

Jebran, P. M., & Gupta, S. (2021). Pre-Diabetic Retinopathy identification using hybridGenetic Algorithm-Neural Network classifier. *Journal of Physics: Conference Series*.

Rosser Jr., Parker, & Vignesh. (2018). Medical applications of drones for disaster relief: A review of the literature. *Surgical Technology International*, *33*, 17–22.

Robakowska, Ślęzak, & Tyrańska-Fobke. (2019). Operational and financial considerations of using drones for medical support of mass events in Poland. *Disaster Medicine and Public Health Preparedness*, *13*(3), 527–532.

Jebran. (2020). Detection of Lesions for Diabetic Retinopathy By using Machine Learning Algorithms. *International Journal of Recent Technology and Engineering*, *8*, 1160–1166.

Sun, G., Tao, X., Li, N., & Xu, J. (2021). Intelligent reflecting surface and uav assisted secrecy communication in millimeter-wave networks. *IEEE Transactions on Vehicular Technology*, *70*(11), 11949–11961.

Thiels, Aho, & Zietlow, & Jenkins. (2015). D.H. Use of unmanned aerial vehicles for medical product transport. *Air Medical Journal*, *34*, 104–108.

Chapter 12
Application of Aerodynamic Shock Wave in Medical Treatment

Kavya J.
ICAR Sugarcane Breeding Institute, Coimbatore, India

Prasad G.
Dayananda Sagar University, Bangalore, India

Bharanidharan N.
Dayananda Sagar University, Bangalore, India

ABSTRACT

Extracorporeal shock wave therapy in orthopaedics and traumatology is a relatively new treatment modality. The advancement of shock wave treatment has been quick in recent years. Shock waves have significantly altered therapy. Shock waves are now the treatment of choice for kidney and urethral stones. Urology has traditionally been the sole medical profession that uses shock waves. Meanwhile, shock waves have been utilised to treat insertion tendinitis, avascular necrosis of the head of the femur, and other necrotic bone changes in orthopaedics and traumatology. In veterinary medicine, another field of shock wave use is the therapy of tendons, ligaments, and bones. The basic theory and applications of shock waves, as well as their history in medicine, are discussed in this study. The goal of utilising shock wave treatment for orthopaedic disorders is to stimulate healing in the tendons, surrounding tissue, and bones. Shock waves have emerged as the preferred therapy for kidney and ureteral stones.

INTRODUCTION

When it comes to shock waves, several disciplines use them, including acoustics and the sciences of sound and matter. They also play an essential part in the domains of aerodynamics, chemistry, and physics, as well as materials science, space science, and biology (Honton, B. & Laperche, C., 2021; Shukla, P et al., 2021). The vast majority of shock wave literature is technical and intended for people with a thorough

DOI: 10.4018/978-1-7998-9534-3.ch012

understanding of physics. Shock waves, on the other hand, are frequently associated with supersonic aircraft. Scientists in fields other than physics may be perplexed by this because the connection to clinically employed shock waves is obscure. Waves in front of a fast-moving item, such as an aeroplane or a bullet, can interfere constructively, creating what's known as a "bow wave." When an object accelerates, the pressure waves in front of it get closer together until they can no longer escape from the source (object) and pile up in front of it, generating the sonic boom that can be heard and felt after a supersonic aircraft has passed. Mach number is defined as the sound velocity divided by the object velocity. Shock waves in fluids, such as those employed in biomedical applications, have a low Mach number (close to one). The term "weak shock wave" refers to this phenomenon. Shock waves utilised in biomedical applications and those created by supersonic planes have certain similarities, but their genesis mechanisms differ (Jadhav, R.S. et al., 2020; Wang, M.-M.& Wu, Z.-N., 2021; Xiong, L et al., 2021).

Figure 1. Sketch of a pressure pulse waveform

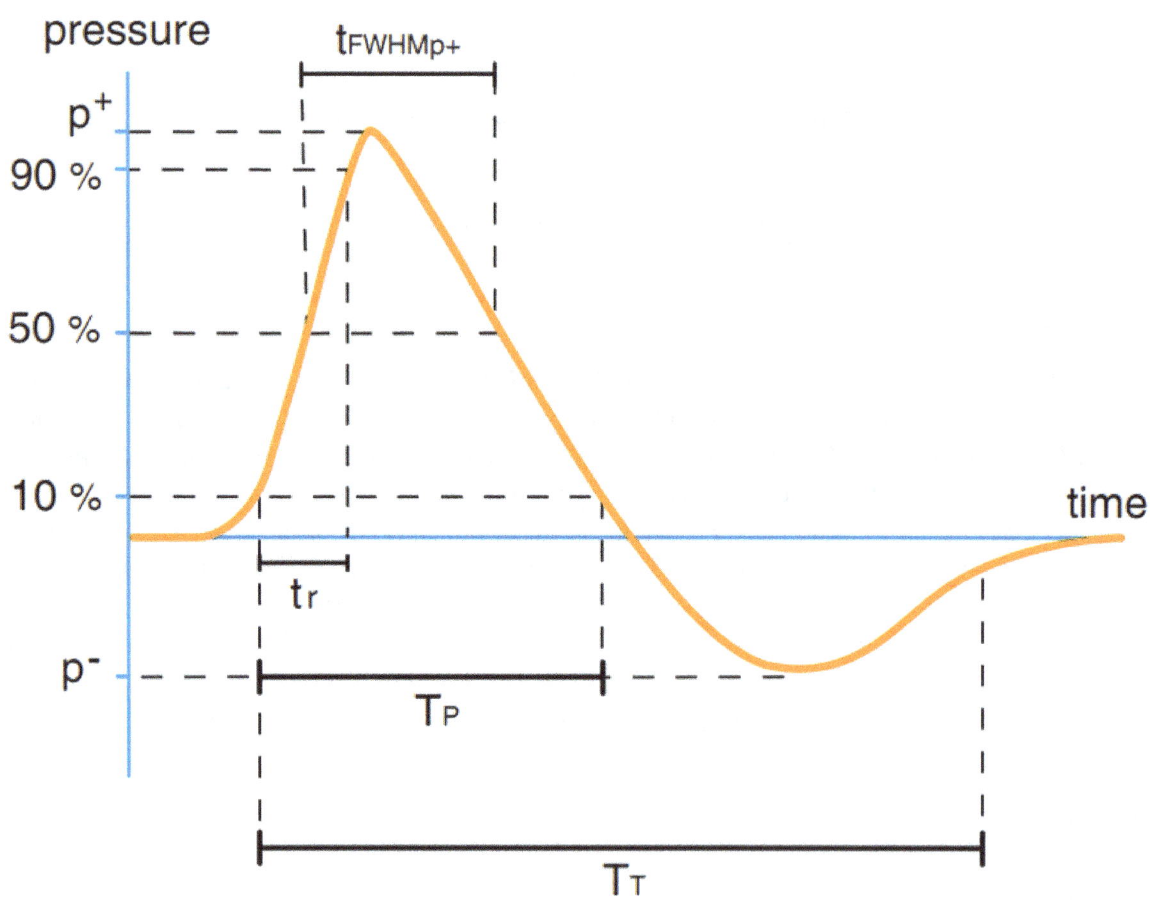

Figure 1 Sketch of a pressure pulse waveform showing the peak-positive pressure (p+), the peak-negative pressure (p−), the rise time (tr), the compressional pulse duration (t FWHMp+), the positive temporal integration limits (TP), and the total temporal integration limits (TT). In physics, the instan-

taneous pressure (p) is determined by subtracting the atmospheric pressure at a given position from the applied pressure. P+ is the highest possible compressional pressure in a pressure field at any given time. To put it another way, the peak-negative pressure is equal to the rarefactional pressure modulus (absolute value) at any given position in the pressure field. Maximum negative pressure or peak-rarefactional pressure are other names for p. It's not uncommon to have pressure recorded as negative even when it has a positive value based on the reference level that's specified as zero: pressure applied perpendicular to a surface. A location with lower air pressure than the surrounding atmosphere could serve as an illustration. The pressure trough that appears after the leading positive pressure pulse is deemed negative in studies dealing with shock wave biomedical applications. This is because the pressure value before the shock wave comes is below the pressure considered negative in these reports.

Shock wave biomedical applications have grown tremendously in the last 25 years and are now widely used in medicine for a variety of safe and efficient treatments. Shock wave lithotripsy (ESWL or SWL), i.e. the noninvasive use of shock waves to break up internal concrements, revolutionised urolithiasis treatment in the early 1990's and stimulated a lot of study in the field. Next came SWL for the treatment of gallstones and stones in the pancreaticoduodenal (CBD) as well as salivary gland ducts (SGDD). For a long time, advances in clinical equipment were made at a glacial pace (Morgan, J.P.M. et al., 2021; Eremina, G.& Smolin, A., 2021; S. G. Mohamed Jebran P, 2020). Ergonomics, user convenience, automation, imaging, and shrinking were prioritised over the fundamental concepts of how shock waves interact with the human body during the development process. Shock waves have found new uses in a variety of medical and biotechnological fields as a result of fundamental research. A growing number of reasons in orthopaedics and traumatology now benefit from extracorporeal shock wave therapy (ESWT) and radial pressure wave therapy (RPWT), such as treating calcium deposits in tendons and tendon inflammation, as well as bone and wound healing. Using shock waves to cure coronary artery disease and treat patients with fibrous plaques in the penis, relieve chronic pelvic pain syndrome, and treat erectile dysfunction and interstitial cystitis are some of the other uses for shock waves in medicine. In addition, shock waves have been examined for their bactericidal properties, and these could have applications in urology for the treatment of chronic bacterial prostatitis, along with other industries. Recent discoveries in filamentous fungus genetic transformation by shock waves may also have far-reaching implications for biotechnology in general. This piece is written with the newbie and experienced in mind. Shock wave biomedical applications cover a wide range of topics, thus readers will have some background knowledge in some areas but need it in others. Researchers in medicine, molecular biology, chemistry, and neuroscience who cooperate with shock wave physicists may benefit from this book. There are a lot of misconceptions in medicine about shock wave physics, therefore it's the physicist's job to clear up any confusion and explain the events that can arise when using concentrated shock waves and radial pressure waves. Despite the fact that there are recommendations for clinical applications, none of the sections is meant to replace specialised training in any way. Short courses should never be used in place of in-depth academic and practical teaching from specialists in the field. Most certified systems on the market can produce good results if they are utilised appropriately, following an adequate procedure, and carefully selecting patients. Because technology changes so quickly, some of the systems and procedures described here may not reflect the most recent state of the art, and it is the reader's obligation to stay up to speed before putting shock waves or radial pressure waves to use in clinical settings.

When you hear about "shock wave acupuncture," you're referring to the practise of stimulating certain receptors with shock waves or radial pressure waves in order to get results comparable to those obtained with needles. Shock wave acupuncture uses the same needles and points as traditional acupuncture.

The study of shock waves has come a long way in the previous two decades. Medical and biomedical applications are mentioned that have promising techniques and advances. Although not a summary of all shock wave research conducted around the world, it is important to note. Thrombus ablation, bone fusion augmentation to cure skull deformities and pain release in neuralgia are some of the new uses for shock waves. Oncological disorders can be treated with shock waves in several ways, including studies on gene transfection, which delivers deoxyribonucleic acid (DNA) into cells, and studies on therapeutic efficacy augmentation by enhancing the lethal effect of shock waves. An ongoing biotechnological problem is transforming filamentous bacteria and fungi. This is true in agriculture, the food and chemical industries, and pharmaceuticals. There is still a need for more efficient methods of delivering exogenous nucleic acid to bacteria and moulds. Bone repair and bacterial biofilm removal are two examples of possible uses.

EXTRACORPOREAL SHOCK WAVES THERAPY

In the noninvasive treatment of musculoskeletal injuries and pain, called extracorporeal shock wave therapy, shock waves generated outside the patient's body are delivered to the affected region in order to trigger the body's mechanisms to initiate natural healing (Schmitz et al. 2015). Shock wave therapy (ESWT) is also known as orthotripsy, extracorporeal shock wave application (ESWA), or shock wave biosurgery even though the name surgery is inappropriate for a noninvasive treatment. Extracorporeal shock wave therapy is referred to as acoustic wave therapy or extracorporeal pulse activation therapy in some publications (rESWT). Despite the fact that the therapeutic device in question generates radial pressure waves rather than shock waves, the term "ESWT" is commonly used in many papers, including this one.

A few pieces of ESWT equipment have a focused shock wave and radial pressure wave therapy head. As a result of its positive therapeutic outcomes, ESWT in the musculoskeletal system has received worldwide acclaim, particularly for treating shoulder-related conditions like tendinitis and non-union of long-bone fractures, as well as heel pain and proximal plantar fasciitis. Patients with diagnoses that are known to respond to shock waves or radial pressure waves may be evaluated for this procedure if other therapy options have been ineffective. There are minimal side effects like tingling, aching, redness, or bruising after an ESWT that lasts shorter than 30 minutes. Depending on the procedure, there may be as few as one session or as many as four. Shock waves can be targeted or not to treat a specific part of the body. Shock wave targeting may be supported by ultrasonography, fluoroscopy, or the patient's feedback, depending on the unique instance. As long as the operation is safe, shock waves or radial pressure waves can be used to relieve pain in the location that's causing it. When used in conjunction with surgery and other traditional treatment modalities, ESWT may be beneficial for a variety of orthopaedic conditions. Most, if not all, ESWT modalities do not yet have their cellular and molecular mechanisms fully elucidated.

An inadvertent osteoblastic response during animal experiments in the 1990s led to shock waves being used in areas other than lithotripsy. Shock waves had an impact on the polymethlymethacrylate (PMMA)-human femoral segment interface in vitro. Extrocorporeal shock wave lithotripters, or specially built shock wave and radial pressure wave generators suspended on articulated arms with three-dimensional movement, are now available from numerous businesses, many of which provide customised versions. The transducers used in these systems can be ballistic, electrohydraulic, electromagnetic, or piezoelectric. The FDA has approved a number of devices for use in conditions where traditional anti-inflammatory therapies like massage, physiotherapy, acupuncture, steroid injections, medicines, or immobilisation devices have failed to provide relief. These FDA-approved devices include: Minimally invasive techniques including selective tissue dissection and drug distribution have been made possible by the development of shock wave sources (Menezes et al. 2012; Rakesh et al. 2012).

Around the world, shock waves and radial pressure waves are successfully used in mechanotransduction to regenerate tissue through a complicated physical and biological process. As an alternative to stem cell therapy for ischemic heart and limb disease, shock waves with an energy flux density (EFD) of roughly 0.1 mJ/mm2 administered at a frequency of 4 Hz have been proposed. In chronic tendinopathies, ESWT is administered to patients, especially when conservative treatments fail (Furia et al 2013). Ischemic heart disease, wound healing problems (Contaldo et al., 2012), and shock waves are among the conditions for which shock and radial pressure waves have been used in clinical trials. Using shock waves to treat bone disorders such avascular necrosis, delayed union, and non-union has been shown to be successful. Shock waves can also be used to treat stress fractures (Russo et al. 2014). As a result, shockwaves and radial pressure waves are being used more and more often to treat many types of pain, including greater trochanteric pain syndrome (inflammation of the groyne area), coccydynia (pain in the area of the coccyx), and more (Marwan et al. 2014). It is also frequently used to treat a variety of other conditions, including calcaneodynia (heel pain), scapulohumeral periarthritis (inflammation of the shoulder's tendons), tennis elbow, soft tissue inflammation, diabetic foot, and non-healing wounds (Rompe et al. 2015). After total knee arthroplasty, rESWT has been utilised successfully to alleviate soft tissue pain syndromes (Gerdesmeyer and Krath 2014). Radial pressure waves may also be a viable treatment for youngsters with calcaneal apophysitis, an inflammation of the heel's growth plate that occurs between the ages of eight and fourteen (Nauck et al. 2014).

Another example of ESWT's broad range of uses is the potential use of shock waves to prevent tooth movement and restore surrounding tissues (Falkensammer et al. 2015). A high energy flux density will be employed to treat pathological calcifications, delayed unions, and avascular necrosis as will be explained in the following section. Lower energies are used on more delicate tissues, such as tendons. ESWT's success is more difficult to gauge than SWL's. Despite numerous studies describing excellent treatment outcomes, proof of the efficacy of ESWT in various settings remains ambiguous.

APPLICATION OF SHOCK WAVES ON THE HUMAN BRAIN

Extracorporeal shock wave lithotripsy, the first clinical application of shock waves, cannot be attributed to a single creator (SWL). Brilliant scientists who happened to be working on the appropriate issue at the right time made contributions to numerous other technical advancements. Unaware of the possibility of shock waves being used for medicinal purposes, it must be taken into account that moving from laboratory tests to clinical prototypes requires a lot of self-confidence, efficient coordination between physicist-engineers-medical physicians and enormous investments. SWL was a game-changer in urology and will go down in history as one of the most significant technological achievements in medicine. A natural next step for researchers was to test whether shock waves might also be used to dissolve calculi in other places of the body after they successfully used them on urinary calculi. Many previously unimagined applications emerged as a result of efforts to improve the equipment's efficiency while minimising injury to the targeted tissues. The interaction between shock waves and living tissue was the focus of several research groups, and the findings of multidisciplinary investigations began to be published.

It is true that sound waves are represented geometrically, much like light rays are, however this simplification is only accurate in a few specific situations. The geometric focus is defined as the point at which imaginary rays originating from the shock wave source or the focusing element (lens or reflector) meet in a single direction. Using a microexplosive shock wave source, Hosseini et al. (2006) investigated how cells respond after being exposed to shock waves. Interesting approaches to cardiovascular therapy and cancer treatment, as well as cranioplasty in close proximity to the brain, were all examined in another research project A 20 mm-diameter metallic reflector half-ellipsoid made up the system. In order to create a shock wave, a Q-switched Nd:YAG laser beam was used to ignite a silver azide pellet (between 1 and 20 mg) located at the focus (F1) closest to the reflector (Hosseini et al. 2005).

Shock wave therapy for orthopaedic problems quickly overtook SWL in terms of patient numbers in many countries. In today's world, shock wave biomedical applications cover such a wide range that detailing the historical evolution of each would be an enormous undertaking.

Figure 2. Schematic of a spark-gap shock wave generator (Loske 2017)

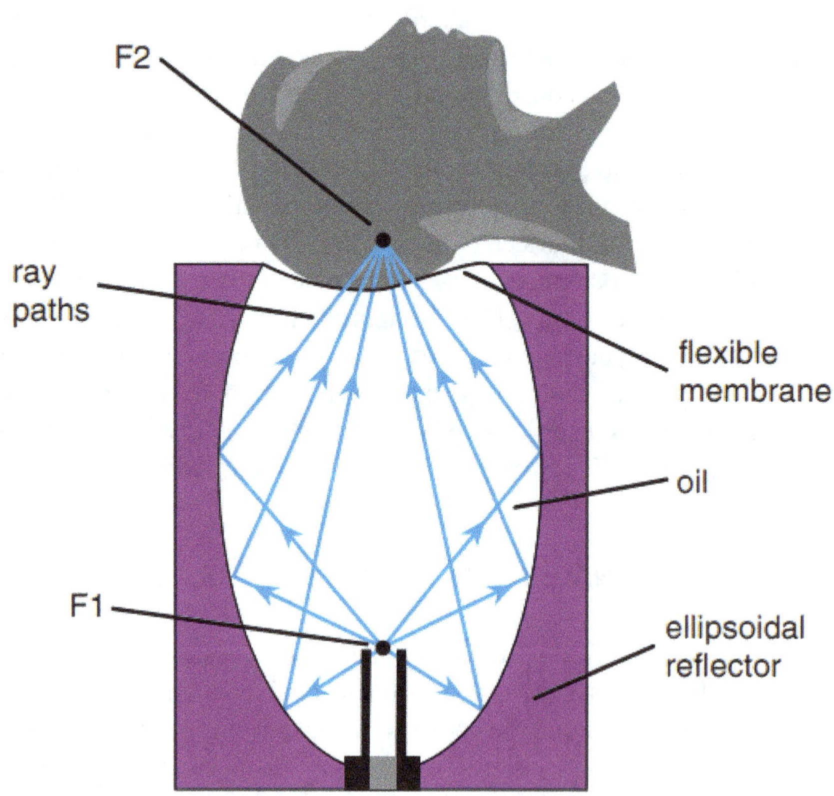

Brain tumours were meant to be destroyed by shock waves created by a high-voltage electric discharge at the inner focus of an oil-filled paraellipsoidal metallic reflector (Figure 2). Electric discharge between two electrodes at the first focus (F1) of a paraellipsoidal reflector filled with oil, similar to modern electrohydraulic shock wave generators, produces a shock wave that is reflected off the reflecting surface and focussed towards the outer focus (F2). The shock waves are transmitted to the patient via a flexible membrane. Because of this, many years elapsed before the spark-gap method was once again proposed to generate shock waves for an extracorporeal use in the medical field.

HUMAN KIDNEY STONE SHOCK WAVE APPLICATION (HOPKINSON EFFECT)

Most countries' healthcare systems struggle with urinary stone formation due to urolithiasis, the condition in which urinary stones form anywhere along the urinary tract. Urolithiasis is on the rise around the world, according to epidemiological statistics from around the world. This is likely due to rising levels of obesity and metabolic syndromes. Up to 10% of Americans are affected with kidney stones. There was an additional rise from 5.2 percent in 1994 to 8.9 percent in 2008 according to the National Health and Nutrition Examination Survey (NHANES) (Scales et al. 2012). Urinary stones affected around 9.7% of German men and 5.9% of German women aged 50 to 64 in 2000, with a recurrence rate of roughly 42%. (Hesse et al. 2003).

Because urinary stones are typically made of brittle materials, compression is a better option than tension when removing them. Shock pulses can cause fracture by converting into reflected tensile waves inside the stone. Whenever a shock wave strikes an acoustically soft interface, such as the border between a medium with high impedance (such as stone) and an area with low impedance (such as urine or soft tissue), a lot of energy is reflected. Tensile refraction occurs when the wave returns in the opposite direction of its original arrival, resulting in a high-amplitude negative pressure pulse (Figure 3). It is known that if the second medium's acoustic impedance is lower than the first, a positive pressure pulse will be received as a negative one. This occurs when incident and reflected waves combine, creating enough tension to cause cleavage, i.e. nucleation and creation of microcracks that can coalesce into larger cracks, resulting in fracture. Shock waves propagate parallel to the failure surface when they strike a flat acoustically soft interface (such as a kidney stone phantom).

Figure 3. Schematic schematic showing spallation of urinary calculi due to shock wave exposure (Hopkinson effect). The superposition of the incoming and reflected waves results in a cleavage plane towards the stone's distal side. Pressure waveforms in real life are irregular in shape and amplitude (Loske 2017)

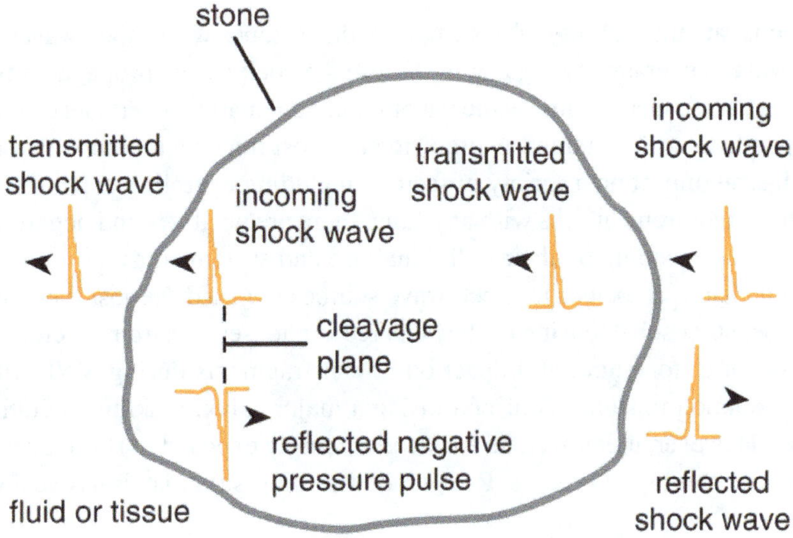

When using shock waves to commute urinary stones without the need of intrusive procedures, this is known as extracorporeal shock wave lithotripsy (litho = stone and tripsy="to crush"). For the time being, it is the only noninvasive treatment option available for the removal of urinary stones. Others include ureteroscopy (URS), which uses pneumatic, ultrasonic, or laser lithotripters to remove ureteral stones, and stone basket retrievers, which involve inserting an endoscope into the urethra and into the ureter to collect the stone basket. pneumatic, ultrasonic, or laser lithotripters are used to remove particularly hard and large kidney stones through a small calibre nephrostomy tract surgically created under radiographic or ultrasound guidance. Retrograde intrarenal surgery (RIRS) uses a laser lithotripter to perform surgery inside the kidney by passing a flexible endoscope through the bladder and ureter into the kidney. Nephrolithotomy is also known as percutaneous nephrolithotomy (SWL can also be used to break up other types of internal stones, such as those found in the pancreas, gallbladder, and salivary glands. As little harm as possible is the purpose of this device's stone pulverisation process.

Figure 4. Shock waves propagated through the water, destroying a kidney stone suspended inside the water tank (Loske 2017)

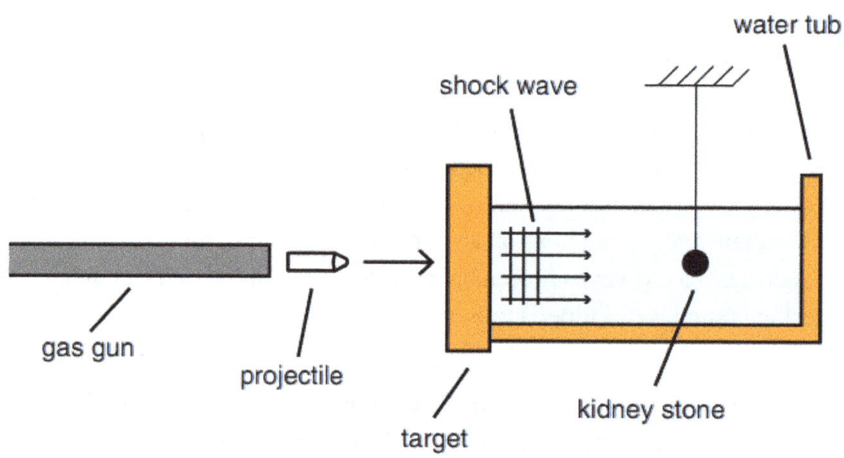

In order to demonstrate the viability of destroying kidney stones with shock waves, excrements were exposed to shock waves generated by a gas gun. Figure 4 Shock waves propagated through the water, destroying a kidney stone suspended inside the water tank. Schematic of an underwater shock wave generator using a projectile to strike a target. A lithotripter's most important component is the shock wave source. Its design has an impact on a variety of factors, including operating expenses, efficiency, tissue injury, and anaesthetic requirements. As with anything, there are positives and negative aspects to shock wave emitters that vary depending on their individual use and system configurations. Either electrohydraulic, electromagnetic or piezoelectric shock wave sources are used in most therapeutic instruments. However, they can be either self-focusing or they can require lenses or hard reflectors to focus the light.

The surroundings of a stone have an impact on how it fragments during SWL. Fluid-filled expansion chambers are common in stones confined inside a major calyx, making cavitation-induced stone commination easier. However, ureteral stone surfaces are rarely exposed to fluid, decreasing the impact of cavitation on the fragmentation process. Retrograde fluid infusion may improve SWL success rates.

For example, Bailey and colleagues (2005) found that inserting an intraurethral catheter with an X-ray contrast agent increased cavitation and aided stone dissolution. There have also been recent proposals for the use of ex vivo produced micro bubbles that contain bisphosphonates that attach precisely to the hydroxyapatite crystals seen in most kidney stones, as well as for diagnostic and lithotripsy purposes. Once the micro bubbles are adhered to the stone's surface, acoustic energy (not necessarily shock waves) can be delivered to the bubbles. Cavitation and stone fragmentation would be aided by the micro bubbles. Because these bubbles preferentially bond to the stone rather than tissue, less tissue injury is envisaged as a result.

To demonstrate that the fragmentation effectiveness of all stone phantoms improved when positioned 10 mm below the geometrical focus F2, closer to F1, well-standardized kidney stone phantoms were subjected to shock waves inside an experimental electrohydraulic shock wave source (Loske 2012). In another portion of the research, lithotripter shock waves were used on rectangular (303014.3 mm) HMT kidney stone models (High Medical Technologies, Kreuzlingen, Switzerland) to compare the shape and size of the craters produced at various energy levels and placements of the stones. Degassed water produced larger craters than non-degassed water when discharged at 20 kV, with F210 mm craters being the largest. Small craters were created by shock waves, confirming that cavitation is the primary mechanism of erosion in this case.

Shock wave radial sources expanded the range of indications for ESWT, despite the fact that they produce radial pressure waves rather than shock waves. Desktop gadgets are prevalent in doctors' offices today for treating a variety of illnesses, such as orthopaedics, dermatology (see Figure 5).

Figure 5. Photograph of shock wave source, designed for orthopedic and traumatic conditions (Loske 2017)

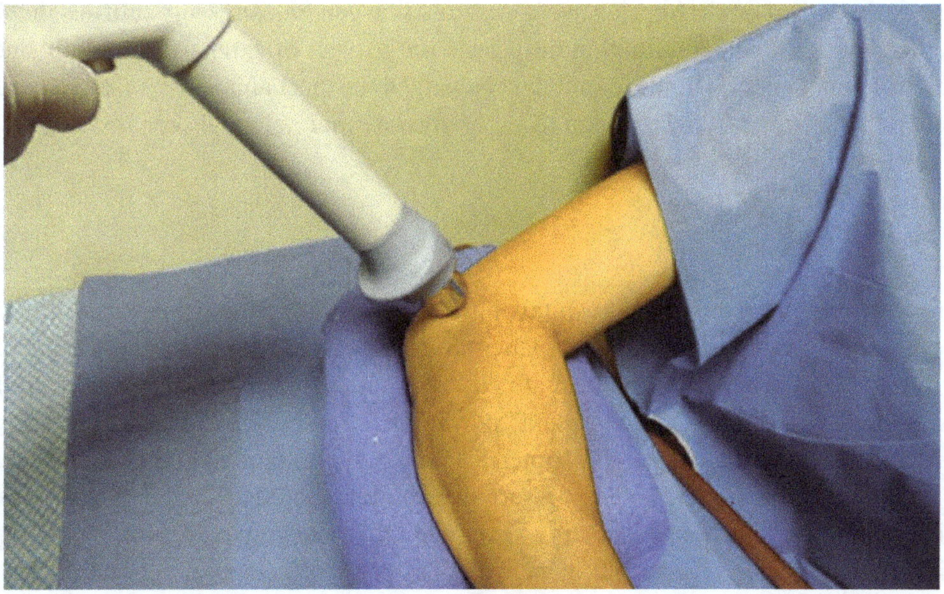

A growing number of sectors are benefiting from shock wave biomedical applications, which complicates the history of the field. Fungi genetic transformation is a noteworthy example. When it comes to producing pharmaceuticals like antibiotics, insulin, and hepatitis vaccine and anticoagulant chemicals from filamentous fungi, the only way to do so is to introduce foreign DNA into their genomes. Standard approaches, however, have low genetic transformation efficiency and poor reproducibility. The use of shock waves to alter fungus has been around for quite some time, but it was only recently discovered that this method works exceptionally well.

SWL'S EVOLUTION AND THE FUTURE

In lithotripsy centres around the world, well-designed case-oriented treatment procedures and careful patient selection will gain popularity, increasing the success rates of SWL (Neisius et al. 2015). It's critical to put SWL back in the hands of skilled urologists if we want to keep up with the growing number of patients with kidney stones. Despite the fact that SWL is a common procedure in many countries, with millions of successful treatments under its belt, researchers are continuously looking for ways to improve fragmentation efficiency and reduce tissue damage and pain (Rassweiler et al. 2013). Design of lithotripters and treatment regimens should be improved in SWL. Incorrect ideas about the causes of urinary stone comminution are still prevalent, as are misunderstandings about treatment parameters like dose, intensity, Shock Wave Lithotripsy energy, and focal area. In today's world, the majority of extracorporeal lithotripters feature attractive multipurpose designs, superior imaging systems, and user-friendly operation; nonetheless, clinical results obtained with newer systems are frequently no better than those obtained with older ones (Preminger et al. 2012; Rassweiler et al. 2014). In addition, there is still no agreement on a number of critical issues. For more than two decades after the first SWL, patients still refer to it as the gold standard due to its high stone-free rate and low need for re-treatment. It's amazing. The great clinical outcomes were no doubt helped by the experienced urologists who were treating patients in the early days of SWL. Shock wave generators that generate pressure profiles that limit tissue injury while improving stone comminution have been the subject of extensive research since they are the most critical component of a lithotripter. Others changed the mechanism they used to generate shock waves or made other changes to their design to accommodate more clinical scenarios.

CONCLUSION

To document treatment settings, many hospitals have an easy-to-use multifunctional lithotripter with easy-to-access software, a high-load capacity patient treatment table with radio translucency, and Trendelenburg positions (supine postures on the treatment table with pelvis higher than the head). Remember that voltage or intensity settings do not represent "power" or "capacity" to comminute urinary stones, as previously mentioned when selecting a lithotripter. The shock wave source's energy density, total energy at the focal volume, focal zone sizes, and pressure distribution should all be taken into account. SWL may cause discomfort. Despite this, there isn't a set process for managing pain. Non-invasive procedures can be carried out using local anaesthetic or intravenous sedation instead of general anaesthesia. Opioids are commonly used in conjunction with sedatives to manage pain during SWL. Additionally, local anaesthetics are injected under the skin and dermal anaesthetics are employed. General anaesthesia has been shown to improve treatment outcomes.

ACKNOWLEDGMENT

We acknowledge all the staff members of Aerospace Engineering, Dayananda Sagar University, Bangalore, India for the constant support and encouragement to carry out the research. I also thank Dr. K.N.B. Murthy (Vice Chancellor), Dr. A. Srinivas (Dean), Dr. BVN Ramakumar (Head of the Department), Dayananda Sagar University, Bangalore, India. I also thank my family members for the understanding and encouragement to preserve the research work. This research received no specific grant from any funding agency in the public, commercial, or not-for-profit sectors.

REFERENCES

Bailey, M. R., Pishchalnikov, Y. A., Sapozhnikov, O. A., Cleveland, R. O., McAteer, J. A., Miller, N. A., Pishchalnikova, I. V., Connors, B. A., Crum, L. A., & Evan, A. P. (2005). Cavitation detection during shock wave lithotripsy. *Ultrasound in Medicine & Biology*, *31*(9), 1245–1256. doi:10.1016/j.ultrasmedbio.2005.02.017 PMID:16176791

Contaldo, C., Högger, D. C., Khorrami Borozadi, M., Stotz, M., Platz, U., Forster, N., Lindenblatt, N., & Giovanoli, P. (2012). Radial pressure waves mediate apoptosis and functional angiogenesis during wound repair in ApoE deficient mice. *Microvascular Research*, *84*(1), 24–33. doi:10.1016/j.mvr.2012.03.006 PMID:22504489

Eremina, G., & Smolin, A. (2021). Numerical modeling of shockwave treatment of knee joint. *Materials (Basel)*, *14*(24), 7678. doi:10.3390/ma14247678 PMID:34947273

Falkensammer, F., Rausch-Fan, X., Schaden, W., Kivaranovic, D., & Freudenthaler, J. (2015). Impact of extracorporeal shockwave therapy on tooth mobility in adult orthodontic patients: A randomized single-center placebo-controlled clinical trial. *Journal of Clinical Periodontology*, *42*(3), 294–301. doi:10.1111/jcpe.12373 PMID:25640577

Furia, J. P., Rompe, J. D., Cacchio, A., Del Buono, A., & Maffulli, N. (2013). A single application of low energy radial extracorporeal shock wave therapy is effective for the management of chronic patellar tendinopathy. *Knee Surgery, Sports Traumatology, Arthroscopy*, *21*(2), 346–350. doi:10.100700167-012-2057-8 PMID:22627667

Gerdesmeyer, L., & Krath, A. (2014). ESWT and knee arthroplasty: radial shock wave therapy in ligament pain after total knee arthroplasty. Multidisciplinary medical applications, 84–96.

Hesse, A., Brändle, E., Wilbert, D., Köhrmann, K. U., & Alken, P. (2003). Study on the prevalence and incidence of urolithiasis in Germany comparing the years 1979 vs. 2000. *European Urology*, *44*(6), 709–713. doi:10.1016/S0302-2838(03)00415-9 PMID:14644124

Honton, B., & Laperche, C. (2021). Why and how do I use Shockwave? [Pourquoi et comment j'utilise le Shockwave?]. *Annales de Cardiologie et d'Angeiologie*, *70*(6), 425–431. doi:10.1016/j.ancard.2021.10.016 PMID:34740397

Hosseini, S. H. R., Kohno, Y., & Takayama, K. (2005). Micro-explosives induced underwater shock waves for medical applications. *Science and Technology of Energetic Materials*, *6*, 411–415.

Hosseini, S. H. R., Menezes, V., Moosavi-Nejad, S., Ohki, T., Nakagawa, A., Tominaga, T., & Takayama, K. (2006). Development of shock wave assisted therapeutic devices and establishment of shock wave therapy. *Minimally Invasive Therapy & Allied Technologies*, *15*(4), 230–240. doi:10.1080/13645700600836315 PMID:16966137

Jadhav, R. S., Gavasane, A., & Agrawal, A. (2020). Improved theory for shock waves using the OBurnett equations. *Journal of Fluid Mechanics*, 929.

Loske, A. M. (2017). *Medical and biomedical applications of shock waves*. Academic Press.

Loske, A. M., Campos-Guillen, J., de Icaza, M., Fernández, F., & Castaño-Tostado, E. (2012) Improved shock-wave-assisted bacteria transformation. In Shock waves. Springer.

Marwan, Y., Husain, W., Alhajii, W., & Mogawer, M. (2014). Extracorporeal shock wave therapy relieved pain in patients with coccydynia: A report of two cases. *The Spine Journal*, *14*(1), e1–e4. doi:10.1016/j.spinee.2013.07.438 PMID:24094989

Menezes, V., Mathew, Y., Takayama, K., Kanno, A., & Hosseini, H. (2012). Laser plasma jet driven microparticles for DNA/drug delivery. *PLoS One*, *7*(11), e50823. doi:10.1371/journal.pone.0050823 PMID:23226394

Mohamed & Jebran. (2020). Detection of Lesions for Diabetic Retinopathy By using Machine Learning Algorithms. *International Journal of Recent Technology and Engineering*, *8*, 1160–1166.

Morgan, J. P. M., Hamm, M., Schmitz, C., & Brem, M. H. (2021). Return to play after treating acute muscle injuries in elite football players with radial extracorporeal shock wave therapy. *Journal of Orthopaedic Surgery and Research*, *16*(1), 708. doi:10.118613018-021-02853-0 PMID:34876172

Nauck, T., Lohrer, H., & Schöll, J. (2014). Paradigm shift: ESWT applied to growth plates: radial shock wave therapy in patients with apophysitis calcanei. Multidisciplinary medical applications, 70–82.

Neisius, A., Lipkin, M. E., Rassweiler, J. J., Zhong, P., Preminger, G. M., & Knoll, T. (2015). Shock wave lithotripsy: The new phoenix? *World Journal of Urology*, *33*(2), 213–221. doi:10.100700345-014-1369-3 PMID:25081010

Preminger, G., Badlani, G., & Kavoussi, L. (Eds.). (2012). *Smith's textbook on endourology*. John Wiley and Sons.

Rassweiler, J., Rassweiler, M. C., Frede, T., & Alken, P. (2014). Extracorporeal shock wave lithotripsy: An opinion on its future. *Indian Journal of Urology*, *30*(1), 73–79. doi:10.4103/0970-1591.124211 PMID:24497687

Rassweiler, J., Rassweiler, M. C., Kenngott, H., Frede, T., Michel, M. S., Alken, P., & Clayman, R. (2013). The past, present and future of minimally invasive therapy in urology: A review and speculative outlook. *Minimally Invasive Therapy & Allied Technologies*, *22*(4), 200–209. doi:10.3109/13645706.2013.816323 PMID:23808367

Rompe, J. D., Furia, J., Cacchio, A., Schmitz, C., & Maffulli, N. (2015). Radial shock wave treatment alone is less efficient than radial shock wave treatment combined with tissue-specific plantar fasciastretching in patients with chronic plantar heel pain. *International Journal of Surgery*, *24*, 135–142. doi:10.1016/j.ijsu.2015.04.082 PMID:25940060

Russo, S. (2014). Avascular osteonecrosis of the femoral head. Multidisciplinary medical applications, 144–161.

Scales, C. D. Jr, Smith, A. C., Hanley, J. M., & Saigal, C. S. (2012). Prevalence of kidney stones in the United States. *European Urology*, *62*(1), 160–165. doi:10.1016/j.eururo.2012.03.052 PMID:22498635

Schmitz, C., Császár, N. B. M., Rompe, J. D., Chaves, H., & Furia, J. P. (2013). Treatment of chronic plantar fasciopathy with extracorporeal shock waves [review]. *Journal of Orthopaedic Surgery and Research*, *8*(1), 31–42. doi:10.1186/1749-799X-8-31 PMID:24004715

Shukla, P., Shen, X., Allott, R., Swanson, P., & Fitzpatrick, M. E. (2021). Response of silicon nitride ceramics subject to laser shock treatment. *Ceramics International*, *47*(24), 34538–34553. doi:10.1016/j.ceramint.2021.08.369

Wang, M.-M., & Wu, Z.-N. (2021). Transition study for asymmetric reflection between moving incident shock waves. *Journal of Fluid Mechanics*, *929*, A26. doi:10.1017/jfm.2021.856

Xiong, L., Liu, Y., Yuan, W., Lin, F., & Pan, Y. (2021). Study of the fracturing behaviour of an electro-hydraulic shock wave in sandstone under static pressure. *Journal of Physics. D, Applied Physics*, *54*(49), 495503. doi:10.1088/1361-6463/ac1cb4

Chapter 13
Diagnostic Categorization and Neurocognitive Prediction Employing Neuroimaging Data Using Deep Learning in Alzheimer's Illness

Srividya Bharadwaja
Dayananda Sagar College of Engineering, India

Smitha Sasi
Dayananda Sagar College of Engineering, India

ABSTRACT

Traditional analytic strategies for investigating neuroimaging biomarkers for neuropsychiatric illnesses have relied on mass univariate statistics, assuming that various brain areas function separately. Machine learning (ML) methods that take into account intercorrelation across areas have recently become a popular and important part of computer-assisted analytical procedures and are now frequently used for the automated diagnosis and analysis of neuropsychiatric illnesses. The goal of this chapter is to provide a detailed overview of CNN and RNN applications in medical image comprehension. The overarching goal is to encourage medical image understanding experts to use CNNs extensively in their research and diagnosis. This chapter describes the development of various novel DL-based approaches and models as well as advancements in high-speed computing techniques, which provide a once-in-a-lifetime chance to anticipate and control Alzheimer's disease.

INTRODUCTION

Alzheimer's disease is a type of dementia marked by memory, cognitive, and behavioral issues. AD affects an estimated 5.5 million people aged 65 and more, and it is the sixth largest cause of mortality in

DOI: 10.4018/978-1-7998-9534-3.ch013

the United States. Improved neuroimaging techniques including as magnetic resonance imaging (MRI) and positron emission tomography (PET) have been developed and implemented to uncover AD-related structural and molecular biomarkers. Due to fast developments in neuroimaging techniques, integrating large-scale, high-dimensional multimodal neuroimaging data has become problematic. As a result, there has been a surge in interest in computer-assisted machine learning approaches for integrative analysis. Linear discriminant analysis (LDA), linear programme boosting method (LPBM), and logistic regression are examples of well-known pattern analysis approaches (LR), Support vector machines (SVM) and support vector machine recursive feature elimination (SVM-RFE) have been utilized and show promise in detecting Alzheimer's disease early and predicting its progression. Appropriate architectural design or pre-processing processes must be pre-defined in order to employ such machine learning algorithms. Feature extraction, feature selection, dimensionality reduction, and feature-based classification method selection are the four processes in the process (Scheltens, 2016). These processes necessitate specialized knowledge as well as many optimization steps, which can be time-consuming. Deep learning, a developing branch of machine learning research that uses raw neuroimaging data to build features using "on-the-fly" learning, is gaining traction in the field of large-scale, high-dimensional medical imaging analysis to address these issues. (Hwang, 2019).

We reviewed various publications where deep learning algorithms and neuroimaging data were utilized to detect Alzheimer's disease early and forecast its progression.

OVERVIEW OF DEEP LEARNING TECHNIQUES

Deep learning is a type of machine learning that learns features through a hierarchical learning process. Methods of deep learning for a variety of domains, categorization and prediction have been used. Including natural language processing and computer vision both of which are show performance breakthroughs. DL is a branch of machine learning that can be used to create models that extract high-dimensional characteristics from data. It has gotten a lot of attention in recent years, notably in the field of image analysis. A number of deep learning architectures have been published in the literature, including CNN, DNN, RNN, AE, Deep Belief Network (DBN), and Probabilistic Neural Network (PNN) (Gulshan, 2016).

Convolutional Neural Network (CNN):

A CNN, also known as a ConvNet, uses learnable weights and biases to apply to distinct regions of an input image, allowing one image to be distinguished from another.

CNN employs convolution instead of basic matrix multiplication in at least one of their layers. It's most commonly used in unstructured datasets. 2D-CNN predicts segmentation maps for a single slice using 2D-convolutional kernels.

Only spatial dimensions such as height and width can be used by 2D-CNN. Context information from adjacent slices cannot be recovered since 2D-CNN only accepts one slice as input. In terms of utility, voxel data from neighboring slices may be sufficient for categorization tasks. By predicting the volumetric patch of neuroimaging data, 3D-CNN, on the other hand, can retain temporal dimensions. Although the capacity of 3D-CNNs to anchor interslice context information improves performance, it comes at a cost in terms of computation time and the number of parameters that 3D-CNNs must utilize. Figure 1 shows CNN Architecture

Figure 1. CNN architecture

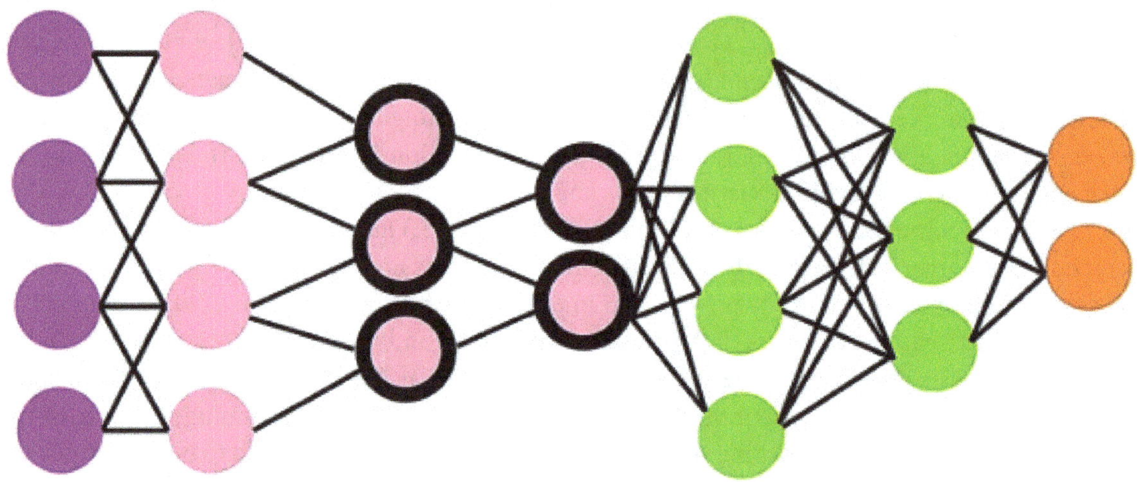

Deep Belief Network (DBN)

DBNs are a form of deep neural network (NN) that consists of a single layer that has a graphical model with both directed and undirected edges. It consists of multiple layers of hidden units, each of which is linked to the next input unit save. DBN is made up of a series of restricted Boltzmann machines (RBM), each of which must communicate with the one before it and the one after it.

The nodes of a single layer do not interact with each other remotely. DBN is used to identify, organize, and originate images, video clips, and motion-capture data. Electroencephalography is a real-life use of an electrophysiological scanning technique for documenting the electrical processes of the brain. The following figure depicts the DBN Architecture

Figure 2. DBN architecture

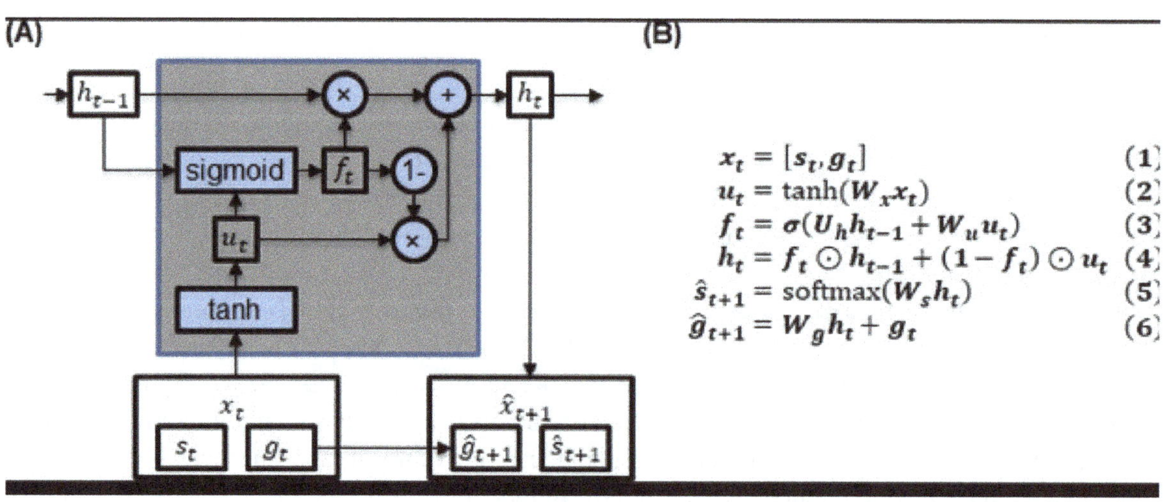

Auto Encoder (AE)

In an unsupervised manner, the AE NN learns to correlate its input to its output. The input code is specified by an internal (hidden) layer. An AE is made up of two basic components: an encoder that turns data into code and a decoder that reverses the process. Sparse AE, denoising AE, and contractive AE are the three most prevalent AE types.

The sparse AE design has more hidden units than inputs, but only a handful of them should be active at any given moment, requiring the model to respond to the statistical features of the training data.

In either approach, denoising AE takes a partially distorted input and trains to recover the original genuine input. Contractive AE also acquires the option to include an explicit regularizes in its goal function, forcing the model to learn a function that is resistant to small input value changes.
The following Figure depicts the AE Architecture.

Figure 3. AE Architecture

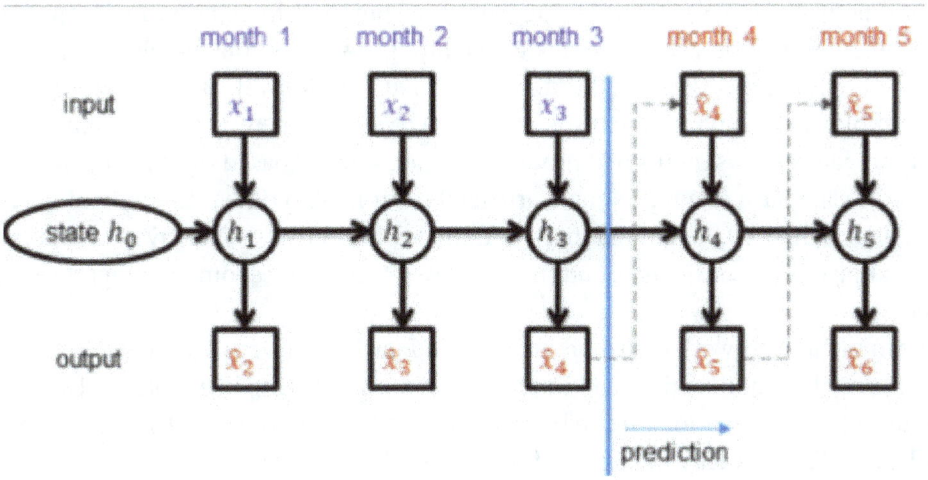

Recurrent Neural Network (RNN)

RNN is for recurrent neural network, and it is a memory network that recalls the past and bases its decisions on what it has learnt in the past. As a result, an RNN can be thought of as an architecture made up of numerous copies of the same network, each of which sends a message to a successor. RNN's Hidden state is its primary and most crucial feature. The hidden state's purpose is to help you remember specific details from a sequence. Every input uses the same parameters since it must do the same task on all inputs (hidden layers) in order to generate the output. In contrast to other NNs, this results in a decrease in complexity parameters. The following Figure depicts the RNN Architecture

Figure 4. RNN Architecture

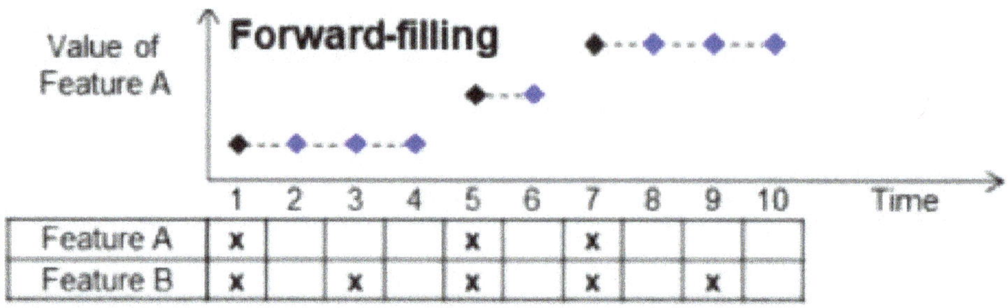

Deep Neural Network (DNN)

Machine learning and artificial intelligence have benefited greatly from deep neural network models. An artificial neural network (ANN) having numerous layers between the input and output layers is known as a deep neural network (DNN). Neurobiology was the source of inspiration for deep neural network models. A biological neuron receives several signals through synapses that touch its dendrites and sends a single stream of action potentials out through its axon at a high level. By categorizing various input patterns, the complexity of multiple inputs is decreased. Artificial neural network models are made up of units that aggregate various inputs and produce a single output, based on this understanding.

Neural networks are built around a simple artificial neuron: a nonlinear function of a weighted average of inputs (such as max (0, value) that tries to mimic brain activity. One layer's outputs become the inputs of the next layer in the sequence, and the next layer's outputs become the inputs of the next layer in the sequence.

DNN refers to a neural network with more than one hidden layer. Every layer in DNN performs certain duties such as embedding, collocating, and so on. In a process, ordering is important. Deep feed-forward NNs are also used in deep feed-forward max (multi-layered perceptron (MLP) is a type of neuron that has multiple layers. There is only one route (forward) for knowledge to travel the network's feedback. MLPs have the ability to cope with a variety of situations. The non-linearly separable relationships between complex non-linearly separable complex non-linearly separable complex non input and output are both important. Internal recurrence and, as a result, input to a a neuron or a layer that has already received and processed data that indication There's a lot of data that's been annotated. The following Figure depicts the DNN Architecture

Figure 5. DNN architecture

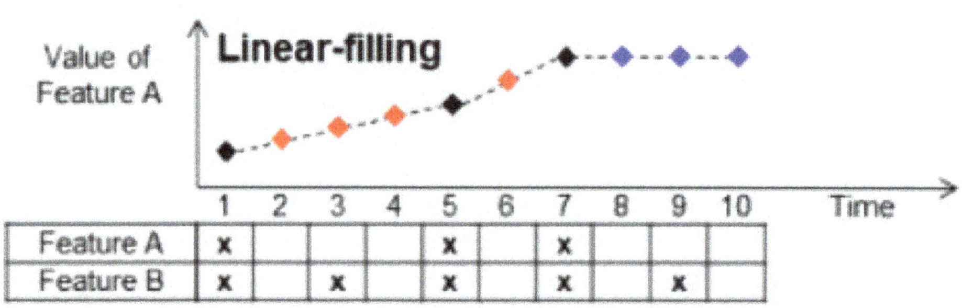

Probabilistic Neural Network (PNN)

PNN is a pattern recognition and classification algorithm. A Parzen window is used to estimate the probability distribution function (PDF) in PNN is a function that is negative. The likelihood of a new input is then calculated. The PDF function is used to calculate the data. Last but not least, to label the new input data, the Bayes rule is utilized. the one having the highest possibility of success. The following Figure depicts the PNN architecture.

Figure 6. PNN architecture

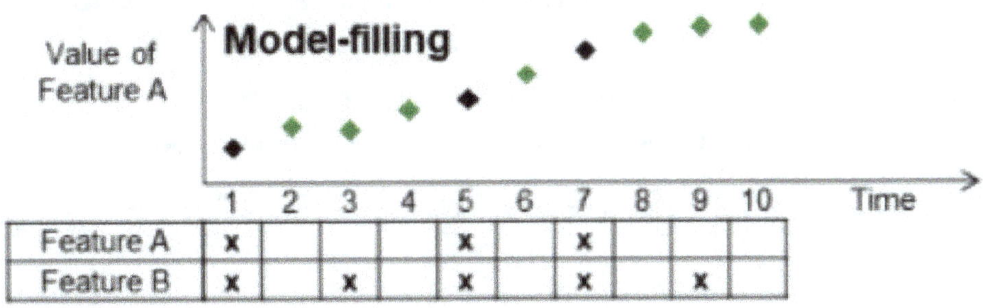

IDENTIFICATION OF ALZHEIMER'S DISEASE USING A CONVOLUTIONAL NEURAL NETWORK MODEL

In this research, the authors proposed a CNN-based approach for classifying AD patients and CN controls using MRI coronal slices spanning the medial temporal lobe. The algorithm was developed and verified on two separate groups with varied races and educational levels. Experiments show that system is fast and accurate, regardless of ethnic and/or demagnification factors (Luo, 2017).

The MTA scale, which is routinely used in clinical practice to validate the prevalence of AD-related neurodegeneration, is used in this method. According to the National Institute on Aging and Alzheimer's Association study guidelines/framework, this scale is also utilized as neurodegeneration evidence for Alzheimer's disease (Liu et al, 2018)

Although information from other regions may be valuable for AD categorization, there is known to be significant inter-subject heterogeneity in exact atrophy patterns19, with MTL-focused atrophy being the most common type.

As a result, trying to add more regions may cause the algorithm to become confused, perhaps leading to misdiagnosis compared to other diseases that have similar atrophy patterns.

METHODOLOGY

The method was used to two datasets in this study: one from the ADNI (Petersen, 2010) and the other from the SNUBH. Participants in ADNI1 and ADNI2 were included if their T1-weighted images were 3.0 T and they were diagnosed as CN or moderate AD (CDR of 0.5 or 1).

Then T1-weighted scans from the SNUBH were used to select AD patients and CN controls. Additional matching for education and cognitive capacity was not achievable since participants from the ADNI were more educated and performed better on the Mini Mental State Examination (MMSE) than those from the SNUBH. (Liu, 2012)

If a participant has multiple MRI scans from different timepoints, choose only one MRI scan based on the participant's age and diagnosis at the time of assessment.

Image Acquisition and Preprocessing

Figure 7. Preprocessing 3D brain images to create 2D coronal slices of the medial temporal lobe

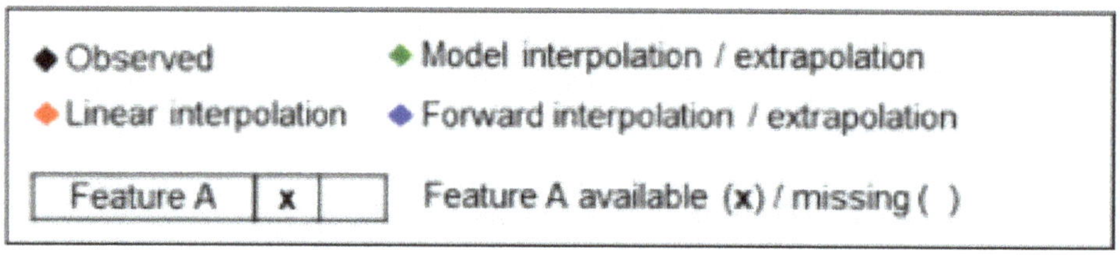

The input whole-brain 3D T1-weighted MRI images are first stiffly transformed to fit a template, then brain extraction is performed (skull stripping). The skull-stripped form of the template is subsequently subjected to a second stiffening process. As soon as the subject image is in the same position as the background image.

DEEP LEARNING MODEL

The outputs from each of the preprocessed coronal slices were then averaged to conduct topic categorization. With a few tweaks37, we used the Inception-v4 architecture as the neural network's backbone. The Inception-v4 neural network is a two-dimensional image categorization neural network that has been shown to be effective.

When a single coronal slice was entered into the Inception backbone architecture, a feature vector of 1024 values representing the convolution results was obtained. Then added three more values to the end of the vector (subject age, sex, and the number of coronal slice being evaluated). After that, the classifier module received the final concatenated feature vector with 1027 values. The module of the Inception-classifier v4 has been replaced with a fully linked layer with 1027 input nodes and two output nodes. Finally, the output of the completely linked layer was fed into a softmax output layer to calculate the probability that an input brain MR image contains A.

Figure 8. A diagram depicts the network architecture

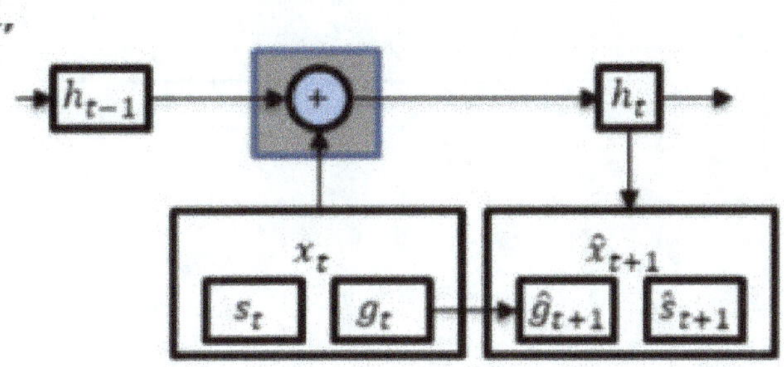

$$x_t = [s_t, g_t] \quad (10)$$
$$h_t = W_h h_{t-1} + W_x x_t \quad (11)$$
$$\hat{s}_{t+1} = \text{softmax}(W_s h_t) \quad (12)$$
$$\hat{g}_{t+1} = W_g h_t + g_t \quad (13)$$

Each patient has one of 30 coronal slices entered into the model separately, with the results of the 30 slices averaged to give an AD likelihood. The architecture of a pretrained network (Inception V4) is the first part of the model, and the last part is the addition of the subject's age, sex, and slice position in the model (a). The Inception v4 components are shown (stem, Inception-A, Inception-B, Inception-C, Reduction-A, Reduction-B)

AD classification is a binary classification issue for predicting the existence of Alzheimer's disease. After each slice image is identified as AD or CN, the results for all slices are averaged.

The inputs are 2D coronal slices xi from a patient's 3D MRI brain scan x, and the output is y, which is a value reflecting the probability of the presence of AD. The expected o's binary cross-entropy loss throughout training.

If xi is a slice from patient x, yi is a true class of xi, and N is the batch size, then yi is a true class of xi. During validation and testing, the mean probability of all input slices (x1, x2,..., xn) for patient x was used to generate the final predicted probability of the occurrence of AD.

Mini-batch stochastic gradient descent with Nesterov momentum and a batch size of 64 was used to optimise all of the models.

$$J(w) = -\frac{1}{N}\sum_{n=1}^{N}[y^n \log\left(f\left(x_i^n, w\right)\right)\hat{y}^n + \overline{\left(1 - y^n\right)\log\left(1 - f\left(x_i^n; w\right)\right)}],$$

During validation and testing, this approach forecasted the subject's class by taking the average of the expected probabilities for each of the 30 slices collected from the subject. The final prediction values for the test sets were estimated using the average ensemble values of the five rounds of fivefold cross-validation for the development set.

Figure 9. Validation and testing

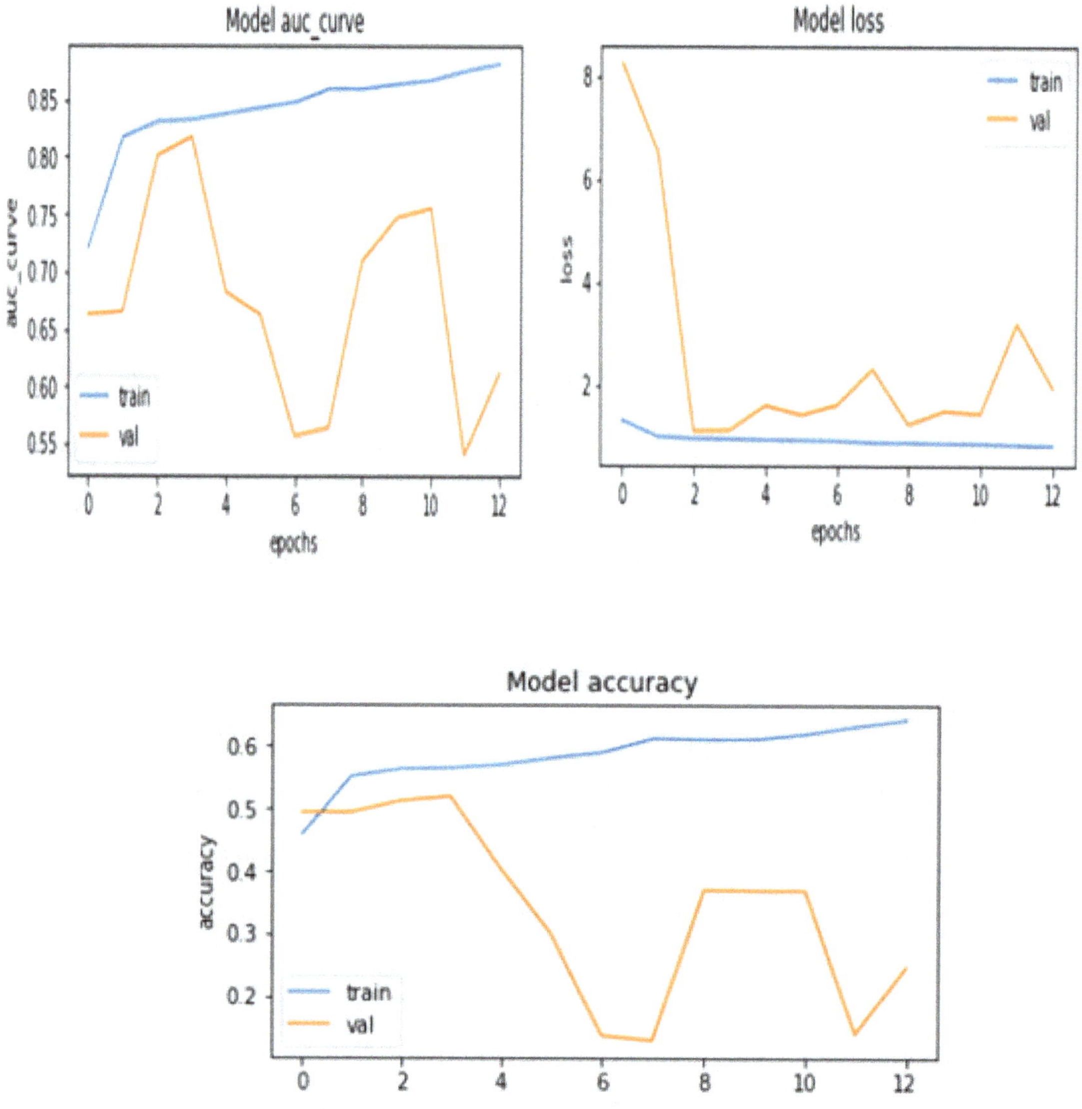

IDENTIFICATION OF ALZHEIMER'S DISEASE USING A RECURRENT NEURAL NETWORK MODEL

Recurrent neural networks (RNNs) are a type of neural network that uses contextual memory to recognize patterns in sequential data. Many sorts of sequential information have been used with recurrent neural networks, including text, audio, movies, music, genetic sequences, and even clinical occurrences. The name "recurrent neural network" is loosely applied to two broad kinds of networks that have a similar overall structure, one with limited impulse and the other with infinite impulse. The behaviors of both types of networks are temporally dynamic. A directed acyclic graph that can be unrolled and substituted with a strictly feedforward neural network is known as a finite impulse recurrent network. Additional stored states are possible in both finite and infinite impulse recurrent networks, and the storage can be controlled directly by the neural network. If another network or graph involves time delays or has feedback loops, it can likewise be used to replace the storage.

Simple feed forward neural networks can be compared to RNNs. Using several inputs to train a simple 'feed forward' network will not modify the bias of the network. Recurrent neural networks, rather than using the standard 'feed forward' architecture, use 'loops' (self-loops, feedback loops, and backward connections) to take into account information received previously and context.

Certain types of imaging, such as ultrasound video, are sequential in nature. Individual 2D images can theoretically be viewed as sequential patterns (if they are turned into a sequence of smaller images). RNNs, on the other hand, are currently more extensively used in areas of radiology that deal with language.

Speech recognition software systems, which radiologists employ to write and transcribe reports, are currently their most popular use in many radiology offices. RNNs have also demonstrated the ability to generate text reports to complement abnormality detection algorithms and have enhanced the process of illness annotation from electronic health record radiological data.

The development of disorder drugs requires early diagnosis of persons at risk of Alzheimer's disease (AD) dementia. Using multimodal AD signs and clinical diagnosis from one or more timepoints, researchers want to anticipate an individual's clinical diagnosis, cognition, and ventricular volume for every month (indefinitely) into the future. To diagnose Alzheimer's disease, researchers created and used a minimal recurrent neural network (minimal RNN) model.

Support vector machine/regression, linear state space (LSS) model, and long short-term memory (LSTM) (Limpton, 2016) model all performed better than minimalRNN with "model filling." Importantly, despite the fact that the training approach used longitudinal data, the trained minimal model performed similarly whether either 1 or 4 input timepoints were used.

The minimalRNN may be less prone to overfitting than other RNN models, such as the LSTM (Ghazi, 2019) model, because it contains fewer parameters. Despite the fact that RNNs are usually trained with feature-complete data, we investigated two "preprocessing" and one "integrative" approach to deal with missing data.

PROPOSED METHOD

The minimal was adapted for forecasting illness development in this technique. Because minimalRNN has fewer parameters and is thus less likely to overfit, it was used instead of LSTM (Junninen, 2004) in this case. Figure 2 depicts the model architecture and update equations. Let xt stand for all variables seen at time t, including the diagnosis st and the other continuous variables gt One-hot encoding was used to represent diagnosis in this case. In other words, diagnosis was represented as a three-dimensional vector. If the first entry was one, the subject was considered a normal control.

If the first entry was one, the subject was considered a normal control. If the participant's second input was one, he or she had minor cognitive impairment. If the third item was one, the person had Alzheimer's disease dementia.

Figure 10. (A) MinimalRNN is a term that refers to a small amount of information. (B) Equations for minimalRNN updates

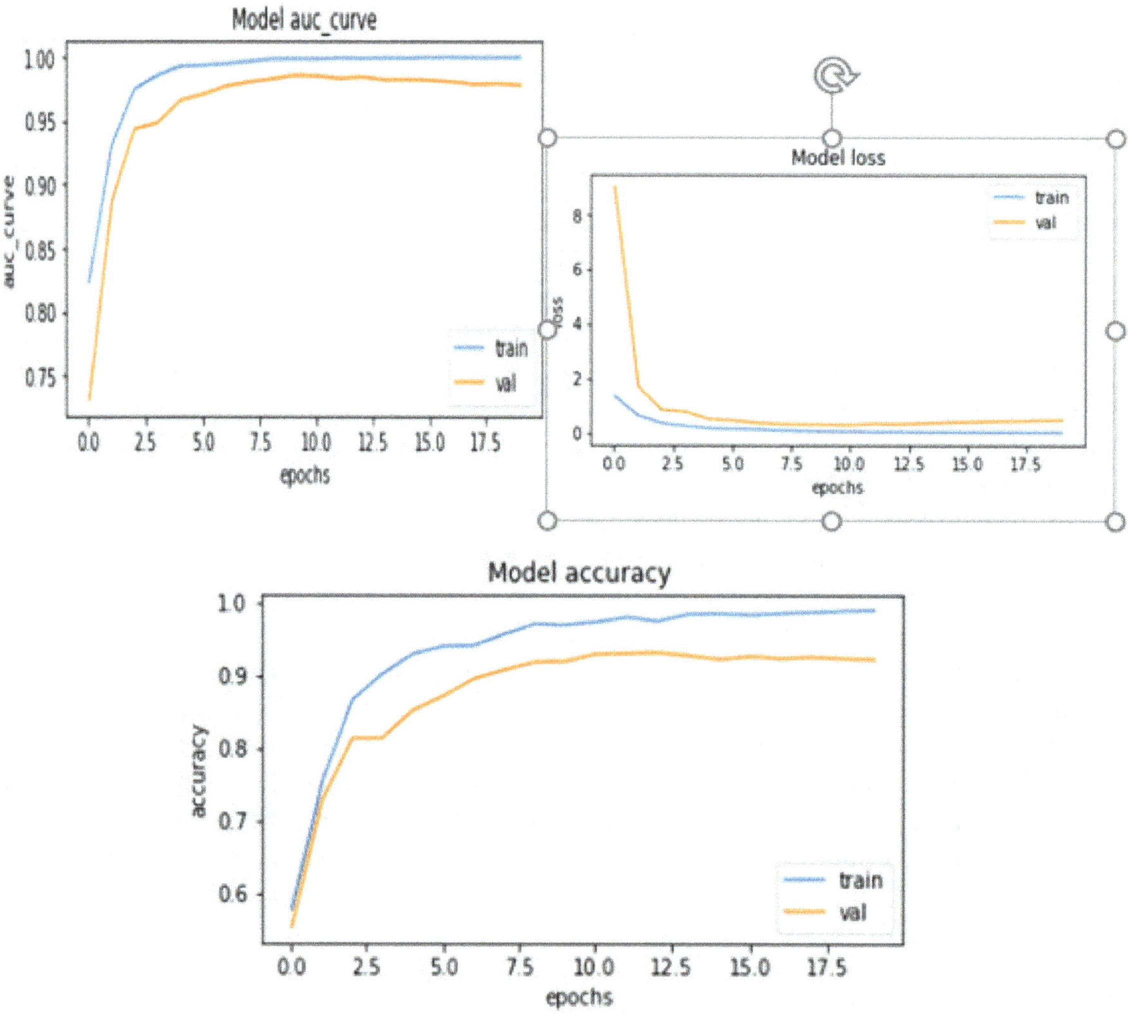

Categorical (i.e., diagnosis) and continuous variables are denoted by st and gt, respectively (Table 1). Each RNN cell's input xt was made up of the diagnosis st and continuous variables gt (Eq. (1)). It's worth noting that st was encoded with one-hot encoding. The modified input (Eq.) and the preceding hidden state (ht) were combined to create the hidden state ht. The contribution of the prior hidden state and present transformed input ut to the current hidden state ht was weighed by the forget gate ft (Eq. (3)). Using the hidden state ht (Eqs. (5) and (6)), the model predicted the next month's diagnostic and continuous variables. The element-wise product and the sigmoid function are denoted by and, respectively. (Pedregosa et al., 2011)

Training with No Missing Data

The RNN training is shown in Figure 11. Given the prior data, the RNN was trained to predict the next observation (xt) (x1, x2,...xt-1). The model parameters were updated using the differences between the anticipated outputs (e.g.) and the ground truth outputs (e.g. x2). The following is how the mistake (or loss L) was defined.

$$L = \sum_{t>1} (CrossEntropy\left(S_t, \hat{S}_t\right) + MAE\left(g_t, \hat{g}_t\right)$$

$$CrossEntropy\left(S_t, \widehat{S_t}\right) = -\sum_{j=1}^{3} S_t^j log \widehat{S_t^j}$$

$$MAE\left(g_t, \hat{g}_t\right) = \frac{1}{23} \sum_{j=1}^{23} | g_t^j - \widehat{g_t^j} |$$

Prediction with No Missing Data

The RNN was used to forecast the progression of Alzheimer's disease in an example subject, as shown in Fig 11 (from the validation or test set). The model's purpose was to forecast future observations based on data from months 1, 2, and 3. The model predictions (and) were fed in as inputs to the RNN (for months 5 and 6 respectively) starting in month 4 to produce subsequent predictions.

Figure 11. RNN prediction model

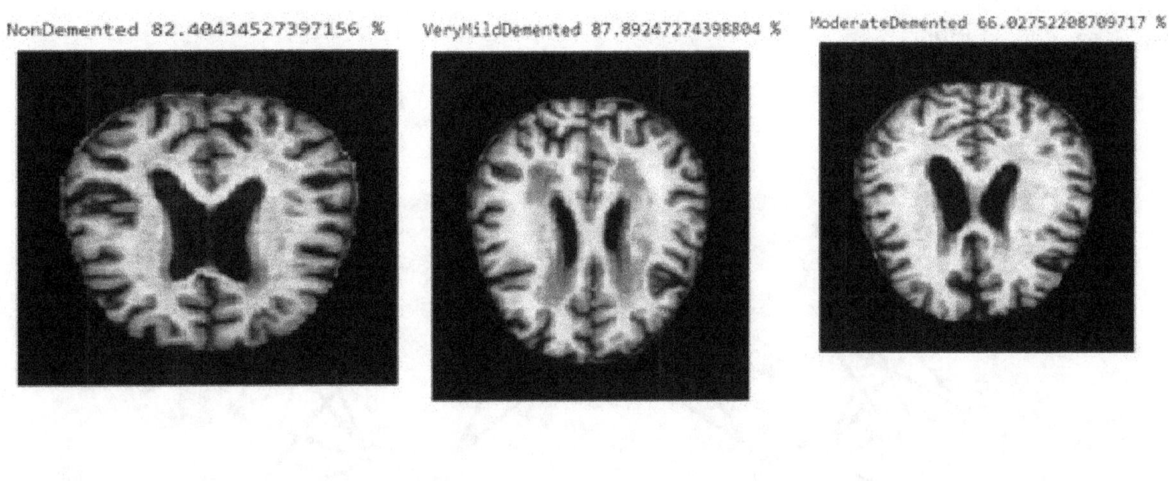

The RNN update equations (Figure 11), which assumed all variables were observed, were likewise hampered by the missing data. To handle missing data, we looked at two "preprocessing" strategies, Forward filling and Linear filling, as well as one "integrative" strategy, Model Filling.

Forward Filling

Imputing the data using the most recent timepoint with accessible data was known as forward filling. Figure 12 shows an example of how missing input data was filled in using forward-filling in time.

Figure 12. Forward filling

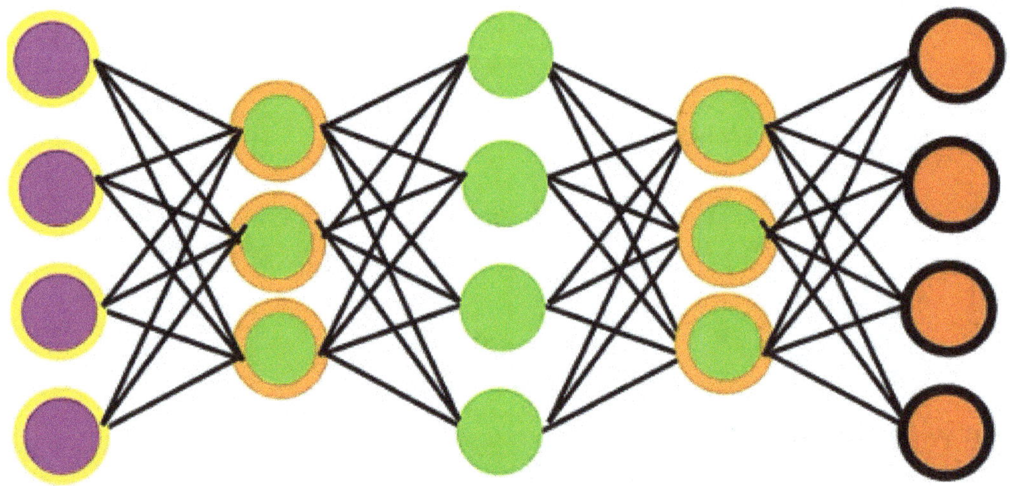

Linear Filling

With available data, the linear filling approach performed linear interpolation between the previous timepoint and the next timepoint. A linear interpolation example is shown in Figure 13.

Figure 13. Linear Filling

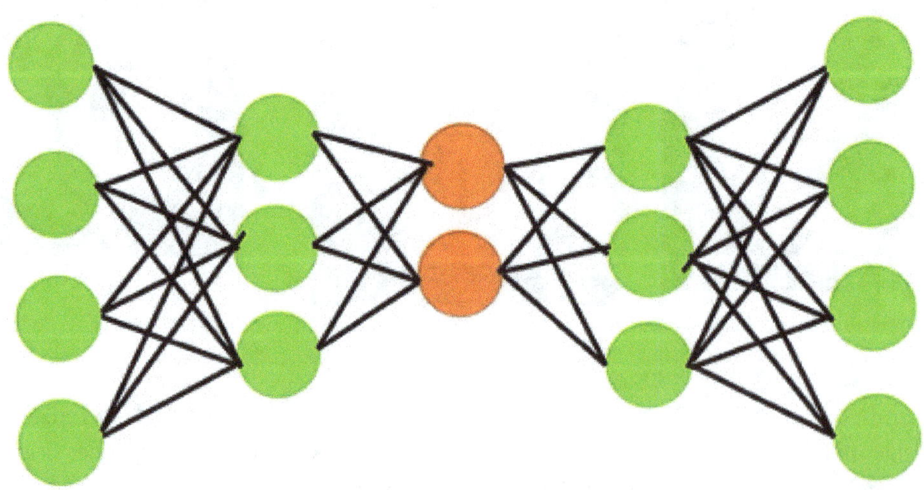

Model Filling

The whole set of characteristics was used for the imputation, which was a potential benefit of modelling filling shown in figure 14

Figure 14. Model filling

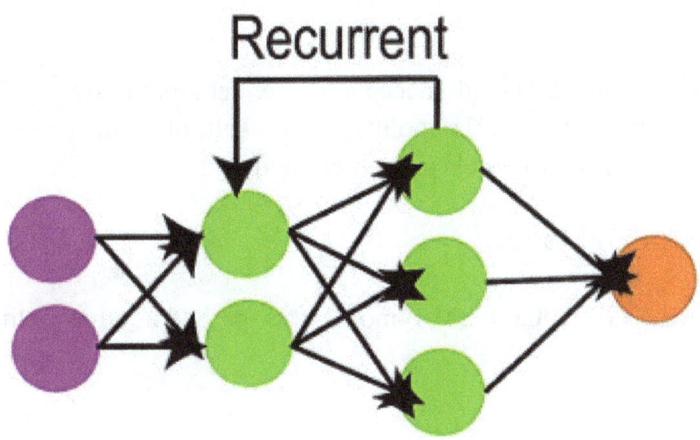

Figure 15. Model filling

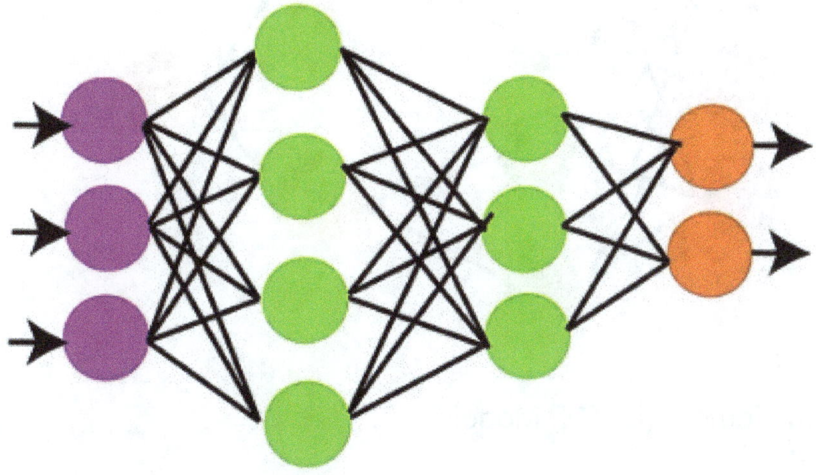

Baselines

This approach considered four baselines: constant prediction, support vector machine/regression (SVM/SVR), linear state-space (LSS) model, and long short-term memory (LSTM) model.

Constant Prediction

All future values would be the same as the last observed values, according to the constant prediction method. There was no need to train the algorithm. While this may appear to be an unnecessarily rudimentary algorithm, we will find that the constant prediction algorithm is highly competitive in terms of short-term forecasting.

SVM/SVR

Because SVM/SVR (McKhann, 1984) only accepts feature vectors of constant length, it can't handle subjects with varying numbers of input timepoints. As a result, utilizing 1 to 4 input timepoints, this strategy trained multiple SVM/SVR models to predict the future.

Linear State Space (LSS) Model

By linearizing the minimal RNN (Happ, 2018) model, this method assumed a linear state space (LSS) baseline (Figure 16).

Figure 16. LSS model

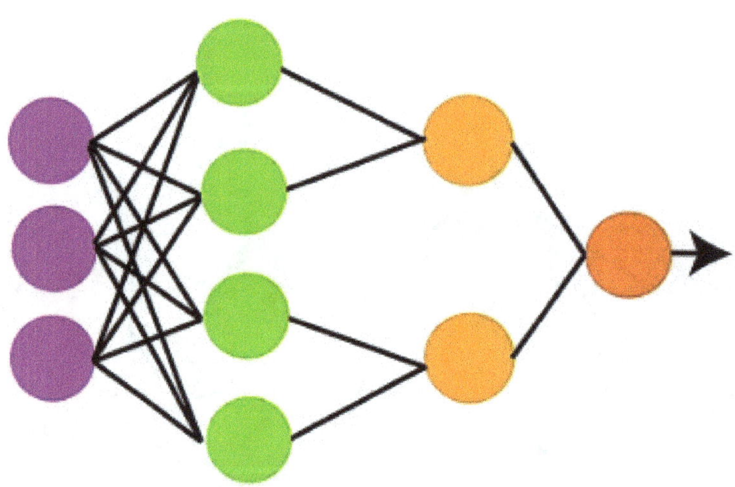

Long Short Term Memory (LSTM) Model

For modelling sequences and temporal trajectories, the LSTM model is commonly employed. When data is restricted, minimalRNN models are preferable to LSTM models because they contain fewer parameters and are less prone to overfitting.

RESULTS AND DISCUSSION

Training the Model

The model is now trained for 100 epochs with a batch size 128. During the training as mentioned earlier 20% of this training data is used for validation. Callbacks are used to know the detailed statistics and also internal states of the model during training. At every given step the callbacks are applied during training. They are set of functions. The list of callbacks is passed to the. fit () method. During each and every stage of training the callbacks are called.

There is an early stop for 50 epochs in the process as there is no much improvement in the accuracy. The increase in the number of epochs is basically assuring the right accuracy after fitting data to the model and training and it is also in order to get good test prediction results.

CNN Model

The performance Metrics of Basic CNN model is shown below.

Figure 17. Performance metrics of CNN model on train data set

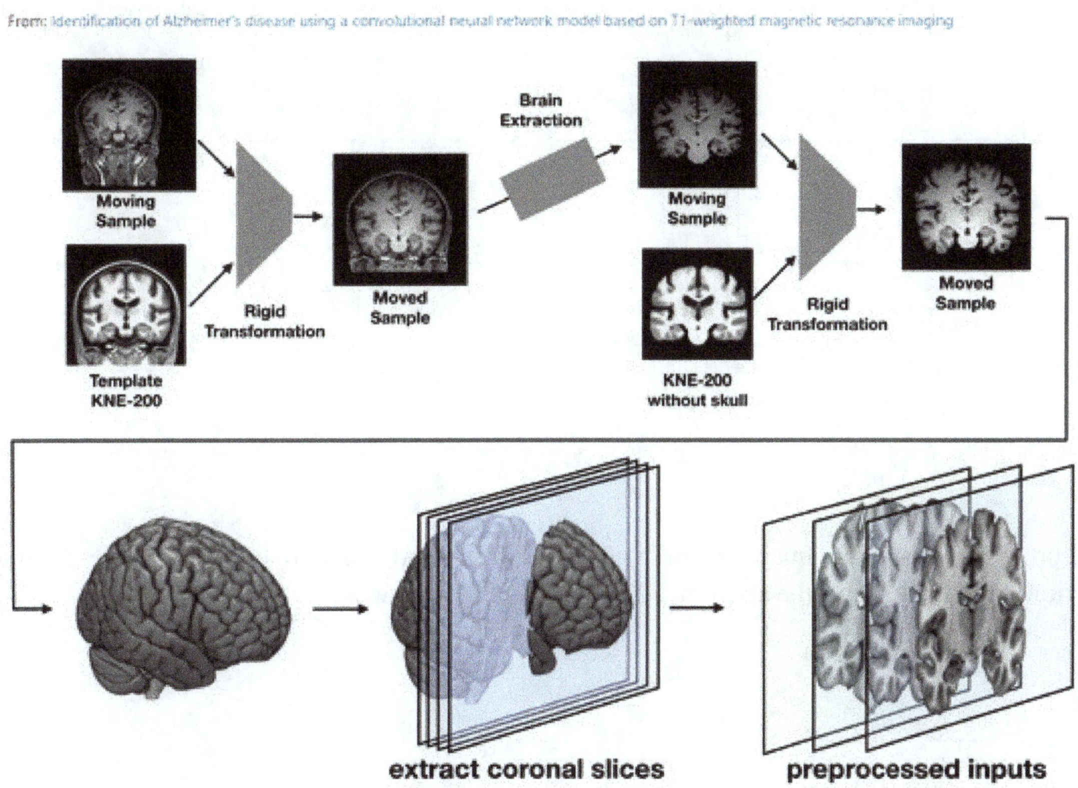

RNN Model

The performance Metrics of RNN Model is shown below. Figure refers to the AUC and Model loss plot and whereas figure is the accuracy curve

Figure 18. Performance metrics of RNN model on train data set

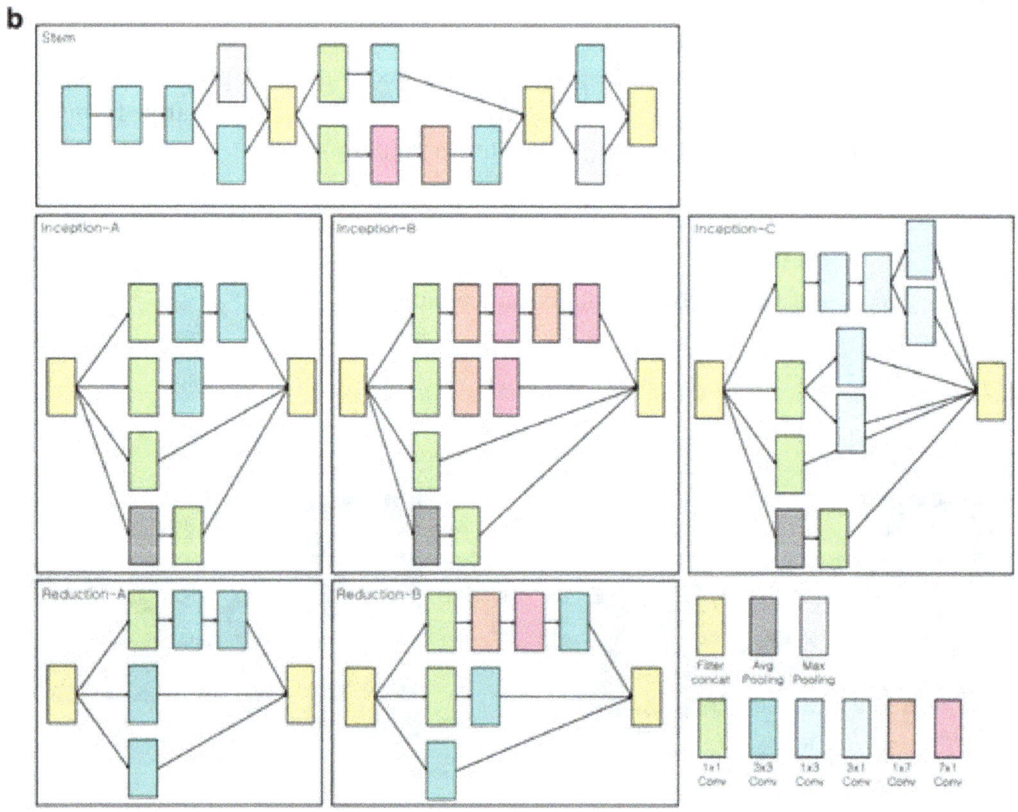

Test

As the process of test a few images from the data set were input and were checked for the accuracy of prediction. Figure 19 shows the abnormal detection on Brain images.

Figure 19. Abnormality on brain Images

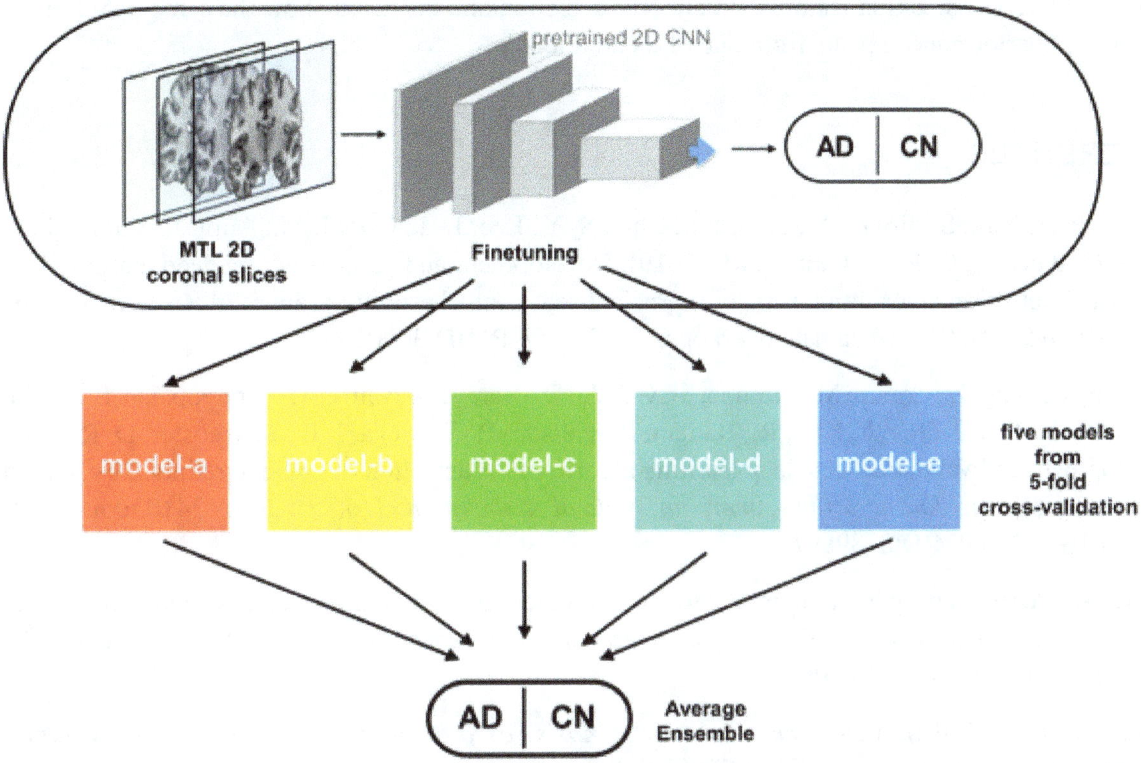

Table 1. Accuracy table of all models

Models	ACCURACY
CNN	70%
RNN	92.29%

CONCLUSION

The aim of the work here was to compare the performance of all the models that were considered in the study. From the results obtained it is evident that RNN has performed better than CNN models. The model gave 92.29% accuracy on the train dataset and 89% on evaluation over test dataset. According to the tests conducted on classifying the test images into the model seems to have performed exceptionally well and has classified the images accurately.

The major factor that affects any model is irregularity in data or the size of the data. Considering the conditions available the model was fit to perform better with those classes which had enough amount of data to train the model with. Data Augmentation did make a change in getting some better performance metrics for the test set considered.

As known the CNN architectures is always the one most preferred when it comes to image classification and live visualization feature extraction or detection and the result show the same upholding the exceptional performance results from one of its architectures.

REFERENCES

Hwang, E. J., Park, S., Jin, K.-N., Kim, J. I., Choi, S. Y., Lee, J. H., Goo, J. M., Aum, J., Yim, J.-J., Cohen, J. G., Ferretti, G. R., & Park, C. M. (2019). Development and validation of a deep learning-based automated detection algorithm for major thoracic diseases on chest radiographs. *JAMA Network Open*, *2*(3), e191095. doi:10.1001/jamanetworkopen.2019.1095 PMID:30901052

Gulshan, V., Peng, L., Coram, M., Stumpe, M. C., Wu, D., Narayanaswamy, A., Venugopalan, S., Widner, K., Madams, T., Cuadros, J., Kim, R., Raman, R., Nelson, P. C., Mega, J. L., & Webster, D. R. (2016). Development and validation of a deep learning algorithm for detection of diabetic retinopathy in retinal fundus photograph. *Journal of the American Medical Association*, *316*(22), 2402–2410. doi:10.1001/jama.2016.17216 PMID:27898976

Esteva, A. (2019). A deep learning model for early prediction of Alzheimer's disease dementia based on hippocampal magnetic resonance imaging data. *Alzheimer's & Dementia*, *15*(8), 1059–1070. doi:10.1016/j.jalz.2019.02.007 PMID:31201098

Li, F. & Liu, M. (2018). *Alzheimer's disease diagnosis based on multiple cluster dense convolutional network*. doi:10.1016/j.compmedimag.2018.09.009

Luo, S., Li, X., & Li, J. (2017). Automatic Alzheimer's disease recognition from MRI data using deep learning method. *Zeitschrift für Angewandte Mathematik und Physik*, *05*(09), 1892–1898. doi:10.4236/jamp.2017.59159

Liu, M., Zhang, J., Adeli, E., & Shen, D. (2018). Landmark-based deep multi-instance learning for brain disease diagnosis. *Medical Image Analysis*, *43*, 157–168. doi:10.1016/j.media.2017.10.005 PMID:29107865

Basaia, S., Agosta, F., Wagner, L., Canu, E., Magnani, G., Santangelo, R., & Filippi, M. (2019). Automated classification of Alzheimer's disease and mild cognitive impairment using a single MRI and deep neural networks. *NeuroImage. Clinical*, *21*, 101645. doi:10.1016/j.nicl.2018.101645 PMID:30584016

Lu, D., Popuri, K., Ding, G. W., Balachandar, R., & Beg, M. F. (2018). Multimodal and multiscale deep neural networks for the early diagnosis of Alzheimer's disease using structural MR and FDG-PET images. *Scientific Reports*, *8*(1), 5697. doi:10.103841598-018-22871-z PMID:29632364

Petersen, R. C., Aisen, P. S., Beckett, L. A., Donohue, M. C., Gamst, A. C., Harvey, D. J., Jack, C. R., Jagust, W. J., Shaw, L. M., Toga, A. W., Trojanowski, J. Q., & Weiner, M. W. (2010). Alzheimer's disease neuroimaging initiative (ADNI): Clinical characterization. *Neurology*, *74*(3), 201–209. doi:10.1212/WNL.0b013e3181cb3e25 PMID:20042704

Liu, Y., Julkunen, V., Paajanen, T., Westman, E., Wahlund, L.-O., Aitken, A., Sobow, T., Mecocci, P., Tsolaki, M., Vellas, B., Muehlboeck, S., Spenger, C., Lovestone, S., Simmons, A., & Soininen, H. (2012). Education increases reserve against Alzheimer's disease-evidence from structural MRI analysis. *Neuroradiology*, *54*(9), 929–938. doi:10.100700234-012-1005-0 PMID:22246242

Chen, T., & Guestrin, C. (2016). XGBoost: A scalable tree boosting system. In *Proceedings of the 22Nd ACM SIGKDD International Conference on Knowledge Discovery and Data Mining, KDD '16*. ACM. 10.1145/2939672.2939785

Pedregosa, F., Varoquaux, G., Gramfort, A., Michel, V., Thirion, B., Grisel, O., Blondel, M., Prettenhofer, P., Weiss, R., & Dubourg, V. (2011). Scikit-learn: Machine learning in Python. *Journal of Machine Learning Research*, *12*, 2825–2830.

Ghazi, M., Nielsen, M., Pai, A., Cardoso, M. J., Modat, M., Ourselin, S., & Sørensen, L. (2019). Training recurrent neural networks robust to incomplete data: Application to Alzheimer's disease progression modeling. *Medical Image Analysis*, *53*, 39–46. doi:10.1016/j.media.2019.01.004 PMID:30682584

Lipton, Z. C., Kale, D. C., Elkan, C., & Wetzel, R. (2016a). Learning to diagnose with LSTM recurrent neural networks. *Proceedings of the International Conference on Learning Representations (ICLR)*.

Junninen, H., Niska, H., Tuppurainen, K., Ruuskanen, J., & Kolehmainen, M. (2004). Methods for imputation of missing values in air quality data sets. *Atmospheric Environment*, *38*(18), 2895–2907. doi:10.1016/j.atmosenv.2004.02.026

Hand, D. J., & Till, R. J. (2001). A simple generalization of the area under the ROC curve for multiple class classification problems. *Machine Learning*, *45*(2), 171–186. doi:10.1023/A:1010920819831

Happ, C., & Greven, S. (2018). Multivariate functional principal component analysis for data observed on different (dimensional) domains. *Journal of the American Statistical Association*, *113*(522), 649–659. doi:10.1080/01621459.2016.1273115

Jo, T., Nho, K., & Saykin, A. J. (2019). Deep learning in Alzheimer's disease: Diagnostic classification and prognostic prediction using neuroimaging data. *Frontiers in Aging Neuroscience*, *11*, 220. doi:10.3389/fnagi.2019.00220 PMID:31481890

Suk, H. I., & Shen, D. (2013). Deep learning-based feature representation for AD/MCI classification. Med. Image Comput. Comput. Assist Interv., 16, 583–590. doi:10.1007/978-3-642-40763-5_72

Liu, S., Liu, S., Cai, W., Che, H., Pujol, S., Kikinis, R., Feng, D., Fulham, M. J., & Adni. (2015). Multimodal neuroimaging feature learning for multiclass diagnosis of Alzheimer's disease. *IEEE Transactions on Biomedical Engineering*, *62*(4), 1132–1140. doi:10.1109/TBME.2014.2372011 PMID:25423647

Suk, H. I., Lee, S. W., & Shen, D. (2015). Latent feature representation with stacked auto-encoder for AD/MCI diagnosis. *Brain Structure & Function*, *220*(2), 841–859. doi:10.100700429-013-0687-3 PMID:24363140

Galasko, D., Hansen, L. A., Katzman, R., Wiederholt, W., Masliah, E., Terry, R., Hill, L. R., Lessin, P., & Thal, L. J. (1994). Clinical-neuropathological correlations in Alzheimer's disease and related dementias. *Archives of Neurology*, *51*(9), 888–895. doi:10.1001/archneur.1994.00540210060013 PMID:8080388

White, L., Small, B. J., Petrovitch, H., Ross, G. W., Masaki, K., Abbott, R. D., Hardman, J., Davis, D., Nelson, J., & Markesbery, W. (2005). Recent clinical-pathologic research on the causes of dementia in late life: Update from the Honolulu-Asia Aging Study. *Journal of Geriatric Psychiatry and Neurology, 18*(4), 224–227. doi:10.1177/0891988705281872 PMID:16306244

Jia, X., Shi, L., Qian, T., Li, Y., Wang, D., Liang, P., & Li, K. (2018). Improved gray matter atrophy detection in Alzheimer disease in Chinese populations using Chinese brain template ". *Alzheimer Disease and Associated Disorders, 32*(4), 309–313. doi:10.1097/WAD.0000000000000264 PMID:30024411

Charletta, D., Gorelick, P. B., Dollear, T., Freels, S., & Harris, Y. (1995). CT and MRI fndings among African-Americans with Alzheimer's disease, vascular dementia, and stroke without dementia. *Neurology, 45*(8), 1456–1461. doi:10.1212/WNL.45.8.1456 PMID:7644040

Petersen, R. C. (2004). Mild cognitive impairment as a diagnostic entity. *Journal of Internal Medicine, 256*(3), 183–194. doi:10.1111/j.1365-2796.2004.01388.x PMID:15324362

Jansen, W. J., Ossenkoppele, R., Knol, D. L., Tijms, B. M., Scheltens, P., Verhey, F. R. J., Visser, P. J., Aalten, P., Aarsland, D., Alcolea, D., Alexander, M., Almdahl, I. S., Arnold, S. E., Baldeiras, I., Barthel, H., van Berckel, B. N. M., Bibeau, K., Blennow, K., Brooks, D. J., ... Zetterberg, H. (2015). Prevalence of cerebral amyloid pathology in persons without dementia: A meta-analysis. *Journal of the American Medical Association, 313*(19), 1924–1938. doi:10.1001/jama.2015.4668 PMID:25988462

McKhann, G., Drachman, D., Folstein, M., Katzman, R., Price, D., & Stadlan, E. M. (1984). Clinical diagnosis of Alzheimer's disease Report of the NINCDS-ADRDA Work Group under the auspices of Department of Health and Human Services Task Force on Alzheimer's Disease. *Neurology, 34*(7), 939–939. doi:10.1212/WNL.34.7.939 PMID:6610841

Lacor, P. N. (2004). Synaptic targeting by Alzheimer's-related amyloid β oligomers. *The Journal of Neuroscience: The Official Journal of the Society for Neuroscience, 24*(45), 10191–10200. doi:10.1523/JNEUROSCI.3432-04.2004 PMID:15537891

Fischl, B. (2012). FreeSurfer. *NeuroImage, 62*(2), 774–781. doi:10.1016/j.neuroimage.2012.01.021 PMID:22248573

Smith, S. M. (2000). *BET: Brain extraction tool. Oxford Centre for Functional Magnetic Resonance Imaging of the Brain, Department of Clinical Neurology, Oxford University, John Radclife Hospital.*

Avants, B. B., Tustison, N., & Song, G. (2009). Advanced normalization tools (ANTS). *The Insight Journal, 2*, 1–35.

Scheltens, P., Leys, D., Barkhof, F., Huglo, D., Weinstein, H. C., Vermersch, P., Kuiper, M., Steinling, M., Wolters, E. C., & Valk, J. (1992). Atrophy of medial temporal lobes on MRI in "probable" Alzheimer's disease and normal ageing: Diagnostic value and neuropsychological correlates. *Journal of Neurology, Neurosurgery, and Psychiatry, 55*(10), 967–972. doi:10.1136/jnnp.55.10.967 PMID:1431963

Szegedy, C., Iofe, S., Vanhoucke, V. & Alemi, A. (2016). *Inception-v4, inception-resnet and the impact of residual connections on learning.* arXiv preprint 1602.07261

Qian, N. (1999). On the momentum term in gradient descent learning algorithms. *Neural Networks, 12*(1), 145–151. doi:10.1016/S0893-6080(98)00116-6 PMID:12662723

Youden, W. J. (1950). Index for rating diagnostic tests. *Cancer, 3*(1), 32–35. doi:10.1002/1097-0142(1950)3:1<32::AID-CNCR2820030106>3.0.CO;2-3 PMID:15405679

DeLong, E. R., DeLong, D. M., & Clarke-Pearson, D. L. (1988). Comparing the areas under two or more correlated receiver operating characteristic curves: A nonparametric approach ". *Biometrics, 44*(3), 837–845. doi:10.2307/2531595 PMID:3203132

Achille, A., & Soatto, S. (2018). Information dropout: Learning optimal representations through noisy computation. *IEEE Transactions on Pattern Analysis and Machine Intelligence, 40*(12), 2897–2905. doi:10.1109/TPAMI.2017.2784440 PMID:29994167

Bianchi, F. M., Maiorino, E., Kampffmeyer, M. C., Rizzi, A., & Jenssen, R. (2017). *An overview and comparative analysis of recurrent neural networks for short term load forecasting*. arXiv:1705.04378

Deng, L., & Dong, Y. (2014). Deep learning: Methods and applications. *Found. Trends® Signal Process, 7*(3–4), 197–387. doi:10.1007/978-981-13-3459-7_3

Erhan, D., Bengio, Y., Courville, A., Manzagol, P.-A., Vincent, P., & Bengio, S. (2010). Why does unsupervised pre-training help deep learning? *Journal of Machine Learning Research, 11*, 625–660.

Goodfellow, I., Pouget-Abadie, J., Mirza, M., Xu, B., Warde-Farley, D., Ozair, S., Courville, A., & Bengio, Y. (2014). Generative adversarial nets. Advances in Neural Information Processing Systems, 2672–2680.

Goyal, P., Pandey, S., & Jain, K. (2018). Introduction to natural language processing and deep learning. In Deep Learning for Natural Language Processing (pp. 1–74). Springer. doi:10.1007/978-1-4842-3685-7_1

Hubens, N. (2018). *Deep inside: autoencoders—towards data science.* Google Scholar.

Le, G.V. (2015). A tutorial on deep learning part 2: autoencoders, convolutional neural networks and recurrent neural networks. *Google Brain*, 1–20.

Chapter 14
An Industry Internet of Things Framework for Epilepsy Detection, Monitoring, and Control

Smitha Sasi
Dayananda Sagar College of Engineering, India

Srividya B. V.
Dayanandasagar College of Engineering, India

ABSTRACT

Epilepsy is long-term neurological seizures of various types, some of which are defined by involuntary repetitive convulsions and have a substantial impact on patients' everyday lives. Several approaches for diagnosing these types of seizures and observing the patient have been proposed in the literature; however, these approaches fall short in terms of ergonomics and proper integration with the health system. The precision measuring that this study looks into shows what an epileptic detection and monitoring tool should be able to do. This chapter describes specific epilepsy detection and monitoring platforms that specify the conditions. The information is gathered from the wearable part of the system.

INTRODUCTION

Inadvertent convulsions are a symptom of epilepsy, a chronic neurological condition.

Around 65 million people worldwide are affected, having not only does it have a significant and dramatic influence on the patient's standard of living, but it also has a significant and dramatic impact on the patient's, but also on their career and social development; The budget of the health-care system is also severely damaged. The availability of diagnostics platforms and weblogs aids in the improvement of sickness anamnesis. These frameworks' main component was designed for two types of epilepsy crises:

DOI: 10.4018/978-1-7998-9534-3.ch014

generalized tonic-clonic seizures (S. Benicezky, 2013) and typical absence seizures, which are the most common. It's challenging to keep track of and manage epileptic episodes.

Despite the increase in anti-epileptic medications, most recent investigations of epileptic seizure detection reveal that drug-resistant epilepsy still lacks an ultimate cure.

Researchers have devised a number of epilepsy and healthcare monitoring systems to identify seizures and keep track of the patient. The majority of these management techniques are simply focused on how to enhance seizure detection and prediction

Wearable Devices (WD) and/or Body Sensor Networks (G Fortino, 2012) are two types of eHealth platforms that have been developed and according to the survey for the identification and/or diagnostics of illnesses in real time (BSN). WD are typically offered for data collection, biological variable measurement, or user input, with Mobile Cloud Computing (MCC) (Thome-Souza, 2014) processing performed locally or Cloud Computing (CC) services requested. CC services are typically in charge of collecting and analyzing model learning and computationally intensive operations, as well as sampling data from sensors. In addition, the CC services provide a presentation layer, which includes user alarms for patients or medical professionals, the patient's relations are informed and even visuals and data analytics for future research (Khelil, 2014).

CoCaMaal, ROCHAS, (M.Chen, 2013) and AACMPE are examples of such platforms. A firm called CoCaMaal (A. Forkan, 2014), or cloud-oriented perspective middleware in environmental aided living, specializes in patient monitoring and event control, such as alerts and accidents.

This technique is limited to thoroughly regulated environments as long as it recommends BSN implementation based on the patient's needs. ROCHAS (Robotics and Cloud-assisted Healthcare System for Empty Nesters) is a second intriguing platform that offers the observation of individuals with disabilities in their own homes, permits to lead life as autonomously as possible with the help of an aid robot. In a series of research examining how open software platforms can function together, an assistance platform for older people was presented.

ACM (Triaxial Accelerometer) (C. Pradhan, 2011) was presented as a solution for epileptic seizure detection, and a wristband with an ACM that is tethered to a smartphone was recommended for MCC-based solutions detect the presence convulsions; however, no additional connections with CC services are planned. The BSN was proposed in, utilizing the localized Smart devices for information analysis and communicating to the health industry personnel with the patient situation. Work that was similar to this was shown in "Health Monitoring and Management Using Internet-of-Things (IoT) Sensing with Cloud-based Processing"

The Internet of Things (IoT) has enabled a plethora of applications, one of which is smart and linked health care. Networked sensors, whether worn on the body or integrated in our living spaces, allow for the collection of detailed information about our physical and mental health. Such data, if collected on a regular basis, consolidated, and efficiently mined, has the potential to reshape the health-care landscape for the better (R F Fischer, 2011).

In particular, data analysis at previously unimagined scales and temporal longitudes, combined with today's intelligent processing algorithms, can: (a) aid in the evolution of medical practice from the current post facto diagnose-and-treat activated concept to a proactive framework for disease prognosis, prevention, cure, and proper effectiveness.

Using a Wrist-Based Wearable Platform to Detect and Predict Seizures

The suggested technology attempts to create comprehensive Multimodal seizure detection approaches are used in this wrist-based device. The purpose is to promote a platform that handles febrile seizures as well as seizures in general, with three main phases: (1) seizure detection, (2) continuous monitoring and data collection, and (3) seizure prediction in the long term. After analyzing existing seizure detection equipment and methods and weighing the benefits and drawbacks of each, it was determined that seizure detection would essentially include the measurement of the following criteria. - motion, electrodermal activity (EDA), skin temperature, and heart rate. The efficacy of seizure detection would be improved if all of the aforementioned factors were measured at the same time.

Skin Temperature Measurement

Because fever is the most common cause of seizure, temperature is an important metric to monitor in the event of febrile seizures. Because a child's brain is more vulnerable to fever than an adult's, febrile seizures are most common in children under the age of six, particularly between the ages of 12 and 18 months. The gadget incorporates a skin temperature sensor (a calibrated thermistor) with an accuracy of 0.1°C because temperature is an important characteristic to assess for identifying a febrile seizure. The sensor is actively checking the skin temperature for any significant changes in temperature.

Heart Rate

Heart rate variations caused by seizures are rather common. Seizure-related cardiac alterations are usually transitory and need not likely to be causing any clinically significant abnormalities in the patient. Because of a suspected link with sudden unexpected mortality in epilepsy, seizure-related cardiac abnormalities have gained more attention in recent years (SUDEP). Extremely high rates that prevent the heart from filling with blood, or pauses in the heart rate, are the most severe.

Reflectance photoplethysmography is used to determine a patient's heart rate (PPG). Light is emitted onto the tissue in reflectance photoplethysmography, and the reflected light is recorded by the detector (a photo diode). Because of the pulsatile blood flow induced by the heart's beating, the detected light reflected from the bodily portion will fluctuate. The time gap between two subsequent peaks of maximal light absorption and reflectance is used to measure heart rate. The LED utilized as a light source in PPG has a wavelength of 570nm and a sampling rate of 30 S/s.

Detection

Video, accelerometers, gyroscopes, magnetometers, and electromyography are commonly used to identify abnormal movement (EMG). To detect rapid, uncoordinated movements that occur during seizures, a system of accelerometer, gyroscope, and magnetometer can be affixed to one of the four limbs of the body.

Electrodermal Activity (EDA)

The sympathetic nervous system's arousal is measured by electrodermal activity, often known as galvanic skin reaction. Galvanometers or ohm-meters in the form of electrodes are used to measure skin conductance or impedance.

The sympathetic and parasympathetic nerve systems make up the autonomic nervous system.

The sympathetic nervous system regulates the human body's response. Your sympathetic activation increases when you're excited or stressed, whether it's physical, emotional, or cognitive. Significant increases in sympathetic activation, which correspond to the activation of specific brain areas, are also observed.

Because the sympathetic nervous system affects only the skin and not the parasympathetic nervous system, Electrodermal Activity (EDA) can be utilized to identify seizures. When the sweat glands are overworked,

The electrical conductivity of the skin changes when it is stimulated. EDA can be used to detect these changes. Electrodes attached to the device's strap/band are used to measure EDA. Electrodes made of stainless steel or silver can be utilized for this. These electrodes deliver a tiny alternating current to the skin. Changes in skin conductance caused by changes in the autonomic nervous system are then measured by the electrodes.

Figure 1. Generalized block diagram

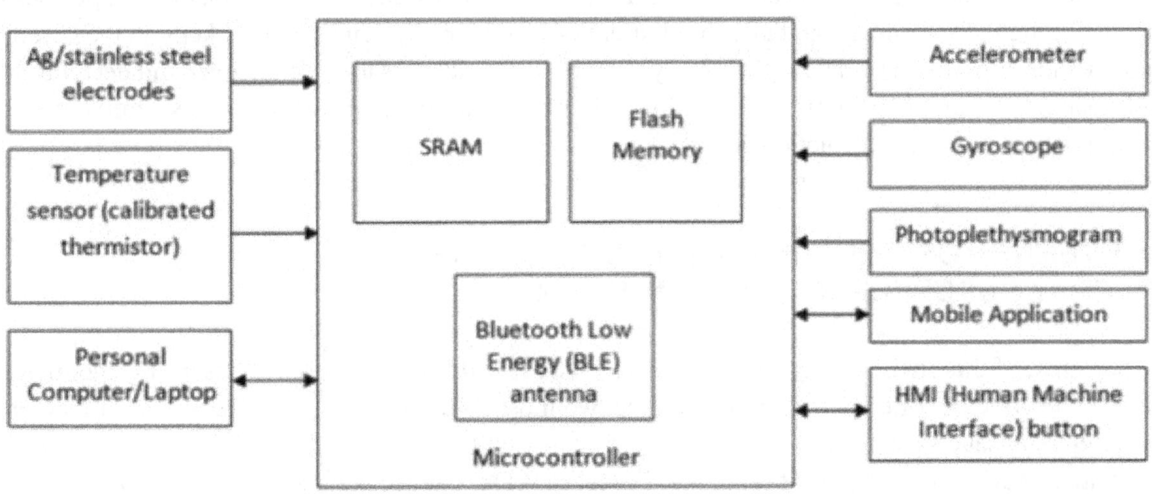

Figure 2. Cloud based server connectivity

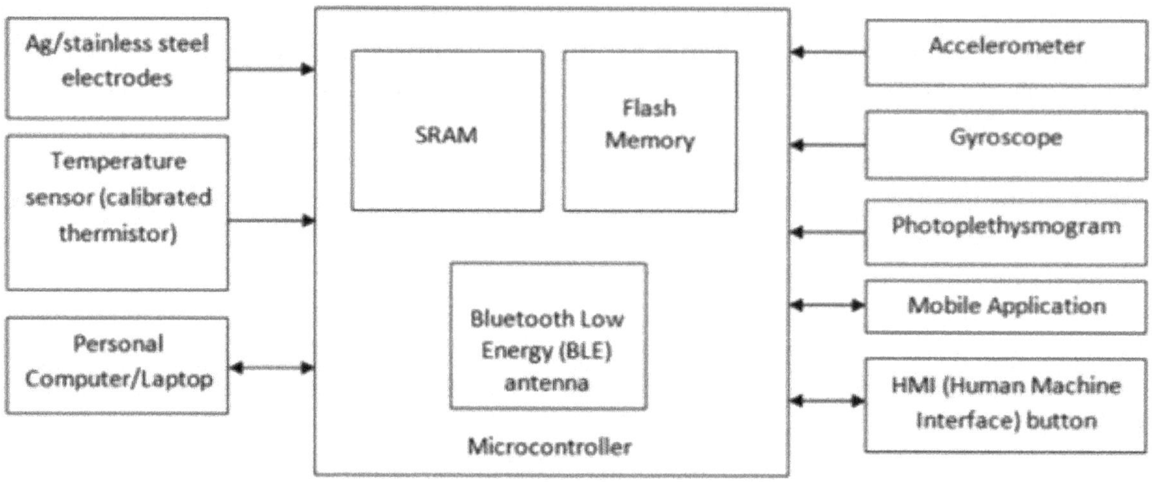

Data Analysis and Seizure Prediction

The suggested concept is a dynamic platform that grows from a seizure detection device to a seizure prediction device by collecting vast amounts of data from people of all ages who suffer from various types of seizures and epilepsy. Patients who suffer from seizures are researched for extended periods of time, including before, during, and after a seizure. For usage by physicians, data is kept on the cloud as can be seen in Figure 2. The data is then analyzed with data analytics tools to uncover and detect trends in the many different physiological signs, allowing the system to adapt and improve seizure detection algorithms based on the information acquired.

AN INTERNET OF THING INFRASTRUCTURE FOR EPILEPSY SUPERVISING AND MONITORING

The objective of this study is to create Internet of Thing based Infrastructure for observing and managing epileptic affected patients, with a focus on the two most common types of epilepsy: focal myoclonic and epileptic absence seizures.

A Patient's Kit (PK) is a pair of Wearable Devices (WDs) connected to a Smartphone by Bluetooth 4.0 Low Energy in this investigation (PK). This solution improves the solution's ergonomic concerns while encouraging patients to use it indefinitely. The WD should feature Triaxial Accelerometer (ACM) and Heart Rate (HR) sensors to identify epileptic convulsions of 2 kinds.

Design Decisions and Requirements

The application of percutaneous WD, like as a wristband for sensory stimulation and a Smartphone, is recommended in this study to help patients continue with their everyday activities. In this investigation, a patient's kit consists of a pair of WDs connected to a Smartphone through Bluetooth 4.0 Low Energy

(PK). This s remedy addresses the user-friendly concerns of the issues while also motivating patients to using indefinitely. The WD should feature ACM and HR (Petersen, 2011) sensory instruments to monitor epileptic convulsions of 2 kinds. The strategies used were determined by two factors: i) the results gained, and (ii) the model's simplicity. They may be designed to execute on any available infrastructure, even smartphones, due to their simplicity.

This method stated that, in addition to data gathering and processing, MCC services (J R Viller, 2016) may be upgraded to include assessment of a localized model and possibly simple thresholding. To accomplish this, The MCC kernel would benefit from gradual delivery/ deployment of trained/tuned models to enable regular reporting and timely responses are even when the Cloud Computing is completely unavailable over Wi-Fi networks. With the goal of maximizing battery life, a combination of MCC and CC, as well as a good balance algorithm to identify where the decisions or calculations should be done.

One of the contributions of this work is to analyze the effectiveness of MCC computation, which minimizes communication actions, and Cloud Computing computations, which reduces time complexity in the Smart devices.

The concept of ontology-driven tasks makes it easier to extend the system, allowing new procedures to be readily conceptualized, distributed, and deployed across any of the accessible compute levels. Dynamic data collecting personalization, on the other hand, relates to the markers for which patients' data should be obtained. The implementation of dynamic data gathering is enabled by the construction of ontology driven tasks, which may be considered as a new task dedicated to a certain set of patients.

The System Abstract Architecture

Consider the following scenario: a full description of the computing devices that can be utilized to execute all of the computations required to distinguish and analyze a specific patient. Assume you have a comprehensive ontology of applications, processes, gadgets, and contexts.

A mediator is used in this technique, who assigns tasks to be accomplished and where they should be completed for each case. As a result, a job sequence for each patient and scenario can be planned and assigned.

In other words, for each patient and scenario, they can construct a unique work completion and task assignment. Both are publicly expressed in the ontology, and this information is available on any computer device, even cellphones.

As a solution for this particularly specialized epilepsy observation and supervision platform, Figure 3 portrays proposed abstract architecture. A PK consists of a WD and a Smartphone with a full app that does sensor sampling and other operations in addition to the ontology and current schedule.

A PK is made up of a WD and a Mobile device; the Smartphone contains a comprehensive app that does sensor sampling and other functions in addition to the ontology and current schedule. Wi-Fi networks are utilized to transmit information samples and to be secured storage in the health industry. Notifications and cautions, on the other hand, should be transmitted using the available connectivity.

Additionally, some venues may be able to accommodate specialized hardware that serves as a federated CC server. When Wi-Fi is accessible, the Smartphone must assign to these systems to reduce the prerequisites for computation and hence extend battery life.

The health system services, both CC and data storage, handle seizure detection, alert production, and notifications, as well as medical staff reporting.

The services required for appropriate epileptic convulsions detection and diagnostic testing are managed by the central Cloud computing services, as shown in the Dmz network, whereas solutions and activities devoted to extracting relevant information's should be done on specific servers pertaining to the individual trauma facility.

The MCC and Monitoring unit are depicted schematically in Figure 3. The proposed architecture for this investigation. In the current scenario, every computing element has exposure to the ontology, the patient's idea of the work, and allotment. The PK can work on its own or in conjunction with the CC services that are provided. The setup that results in the longest battery life will be chosen wherever possible.

Figure 3. The MCC and monitoring unit

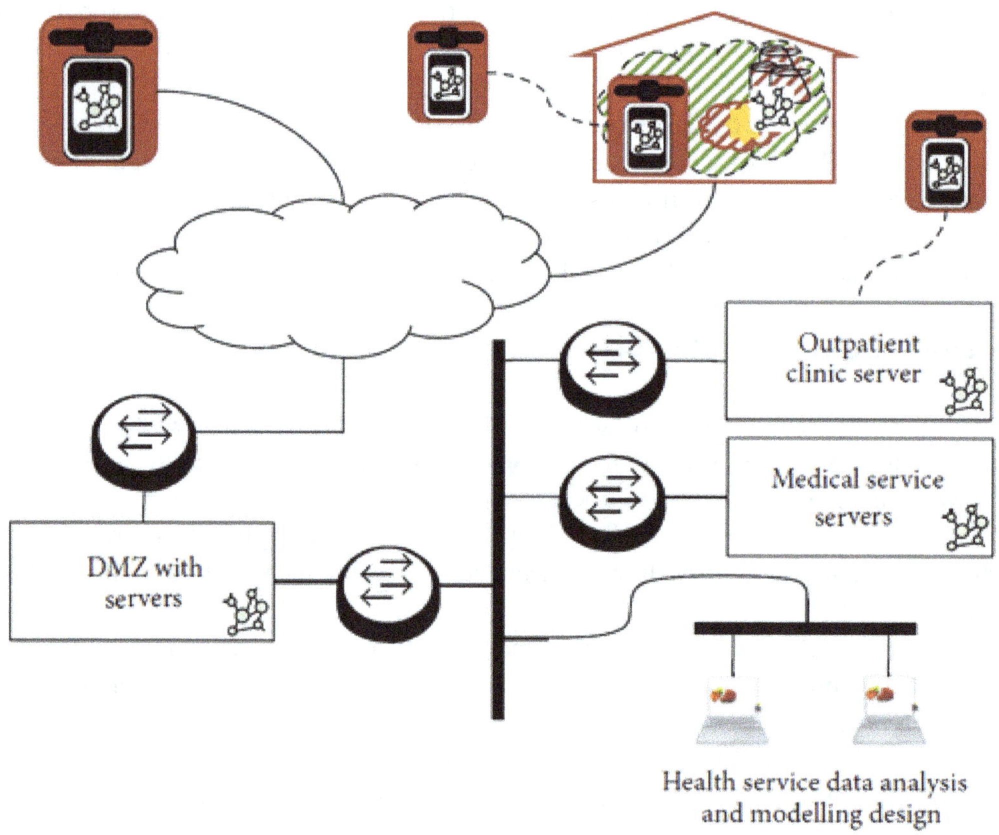

Figure 4. a) The PK scheme (b) The MCC structure

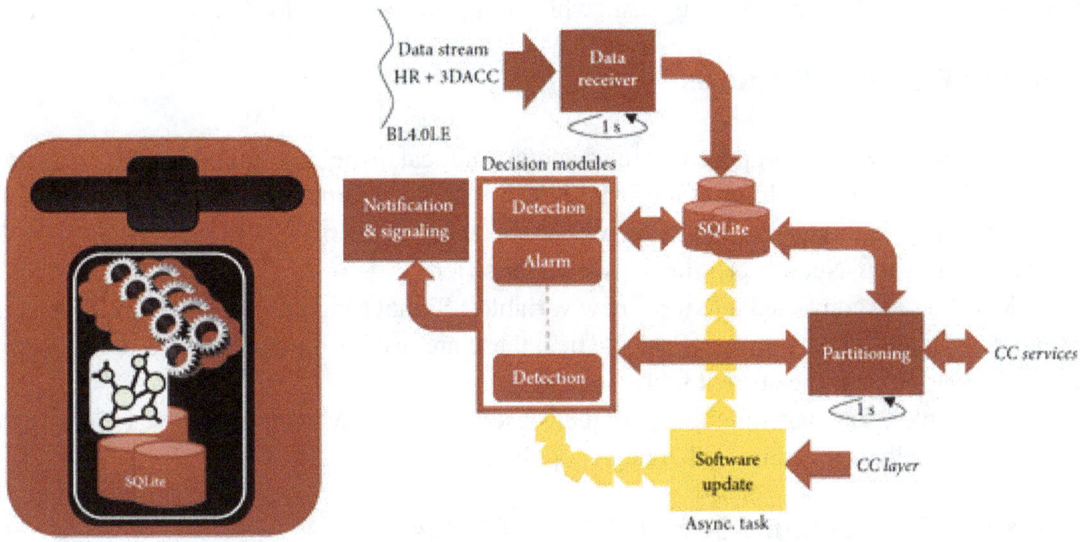

(a) The patient's kit scheme (b) The MCC architecture

The various services refer to the software's ability to I accept and send data from the WD and transmit it to the CC layer, (ii) receive and send notifications and alarms, and so on.

MCCC Architecture

MANET is the appropriate architecture for this proposed approach. Because of its local storage capacity and data processing, the MANET architecture enables a high level of autonomy. In addition, queries to cloud services that need a large amount of processing power are permitted.

Consequently, the cloudlet solution is unsuitable for only one functional that can be associated with the MCC layer, and most importantly, each patient's data is completely independent of one another; this last fact implies that MCC synchronization among MCC layers is excessive, reduces computational requirements of this layer. The Smartphone is envisioned as a service node that is in charge of storing real-time data and its transformations, as well as performing limited computing activities.

Figure 4 (b) shows the planned architecture in detail. On a continual basis, a timer dispatches two key jobs, the Data Receiver and the Partitioning activities.

These jobs are in charge of interacting with the architecture's exterior layers as well as the computer decision models (Decision Modules). The Data Receiver job collects information from the bracelet and stores it in an SQLite database.

This task takes as input a block of measurements taken in the bracelet over the course of one second, which are safely saved in the SQLite database or data repository. The Partitioning job is also responsible for offloading; its objective is to partition the data and request CC or MCC services using raw or processed data.

This job runs sliding windows on unprocessed data, asking services for computing data transformations and implementing decision models based on data whenever there is unprocessed data. The job will request services from the MCC or the CC, saving intermediate data in SQLite, if necessary, based on the energy efficiency information. Furthermore, the Partitioning task should be split into two parts: the windowing service and the job scheduling task, which is also responsible for CC/MCC service requests.

Detection of Epileptic Seizures

Two types of models have been proposed for the detection of focal myoclonic epileptic seizures: primarily Genetic Fuzzy Finite State Machines (GFFSM) (J. R. Villar, 2016) implemented for epileptic recognition, and secondarily feature extraction using a Distance based Principal Component Analysis (DPCA) step accompanied by a K-Nearest Neighbor (KNN) classifier.

The ACM values are converted into three new variables: Signal Magnitude Ratio (SMA), Amount of Movement (AoM), and Time Between Peaks (TbP), these are used as input variables to the fuzzy rule system, in association with the current fuzzy state.

If a good variable fuzzy partitioning technique is used, the GFFSM approach yields highly generalized systems that really can handle with a huge population.

A Robust and Fast Seizure Detector for IoT Edge

This research proposed by using the discrete wavelet transform, statistical feature extraction, and a naïve Bayes (NB) classifier are used to detect seizures. The system that has been proposed Simulink R was used to create and test the model. Thing Speak and commercially available microcontrollers. The results of the experiments demonstrate shows the proposed approach lowering latency by 44% when compared to the current system a cloud-based IoT system that generates a classification accuracy of 98.65%.

Figure 5. Proposed seizure detection framework

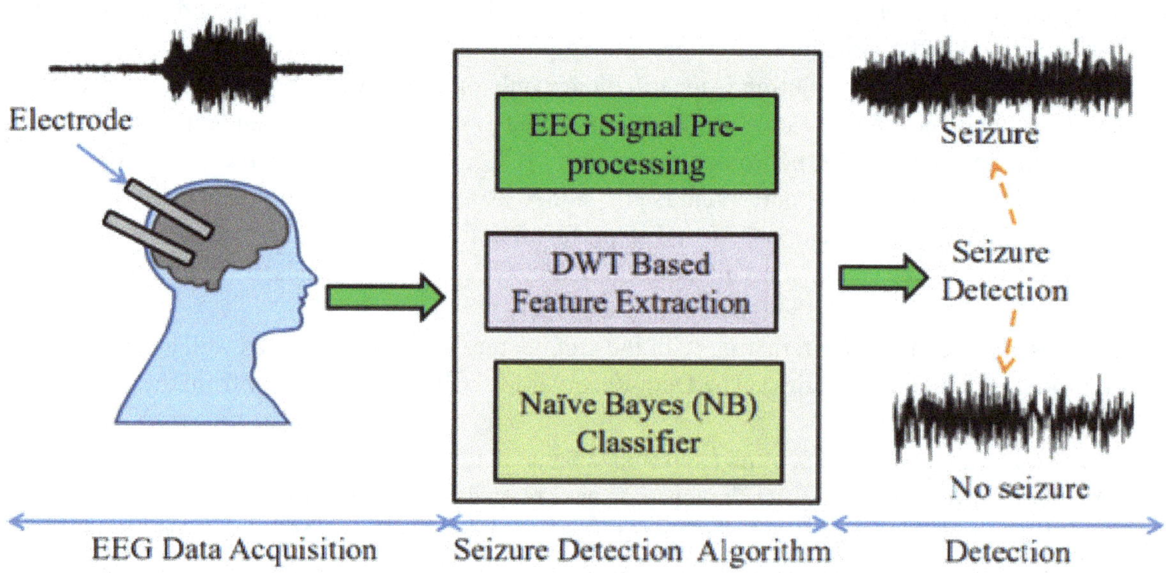

The Main Contribution of this research:

The suggested seizure detection method employs the DWT, statistical characteristics, and a naive Bayes classifier. DWT is used to localize the Temporal Frequency (TF) of the Electroencephalogram (EEG) signal. The statistical features have a lot of potential for separating seizure from non-seizure behavior, and the naive Bayes classifier enhances classification accuracy.

Cloud computing has a lot of processing power and storage, but it has a long reaction time, whereas edge computing has a lot of computational power and storage but a fast response time. To cope with a patient's urgent health circumstances, Internet of Medical Things (IoMT) apps require a quick response time and an acceptable computation capacity.

In comparison to cloud-IoT frameworks, the suggested edge-IoT framework minimizes latency and enables universal connectivity with ambient intelligence. The patient's healthcare data can be accessed from anywhere and at any time in the edge-IoT architecture for remote consultation.

EDGE-IOT PERSPECTIVE

Figure 6. Architecture of the proposed system in the edge-IoT perspective

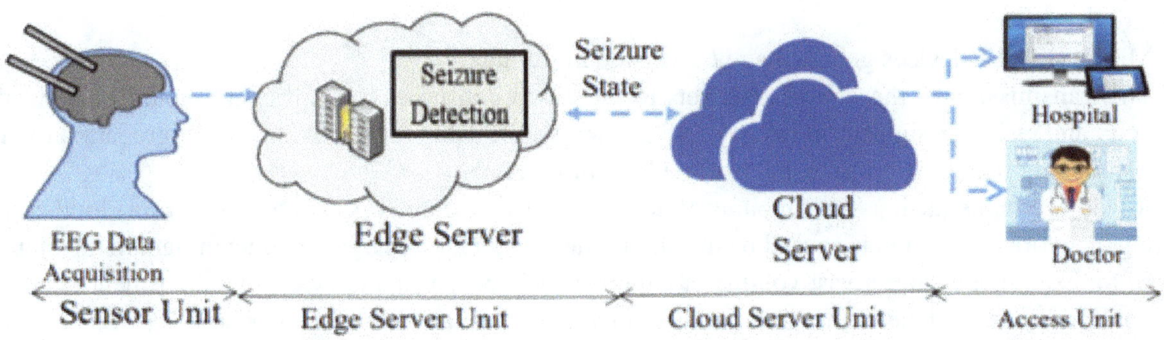

Sensor Unit

The large IoT network contains vast number of sensors and devices. The sensor unit is critical for the IoT since it consumes the majority of the resources. Due to its low capacity, the sensor unit cannot fulfil the majority of these requirements. The sensor unit is in charge of collecting EEG data. When the data collection is finished, it is transferred to the edge server for processing.

Edge Server Unit

In typical cloud-based IoT, the cloud handles the majority of computations. Edge computing meets the majority of resource requirements, such as EEG data interpretation and data storage.

Processing and temporary data storage are done on the computer. edge servers, which boost data processing and archiving performance. The proposed technique is utilized to detect seizures by analyzing and processing EEG data. This gadget can also be used as a temporary storage site for the patient's EEG data. The information pertaining to the patient's seizure status is transferred to the cloud when a seizure is detected

Only relevant data is delivered to the cloud through the edge servers.

Cloud Server Unit

Cloud servers are installed remote from end devices in edge computing, allowing for high processing and big data storage. Edge nodes can meet the computational needs of IoT devices devices in real-time services since IoT devices do not require a lot of processing power. Furthermore, by offloading computation processes, power consumption has been greatly lowered.

Access Unit

Health practitioners may access cloud data from anywhere at any time, enabling remote health services and providing universal connectivity to IoT devices. A notification will be sent to the doctor in the event of a health abnormality. After examining the patient's medication history, the doctor will prescribe the appropriate dosage.

Seizure detection at the edge of the Internet of Things has the following advantages over cloud-based seizure detection:

Millions of IoT devices generate a massive amount of data.

The transmission of these large data sets to the cloud consumes a significant amount of network capacity and results in significant latency. IoT gateways shift data pre-processing and aggregation to the edge, reducing transmission time and bandwidth requirements.

IoT devices generate massive amounts of data that must be stored on a storage server. In cloud computing, network congestion is caused by the simultaneous storage of large amounts of data in the cloud. EEG, for example, creates a vast volume of data that must be saved and evaluated in a timely manner. The performance of cloud computing-based storage is inadequate due to network traffic. The network traffic can be decreased by transferring storage demand to other edge storage nodes in edge computing.

The DWT Based Seizure Detection Approach

The DWT is used to first deconstruct EEG signals, and then the decomposed signals are fed into the feature extraction unit. The extracted features are delivered to the NB classifier for classification once feature extraction is complete.

Figure 7. Architecture of the proposed seizure detection approach

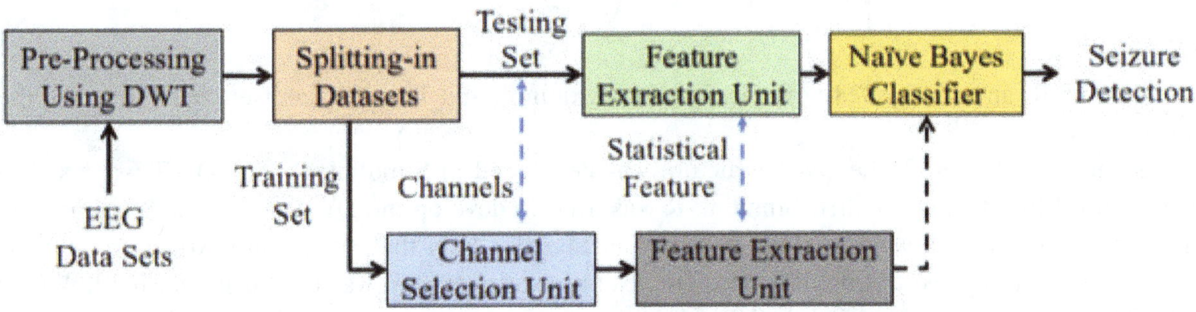

Variance and Standard Deviation

The dispersion of data from its main value is measured by variance and its square root (standard deviation. The energy of the kth epoch is denoted by

$$Energy = \sum_{K=1}^{L} (A_k)^2$$

where Ak is the amplitude of the kth sample and L is the epoch's total number of samples

Naive Bayes (NB) Classifier

Based on Bayesian theory, the Naive Bayes classifier requires less data for training. The NB classifier's algorithm is as follows:

Consider an n-feature attribute vector z. For the attribute z, the posterior probability of the class Cp is derived as follows:

$$P\left(C_p|z\right) = \frac{P\left(z|C_p\right)P\left(C_p\right)}{p\left(z\right)}$$

where p(Cp) is the class's prior probability, p(z) is the attribute's prior probability, and p(cup) is the probability of z for a particular class. Conditional independence is used in Naive Bayes models, where zi is independent of Zu for a given class Cp. The equation above can be represented as:

$$p\left(C_p|z\right) = p\left(C_p\right)\prod_{i=1}^{n} p(z_i \mid C_p)$$

The attribute is assigned a class label based on the highest posterior probability, which is specified by the equation below.

$$p\left(C_1\right)\prod_{i=1}^{n}p\left(z_i|C_1\right) > p\left(C_2\right)\prod_{i=1}^{n}p(z_i \mid C_2)$$

Simulink R, an ATmega328P microcontroller (Arduino), and Thing Speak were used to create the suggested system.

As shown in Figure 8, the DWT structure was developed in Simulink R. The DWT was used to decompose EEG datasets at first. Simulink R was used to develop the DWT structure. A training set and a testing set were created from the decomposed signals. After that, the feature extraction unit was fed both the training and testing data sets. The feature extraction unit was built using a Simulink user specified function. The naïve Bayes (NB) classifier was used to process the statistical characteristics extracted from the feature extraction unit. A Simulink function was used to build the NB classifier's structure. The classifier was trained using the training data sets. The detection was based on the class with the highest posterior probability.

To save the data in the cloud, Thing Speak, an open data platform, was used. Simulink sends a notification to Thing Speak when it detects a seizure.

Figure 8. DWT structure with Simulink R

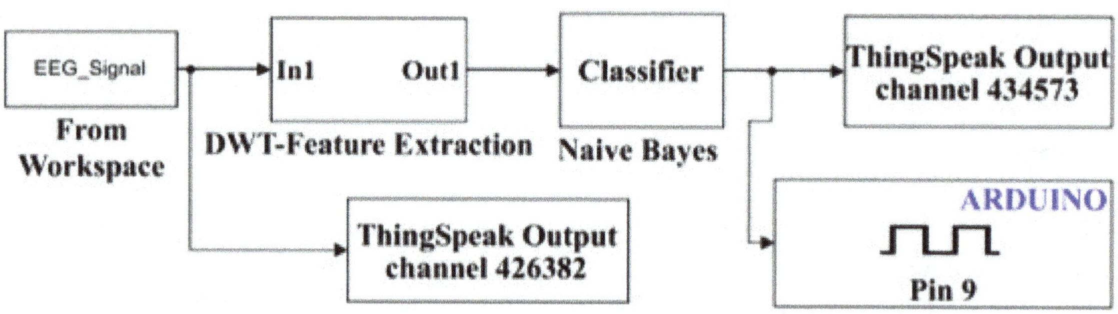

ACCURACY COMPARISON WITH EXISTING SYSTEMS

The experimental analysis of various image processing and Artificial Intelligence techniques with respect to accuracy for classification of epilepsy-based disorders is shown in Table 1

Table 1. Accuracy comparison with existing systems

Methods	Accuracy (%)
Support Vector Machines	78.74
Neural Network	95
Weighted Permutation Entropy	96.5
Feature Extraction, k-NN classifier	97.08
DWT and Naïve Bayes Classifier	98.65

The DWT and Naïve Bayes Classifier technique gives a higher accuracy, as can be seen in Table 1.

Table 2 highlights the Main epileptic detection platforms and possible solutions published so far. A detailed description with some concerns with respect to the relevant factors is elaborated

Table 2. Survey study of various techniques for detection of epilepsy

Self-tracking via brain-mobile-cloud interface,	CC services are used in conjunction with EEG (G. Bajwa, 2013) sensory equipment connected to a smartphone that does some data processing. However, because this is a brief communication, the answer is not detailed.
Detection of generalized tonic-clonic seizures by a wireless wrist accelerometer: a prospective, multicenter study	This is primarily a research project aimed solely at detecting tonic-clonic epileptic episodes. For obtaining offline models, AWD without wireless transmission saved data and several machine learning approaches were used
EpiCare - a home care platform based on mobile cloud computing to assist epilepsy diagnosis	The Android software in EpiCare (D. Callegari, 2014) collects data from an EEG electrode cap and runs on a Smartphone device. This hardware makes this method extremely efficient, but it is also quite uncomfortable. The essential point is that the study is focused on SUDEP, As a result, sleeping with a cap is possible. A CC/MCC hybrid approach is developed., implying that intelligent task delivery and allocation should be carried out but without presenting a realistic method.
Myepipal, Mobile application for managing, monitoring and predicting epilepsy patient,	MyEpiPal(N. A. Marzuki, 2016) is a patient-monitoring app that also facilitates caregiver-patient contact and allows for self-management. This means that, while it makes use of the Smartphone's sensory capabilities, the main purpose is to assist the patient in daily activities. Although the measures can aid in the prediction of the development of a seizure, it is included in this comparison because it is not an epilepsy detection platform.
Miniaturized wireless Electrocardiogram (ECG) (F. Masse, 2013) monitor for real-time detection of epileptic seizures	This article describes the creation of an ad hoc epilepsy detection ECG wireless intelligent sensor that comprises multiple detection methods and is connected to a local computer via a network. Ergonomic problems and battery longevity were among the many critical factors investigated. To send alerts, receive configuration commands, and start/stop HR recording so that it can be downloaded, the WD connects to the local computer. There is a rather detailed explanation of both the criteria and the hardware choices.
An automatic prediction of epileptic seizures using cloud computing and wireless sensor networks	The data from an EEG cap connected to a Smartphone is sent to CC services. When a seizure is identified in the cloud, the notification system sends out GPS coordinates. The platform's ergonomics, battery life and autonomy, as well as its economic considerations, have not been examined.
Free Epilepsy Smart-Phone App (T E Society, 2013)	The Epilepsy Society of the United Kingdom has released an app for Android and iPhone that incorporates a Web-based seizure journal, medication monitoring, and other features. This is a stand-alone service, and the data it collects is not shared with any health-care provider.
Epilepsy seizure detection app for wearable technologies	An independent mobile solution is available, which is based on a commercial Smartwatch (MIO Alpha) (S. Sareen, 2016) that is connected to an Android phone. Data collection and processing, as well as epileptic seizure detection modules, are all handled by the app. The method solely considers thresholds and ignores intelligent modules; this methodology is ineffective for this type of detection. (A. Ulate-Campos-2016)

CONCLUSION

This study investigated the solutions described in the literature for epileptic tonic-clonic seizure detection and monitoring. The great majority of approaches supports various distinguishing characteristics, including establishing ergonomic ways, supporting everyday life, providing cost-effective solutions, storing sampled data, and providing intelligent CC services. Adding real-time response or taking into account multiple services based on MCC size. This study considers each of these variables while designing an IoT platform for epileptic seizure detection and monitoring. One of the approaches is based on a wristband connected to a smartphone that implements MCC services and also has access to CC services. The overall goal is to identify seizures, store sensory system information, generate warnings and notifications, and apply machine learning techniques to the data to create the best models to detect or visualize the data.

REFERENCES

Andrzejak, R. G., Lehnertz, K., Mormann, F., Rieke, C., David, P., & Elger, C. E. (2001, November). Indications of Nonlinear Deterministic and Finite-dimensional Structures in Time Series of Brain Electrical Activity: Dependence on Recording Region and Brain State. *Physical Review E: Statistical, Nonlinear, and Soft Matter Physics*, *64*(6), 061907. doi:10.1103/PhysRevE.64.061907 PMID:11736210

Bajwa, G., Dantu, R., Issadeen, M. F. M., & Joseph, R. M. (2013). Selftracking via brain-mobile-cloud interface. *Proceedings of the AAAI Spring Symposium Series.*

Bayindir, R., Yesilbudak, M., Colak, M., & Genc, N. (2017). A Novel Application of Naive Bayes Classifier in Photovoltaic Energy Prediction. *Proceedings of the 16th IEEE International Conference on Machine Learning and Applications*, 523–527. 10.1109/ICMLA.2017.0-108

Beniczky, S., Polster, T., Kjaer, T. W., & Hjalgrim, H. (2013). Detection of generalized tonic-clonic seizures by a wireless wrist accelerometer: A prospective, multicenter study. *Epilepsia*, *54*(4), e58–e61. doi:10.1111/epi.12120 PMID:23398578

Borcea, C., Ding, X., Gehani, N., Curtmola, R., Khan, M. A., & Debnath, H. (2015). Avatar: mobile distributed computing in the cloud. *Proceedings of the 3rd IEEE International Conference on Mobile Cloud Computing, Services, and Engineering, Mobile-Cloud 2015*, 151–156. 10.1109/MobileCloud.2015.22

Callegari, D., Conte, E., & Ferreto, T. (2014). EpiCare - a home care platform based on mobile cloud computing to assist epilepsy diagnosis. *Proceedings of the 4th International Conference on Wireless Mobile Communication and Healthcare, MOBIHEALTH 2014*, 148–151. 10.4108/icst.mobihealth.2014.257379

Daoud, H. G., Abdelhameed, A. M., & Bayoumi, M. (2018). Automatic Epileptic Seizure Detection Based on Empirical Mode Decomposition An Deep Neural Network. *Proceedings of the IEEE 14th International Colloquium on Signal Processing Its Applications*, 182–186. 10.1109/CSPA.2018.8368709

Deshmukh, S., & Shah, R. (2016). Computation offloading frameworks in mobile cloud computing: a survey. *Proceedings of the 2016 IEEE International Conference on Current Trends in Advanced Computing, ICCTAC 2016*, 1–5. 10.1109/ICCTAC.2016.7567332

Direito, B., Teixeira, C., Ribeiro, B., Castelo-Branco, M., Sales, F., & Dourado, A. (2012). Modeling epileptic brain states using EEG spectral analysis and topographic mapping. *Journal of Neuroscience Methods*, *210*(2), 220–229. doi:10.1016/j.jneumeth.2012.07.006 PMID:22850556

Dolgin, E. (2018). *This Seizure-Detecting Smartwatch Could Save Your Life*. https://spectrum.ieee.org/the-human-os/biomedical/diagnostics/this-seizuredetecting-smartwatch-could-save-your-life

Doukas, C., & Maglogiannis, I. (2011). Managing wearable sensor data through Cloud Computing. *Proceedings of the 2011 3rd IEEE International Conference on Cloud Computing Technology and Science, CloudCom 2011*, 440–445. 10.1109/CloudCom.2011.65

Engel, J. Jr. (2001). A proposed diagnostic scheme for people with epileptic seizures and with epilepsy: Report of the ILAE task force on classification and terminology. *Epilepsia*, *42*(6), 796–803. doi:10.1046/j.1528-1157.2001.10401.x PMID:11422340

Fernando, N., Loke, S. W., & Rahayu, W. (2013). Mobile cloud computing: A survey. *Future Generation Computer Systems*, *29*(1), 84–106. doi:10.1016/j.future.2012.05.023

Fisher, R. S., Van Emde Boas, W., & Blume, W. (2005). Epileptic seizures and epilepsy: Definitions proposed by the International League Against Epilepsy (ILAE) and the International Bureau for Epilepsy (IBE). *Epilepsia*, *46*(4), 470–472. doi:10.1111/j.0013-9580.2005.66104.x PMID:15816939

Forkan, A., Khalil, I., & Tari, Z. (2014). CoCaMAAL: A cloud-oriented context-aware middleware in ambient assisted living. *Future Generation Computer Systems*, *35*, 114–127. doi:10.1016/j.future.2013.07.009

Forkan, A., Khalil, I., & Tari, Z. (2014). CoCaMAAL: A cloud-oriented context-aware middleware in ambient assisted living. *Future Generation Computer Systems*, *35*, 114–127. doi:10.1016/j.future.2013.07.009

Fortino, M. P., & di Fatta, G. (2012). BodyCloud: integration of cloud computing and body sensor networks. *Proceedings of the 4th IEEE International Conference on Cloud Computing Technology and Science (CloudCom '12)*, 851–856. 10.1109/CloudCom.2012.6427537

Hasan, R., Hossain, M. M., & Khan, R. (2015). Aura: An IoT based cloud infrastructure for localized mobile computation outsourcing. *Proceedings of the 3rd IEEE International Conference on Mobile Cloud Computing, Services, and Engineering, MobileCloud 2015*, 183–188. 10.1109/MobileCloud.2015.37

Hosseini, M. P., Pompili, D., Elisevich, K., & Soltanian-Zadeh, H. (2017, December). Optimized Deep Learning for EEG Big Data and Seizure Prediction BCI via Internet of Things. *IEEE Transactions on Big Data*, *3*(4), 392–404. doi:10.1109/TBDATA.2017.2769670

Huang, D., Zhang, X., Kang, M., & Luo, J. (2010). MobiCloud: building secure cloud framework for mobile computing and communication. *Proceedings of the 5th IEEE International Symposium on Service-Oriented SystemEngineering, SOSE 2010*, 27–34. 10.1109/SOSE.2010.20

Huerta-Canepa, G., & Lee, D. (2010). A virtual cloud computing provider for mobile devices. In *Proceedings of the 1st ACM Workshop on Mobile Cloud Computing and Services: Social Networks and Beyond (MCS '10)*. ACM. 10.1145/1810931.1810937

Khelil, A., Shaikh, F. K., Sheikh, A. A., Felemban, E., & Bojan, H. (2014). DigiAID: A wearable health platform for automated self-tagging in emergency cases. *Proceedings of the 4th International Conference on Wireless Mobile Communication and Healthcare, MOBIHEALTH2014*, 296–299. 10.4108/icst.mobihealth.2014.257541

Kumar, Y., Dewal, M., & Anand, R. (2014, October). Epileptic Seizures Detection in EEG Using DWT-based ApEn and Artificial Neural Network. *Signal, Image and Video Processing*, *8*(7), 1323–1334. doi:10.100711760-012-0362-9

Liu, F., Shu, P., & Jin, H. (2013). Gearing resource-poor mobile devices with powerful clouds: Architectures, challenges, and applications. *IEEE Wireless Communications*, *20*(3), 14–21. doi:10.1109/MWC.2013.6549279

Marzuki, N. A., Husain, W., & Shahiri, A. M. (2016). Myepipal, Mobile application for managing, monitoring and predicting epilepsy patient. In *Proceedings of the International Conferenceon Advances in Information and Communication Technology*, (pp. 383–392). Springer.

Masse, Bussel, Serteyn, Arends, & Penders. (2013). Miniaturized wireless ECG monitor for real-time detection of epileptic seizures. *Transactions on Embedded Computing Systems, 12*(4).

Othman, M., Madani, S. A., & Khan, S. U. (2014). A survey of mobile cloud computing application models. *IEEE Communications Surveys and Tutorials*, *16*(1), 393–413. doi:10.1109/SURV.2013.062613.00160

Puthal, D., Obaidat, M. S., Nanda, P., Prasad, M., Mohanty, S. P., & Zomaya, A. Y. (2018, May). Secure and Sustainable Load Balancing of Edge Data Centers in Fog Computing. *IEEE Communications Magazine*, *56*(5), 60–65. doi:10.1109/MCOM.2018.1700795

Roman, U. K. D., & Lausen, H. (2005). *The Web Service Modeling Ontology Wsmo*. Final Version. http://www.wsmo.org/TR/d2/v1.1/

Salem, O., Naseem, A., & Mehaoua, A. (2014). Epileptic Seizure Detection from EEG Signal Using Discrete Wavelet Transform and Ant Colony Classifier. *Proceedings of the IEEE International Conference on Communications*, 3529–3534. 10.1109/ICC.2014.6883868

Samie, F., Paul, S., Bauer, L., & Henkel, J. (2018). Highly Efficient And Accurate Seizure Prediction on Constrained IoT Devices. *Proceedings of the Design, Automation Test in Europe Conference Exhibition*, 955–960. 10.23919/DATE.2018.8342147

Sareen, S., Sood, S. K., & Gupta, S. K. (2016). A cloud-based seizure alert system for epileptic patients that uses higher-order statistics. *Computing in Science & Engineering*, *18*(5), 56–67. doi:10.1109/MCSE.2016.82

Sareen, S., Sood, S. K., & Gupta, S. K. (2016). An automatic prediction of epileptic seizures using cloud computing and wireless sensor networks. Journal of Medical Systems, 40(11). doi:10.100710916-016-0579-1

Satyanarayanan, M., Bahl, P., C'aceres, R., & Davies, N. (2009). The case for VM-based cloudlets in mobile computing. *IEEE Pervasive Computing*, *8*(4), 14–23. doi:10.1109/MPRV.2009.82

Sayeed, M. A., Mohanty, S. P., Kougianos, E., & Zaveri, H. (2018). An Energy Efficient Epileptic Seizure Detector. *Proceedings of the IEEE International Conference on Consumer Electronics (ICCE)*, 1–4.

Sayeed, M. A., Mohanty, S. P., Kougianos, E., & Zaveri, H. (2018). A Fast and Accurate Approach for Real-Time Seizure Detection in the IoMT. *Proceedings of the IEEE International Smart Cities Conference (ISC2)*. 10.1109/ISC2.2018.8656713

T. E. Society. (2013). *Free Epilepsy Smart-Phone App*. https://www.epilepsysociety.org.uk/free-epilepsy-smartphone-app#.WC1jamSLR8c

Teohari, V.-M., Ungureanu, C., Bui, V., Arends, J., & Aarts, R. M. (2014). Epilepsy seizure detection app for wearable technologies. *Proceedings of the European Conference on Ambient Intelligence*.

Villar, Vergara, LaCal, Menendez, & Sedano. (2016). Pre-clinical study on the detection of simulated epileptic seizures. *International Journal of Uncertainty, Fuzziness and Knowledge-Based Systems, 24*(2), 33–46.

Xie, S., & Krishnan, S. (2013). Wavelet-based sparse functional linear model with applications to EEGs seizure detection and epilepsy diagnosis. *Medical & Biological Engineering & Computing*, *51*(1-2), 49–60. doi:10.100711517-012-0967-8 PMID:23054383

Yu, W., Liang, F., He, X., Hatcher, W. G., Lu, C., Lin, J., & Yang, X. (2018). A Survey on the Edge Computing for the Internet of Things. *IEEE Access: Practical Innovations, Open Solutions*, *6*, 6900–6919. doi:10.1109/ACCESS.2017.2778504

Zaveri, H. P., Williams, W. J., Iasemidis, L. D., & Sackellares, J. C. (1992). Time-frequency Representation of Electrocorticograms in Temporal Lobe Epilepsy. IEEE Transactions on Biomedical Engineering, 39(5), 502–509. doi:10.1109/10.135544

Chapter 15
Quantum AI and IoT Cognitive Disease Data Security to Evade Quantum Computing Attacks

Pavan Manjunath
Jain University, India

Harish Sudarsanan
Solution Architecture, India

Pritam Gajkumar Shah
Jain University, Australia

ABSTRACT

The aim of the chapter is to provide the enormous profits of the IoT systems (or) devices vulnerable to highly capable intrusions of different attackers. The vital security necessities such as authorization and authentication do not satisfactorily meet the requirements, and prevailing events are not capable of securing the IoT innovative healthcare environment from data gaps of the system security. With the number of IoT application domains growing to incorporate smart homes, mobile healthcare, autonomous intelligent healthcare communication, and smart cities in day-to-day human life, the significance of an attack in the IoT intelligent healthcare networks will become serious. As there are many issues in applying present cryptographic principles to resource-constrained IoT sensor devices, the recommended new security features solutions come with a compromise between security, feasibility, and performance. These research topics focus on evolving lightweight cryptographic results that specifically implement the post-quantum McEliece cryptography algorithm to encrypt the IoT intelligent healthcare device data, which is integrated into the classical blockchain with hashing function SHA-512. The evolving quantum computing integration with AI is together a transformational technology. The AI requires quantum computing power to attain substantial advancement to analyze the enormous data set faster, specifically the mental medical images or patient data.

DOI: 10.4018/978-1-7998-9534-3.ch015

INTRODUCTION

An IoT environment is a set of devices that lets designers extend the IoT applications; all the data is collected remotely with a secure connection (Tripathi, 2017). An IoT environment accomplishes the links of the different devices and permits designers to build newer mobile applications (Raj, 2017). The IoT is the best new reality shifting our everyday lives in healthcare organizations. It assurances to transform the modern healthcare system by enabling more tailored to the health care end-users, protective, and two-way health care system.

The improvements in statistical data and inter-communication knowledge have led to the evolution of the IoT (Bektaş, 2018). In the current healthcare setup, the IoT components convey the suitability of physicians or doctors and patients. Since they are helpful in numerous medical areas, they can collect or monitor real-time patient health status, patient data management, and healthcare hospital management system such as bed allocation to the patients (Bisht, 2021). The body sensor network plays vital devices and is one of the leading machinery of IoT health care application developments. A remote patient in villages can be put into the observation using smaller sensors and lightweight wireless sensor nodes; security is vital for such a system. Expanding this domain in the more intelligent healthcare applications without allowing for protection makes patient confidentiality risky (Chien,2017). The speedy improvement in ground-breaking physical smaller entities equipment has incorporated substantial accomplishments in health care application expansion for wireless sensor-based highly circulated health care communication architecture (Worgan, 2015). During the COVID-19 pandemic, these contactless systems were most of the health care equipment's becoming contactless system. The effectiveness of data retrieval from intelligent IoT devices on hourly or minute essential is very critical. The real-time health care IoT built services have been refined and set up in health care monitoring of the patient's day-to-day life.

Nevertheless, while the IoT-oriented methods progress the way for expanding very collaborating applications, some newer threats or risks might arise from these prospects. For example, Hello Barbie, an innovative IoT-built marketable product for children, exposes a possible confidentiality data risk that permits multiple web cyber-attackers to undercover agents on consumers' or patients' private data (Zhou,2020). The attack targeted particular functionalities, specifically voice communication and the camera, which provides the process of the IoT product and its collaborating health care applications. The health care system interaction with the cognitive diseases patient flow process, as shown in figure 1.

Figure 1. The Internet of Things (IoT) system in the health care system

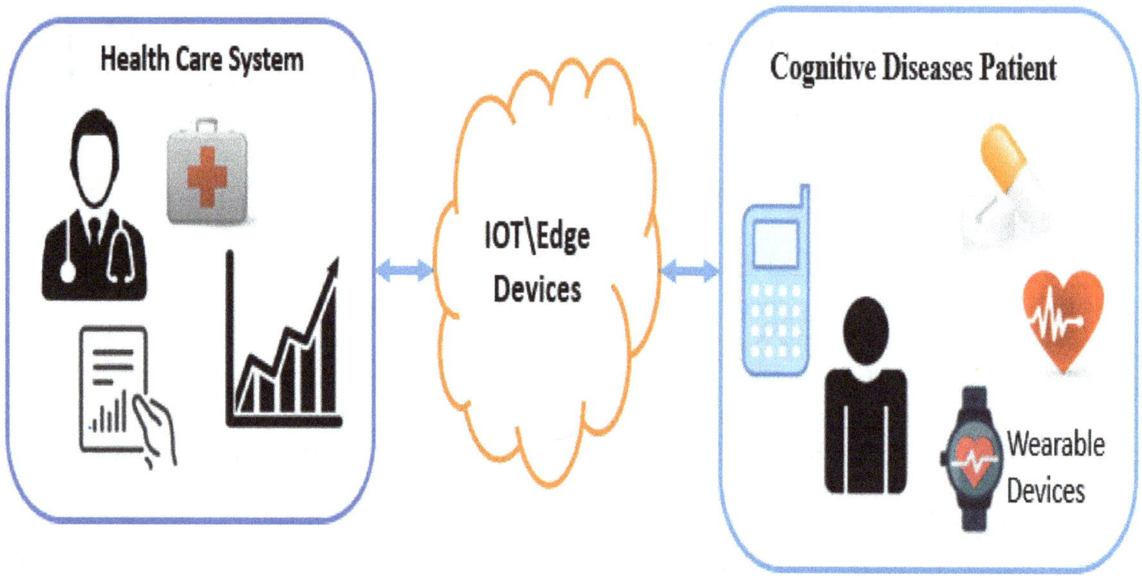

Newly evolved intelligent health care communication systems have attracted a lot of attention from industries and research institutions. As per the estimation so far, the yet to come to IoT (Rashid,2021) will benefit diverse regions of society, including the health care domain, manufacturing industry, transportation, banking, agriculture, government, and logistic sectors. On the other hand, there is no ambiguity that present networks technologies must unquestionably grow to keep up with the IoT applications. In line with the speedy upsurge in the human population, there is a need for an effective intelligent health care communication system (Wu,2018). So we proposed a new framework that solves the drawback of a current smart customer health care communication IoT system security issues and for the classical blockchain and integrated with the Quantum AI for processing the customer's data (Yelizarov,2020). So our system handles all the data securely transferred between the client and healthcare center data communication while transferring from one device to other objects (Sharma,2019). The data is transmitted securely via blockchain, and our proposed research work will also overcome the drawbacks of the classical blockchain facing quantum attacks (Corchia,2019). In our future research work, we use the Quantum Computing integration with AI, where Quantum AI can assist in achieving results that are unlikely to accomplish with outdated systems. Figure 2 showcase the wider varieties of the human handle miniature sensor devices, which give a minute by minute information to the respective healthcare system.

Figure 2. The edge devices (or) sensor connected to the Internet of Things (IoT) health care system

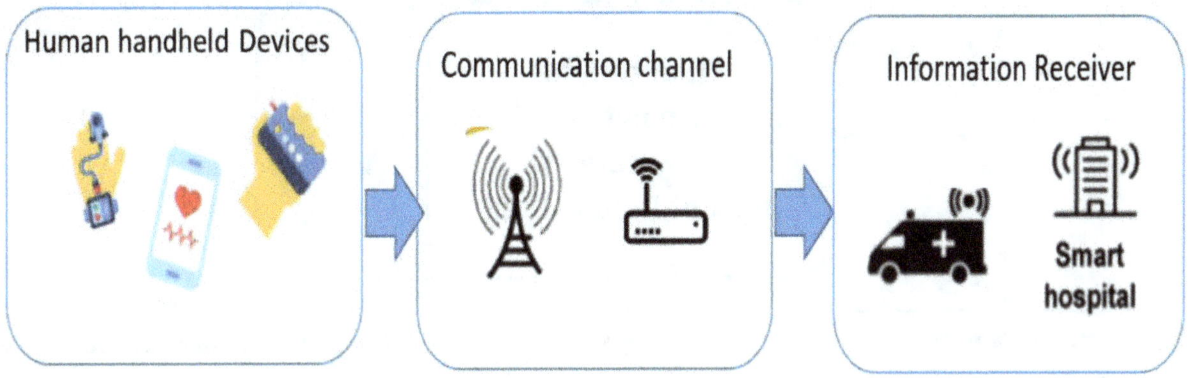

WHAT IS QUANTUM AI?

The Quantum AI application or system uses the quantum computing process to compute the higher level of ML algorithms concepts. Acknowledgments to the computational advantages of the Quantum computing procedure, Quantum AI will aid in attaining outcomes that are not possible to achieve with a classical system. The AI process is faster at forecasting behavior than the human-begin mind (Gupta,2017). The AI domain can also progress significance systems; we cannot say or predicate the valuable assistance given to the health care system. Significantly sooner or later, there could be extraordinary purpose quantum computing computers with 40 to 50 high-quality qubits. As Quantum computing is still in the initial stages, there have been numerous revolutions and innovations. As shown in figure 3, Quantum AI plays a very critical role.

The more extensive bio-medical data images are analyzed and interrupted within fewer minutes than our traditional system. The IoT system will collect all the health care data from the patient's home or an individual user and the information processing done by the Quantum computing system. This system will process the data faster and send the interpreted data reports within a few minutes to the physician (Ablayev,2019). The system will play a vital role where the patients have no access to the hospital in remote locations. Even getting connected to the Internet is a more significant issue, as every user or individual has mobile with the Internet. The patient's data are the handheld sensor device to monitor the status of their body, and the user can capture the image from the mobile. Such images are sent or transferred via IoT or edge devices; the advantage of such a system is as the patient can be treated at the right time. In such as case, Quantum AI plays a vital role in health care or any other domain.

Figure 3. The Internet of Things (IoT) with the Quantum AI health care system Analytics

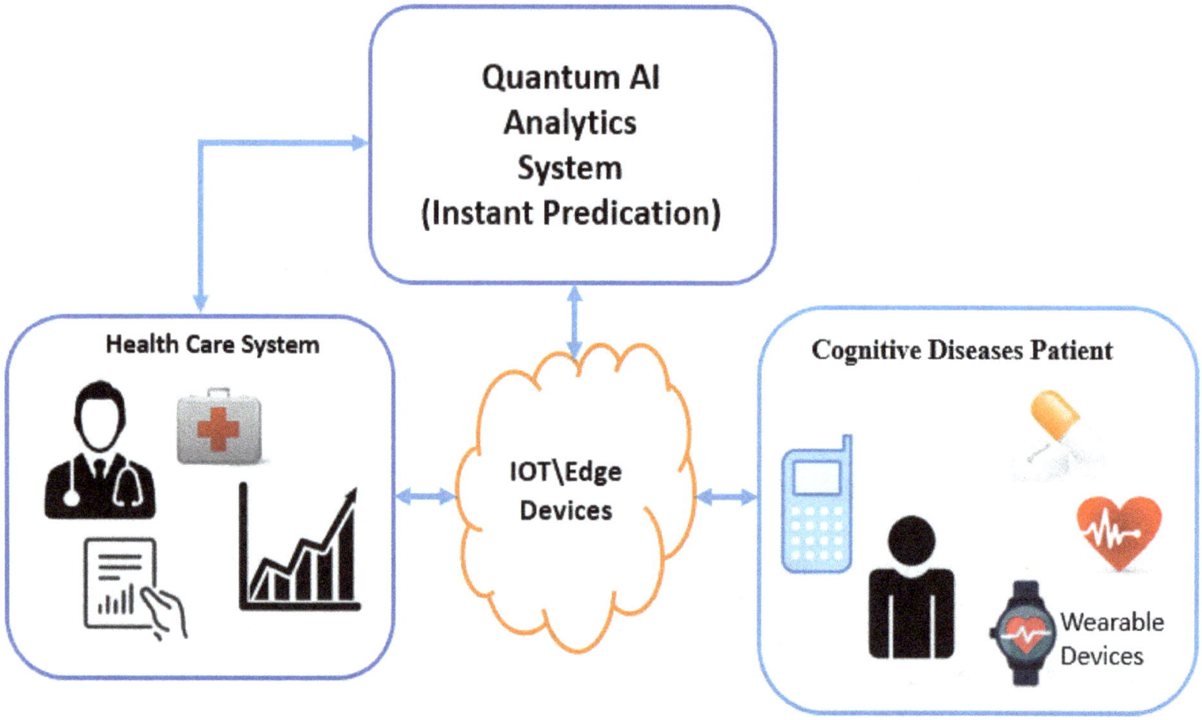

QUANTUM COMPUTING ATTACKS ON THE HEALTH CARE CORE WORKING IOT SYSTEM?

By experimentalizing each feature and self-sufficiently classifying susceptibilities, the system safeguards from vulnerable attacks, and private health care user data is not misused (Bogdanov,2019). The QC can transform the health-related treatment of patients. The QC will help to detect acute diseases by recognizing and predicting failures. There is a more significant threat related to the healthcare IoT data system or banking system, most susceptible to cyber-attacks. In the case of the healthcare IoT component or sensors, excessively absent unproductive safeguard of the customer data. In recent years the invention of the quantum computing system can break any encryption or decryption method (Tang,2017). Health care organizations require a false proof system to protect the data securely and safeguard the data of the health care system from any cyber-attacks or Quantum attacks. The main biggest problem threat or issue in the healthcare system is the data breaches that have originated in identity theft. In such a case, a robust mechanism to battle the security issues gaps in the present healthcare business. If the healthcare patient data are accessible over the public network area, any web attacker may change, interrupt, or even view the source and target streamflow data (Kumari,2020).

The Quantum computing process will evade the security mechanisms and be susceptible to newer types of different cyberattacks. The practical issues are in chip cards and complex high-tech systems such as innovative health care (or) robotic control systems. They can disrupt the cryptographic configurations extensively used in IoT stream data flow message systems (Thompson,2020). Utilizing the arrival of high-end quantum computing computers, newer quantum or post-quantum encryption algorithms are undergoing intensive development that can protect the data variabilities from any cyber-attack issues. With the security of the IoT devices and other cryptographic tools, it is essential to upsurge in the mathematical research area to build secure cryptography of tomorrow, which is unbreakable, unaffected by quantum attacks or any other attacks (Kudyshev,2020).

SMART HEALTHCARE AND PATIENT MONITORING USING IOT

The IoT has been deployed successfully across different parts of our human life. One of the most mainly developing and demanding health care applications. The IoT will affect the medical world, starting from remote area health and monitoring services in any part of the location, aided living and elderly care to detecting and managing chronic diseases, and providing tailored medication (Akkaş,2020).

The analysis and monitoring each individual's health is an essential critical task in the healthcare organization. As in the COVID-19 time, as each individual has minimal time to move out of their house, each individual is not visiting hospitals or any health care, which influence and possibly might lead to various health factors issues in one instantaneous time. Primarily, most healthcare organization systems can predict, diagnose, and give instant treatment for the patients. Customers or people busy in their day-to-day routine work can help them monitor their health conditions on the everyday regular time intervals. Numerous studies and research acritical show that primary prediction and treatment is the best way to cure health issues because initial diagnosis will assist and ready to act by the patients to know the health issues status and act on these issues accordingly. The healthcare issues existence a global trading issue more predominantly, countries like India (or) non-developing nations being an utmost colonized nation. The upsurge of the technology usage, such as AI, Machine nearing or IoT, Blockchain in the healthcare industry. There is a vital need to develop an intelligent, faster, and uninterrupted health monitoring system that can communicate between multiple sensor devices (or) network systems. The newer technologies or applications will constantly monitor the patient and physician without any interruption. The tracking of daily health condition of patients and recording each patient sensitive data set values comprising critical medical information data values, as the new technologies will play and vital in the health care organization (Budida, 2017).

The health monitoring IoT consists of multiple edge computing devices. Each physical entity is inter-linking with numerous sensors components devices, such as microcontrollers systems (or) different sensors. Thus the sensor edge device is installed at the patients' homes in their bodies to analyze every activity of the patients' day-to-day tasks. Moreover, it allows building an appropriate framework with correct protocol stacks, which support them cooperating and communicating between the health care organization and the patients. IoT built healthcare system (or) any other industries, there are multiple sensors devices from the collective, analyses, and each other converse in real-time medical data over the cloud systems. All the data are stored collectively to do data analysis much faster. This innovative data achievement example allows uninterrupted and ubiquitous medical image information access from multiple interconnected components over the IoT. As each of the sensors, features, or edge devices used in IoT has minimal battery power, it is optimal to minimalize the power consumption from each object or component to improve the life of the intelligent healthcare application system (Kodali, 2015). The IoT is a flawless model for data transfer. Still, there are few constraints from a security point of view. On the other side, implant various entities with actuators, sensors, and mini microprocessors, which calculate and communicate over a wider internet area. The intelligent healthcare system explores the values of

IoT for life-saving telemedicine in a very remote location and the remote diagnosis, day-to-day patient monitoring, and treatment. The IoT-based healthcare monitoring model for real-time patient observation by computing biomedical signals in real-time using the AI or ML concepts or quantum AI and hardware's to process a more extensive set of medical images data in the faster phase. The multilayered health care framework improves the efficacies of bio-sensor-based data collection in a much more effective way, along with aggregating the data sets values. Thus it also helps to strategy an efficient real-time result related support system in case of very critical intensive condition of the patient and allows the health care organization to monitor constantly (Jangra, 2018).

A well-organized health care system model, where the doctor can monitor the real-time health of the patient from an isolated location through the effective use of the latest technology, will address this scarcity of healthcare personnel or the doctors in the developing nations scenario. The vital health parameters like ECG, BP, the HBT, GSR, and the GLD of the patient are collected in real-time and assessed through intelligent healthcare devices, as sensor plays a critical role in getting the data. The dataset is additionally transferred wirelessly through Zigbee IEEE 801.15.4 technology for detailed analyses using data analytics (Akshat, 2019). The IoT has given the more creative healthcare setup process a vast advantage. Where even remote locations, users can access the health care system. In the IoT computing process, it plays a vital role in the intelligent healthcare system, thus influencing better vision for the healthcare industries. The system will improve the monitoring of the patient care on the day to day for a longer duration without admitting into hospital, and it will also save the hospital expenses. As per the research, the framework allows more sensors to monitor the patient's symptoms continually and take appropriate action accordingly. The data collected will be monitored by the edge devices, transferred via network gateway through Bluetooth, and then to the cloud computing services over the web-internet. This allows the doctor or physician to identify and monitor each patient's health problems, which can be resolved using the IoT Cloud computing method process (Jaiswal, 2018).

MACHINE LEARNING AND ARTIFICIAL INTELLIGENCE TO IMPROVE DISEASE DETECTION, TREATMENT, AND OUTCOMES

Every year by year, the costs of developing nation or developed nations hospitals charge expensively. Most of the patients who suffer from cognitive health issues are not diagnosed earlier or at the time of admission. The Initial detection and antibiotic handling of mental health issues (sepsis) are essential to progress outcomes for these patients. Even if a few hours is a delay in the treatment, there is a higher chance of mortality. The author predicts cognitive health issues (sepsis) within 12 hours of its diagnosis using vitals and blood tests regularly taken in the ICU. The data analysis is performed using different technologies such as ML or AI algorithms such as XGBoost, CNN-XGBoost, CNN-LSTM, CNN. The XGboost gives an accurate result (Sarafrazi, 2017).

As there are more extensive data values, petabytes of data are saved in healthcare databases, such as clinical experiments, medical pharmaceuticals, and educational research records data systems. The thousands of unstructured and structured datasets are uninterruptedly streaming from patients' wearable sensors devices such as continuous glucose monitoring devices and blood pressure (Ara,2017). The current process of the ML diabetes predicting management applications framework is helping many remote location patients to recover from the health issues and lives by having faster access to advice and consultation and significantly quicker information from doctors s. The beginning of digital sensor devices and highly sophisticated ML analytics tools has attracted old-age companies into the digital data analyses revolution (Park,2014).

SECURITY ISSUES WITH THE IOT HEALTH CARE SYSTEM

In this section, we provide insights into the limitations of the current traditional blockchain and intelligent healthcare communication IoT system. The conventional security methods cannot offer a safer, innovative healthcare communication system and securely save the data values in the big data lake (Bhatt,2020) for analysis purposes. The significant problems in intelligent healthcare communication systems are data accurateness, trust, and trustworthiness of communication data in the communication network; in the past few years, the newly developed (or) classical blockchain application could able to safeguard the user data information's (or) patients information data communication (John,2020) between the doctor or health care system(Mehndiratta,2020). Blockchain technology works for the bitcoin crypto conversation (Zhou,2014), which is newly used to build assurance and trustworthiness in peer-to-peer networks (Lian,2019). It has similar topologies as intelligent health care communication systems. Still, quantum computing is looming as a significant threat to the classical blockchain (Sojuyigbe,2015), which can be easily breakable by using quantum computation. In our research, we are using the classical blockchain concepts to build a blockchain that will resist quantum attacks (or) any other unknown future attacks. These limitations can be overcome by encrypting the classical blockchain data (Arias,2015) values using the post-quantum McEliece cryptography algorithm (Bardis,2015).

OVERCOME THE SECURITY ISSUES IN THE IOT HEALTH CARE SYSTEM

The blockchain with post-quantum McEliece cryptography algorithms will be used in intelligent health care communication IoT systems, where blockchain is currently being adopted. The aim is to study blockchain (Agrawal,2020) as a potential solution to secure the information data generated from IoT sensors. The Operator or hackers while transferring the data over the network (Odin,2019).

The dataset is encapsulated in blocks for each row value when the user data (or) IoT sensor data information is generated. For each block, a hash dataset is created on the data values. Further on, the hashed data values are encrypted using the proposed "Post-Quantum-McEliece-Cryptosystem algorithm" (S. Gupta, 2020). The framework is shown in figure 1. Then once the data values are encrypted into the blocks, they will be transferred over the Internet to the target system. At the destination system, the data values are decrypted into the plain text file. In our research, the focus is to safeguard the data as much as secure the data values. As the data values are first hashed and then encrypted, it makes the attacker into misperception state mode, making it more difficult to breach the encrypted and hashed blockchain data.

Figure 4. Proposed framework of the Internet of Things (IoT) sensor encrypted data encapsulated into the classical block chain of the Patient data in the health care system

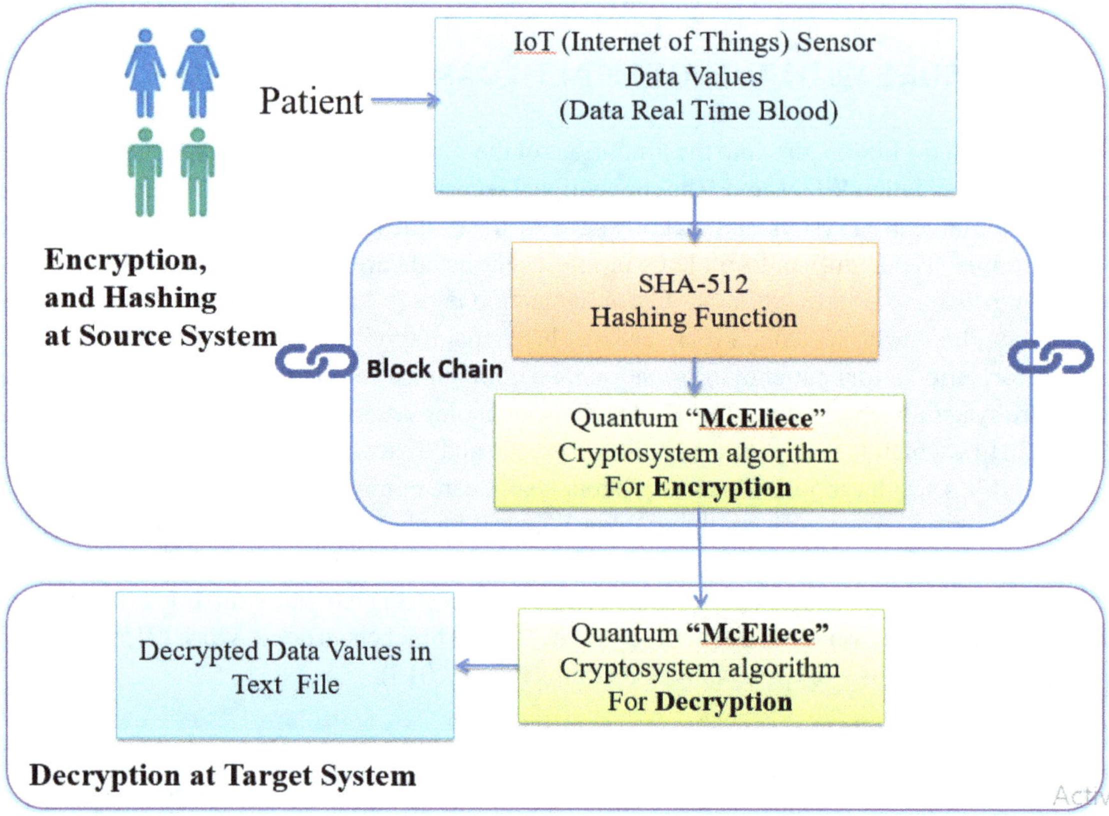

The newer area of post-quantum cryptography is presently in the evolving stage where a lot is trendy happing in this domain, and this can safeguard the health care customer data while transiting over the web internet much securely and also safeguard the whole health care system from any web attacker, the benefits and drawbacks of the presently appropriate algorithms, but as new enhancements and algorithms are developing, they need to be very well gauged to get the precise result out of it. A study of safe quantum algorithms for advanced data security can also be applied as the quantum computing system progresses (S. Gupta, 2018). On the other side, the proposed research can be further investigated concerning a particular application that is both time and mission-critical in order to offer more justification for the applicability of the proposed system on practical grounds. Apart from this, the quantum AI models can be used to predict intruder attacks and analyze the encryption and decryption process and the processing of the encryption and decryption, which can be faster while using the Quantum hardware (S. Gupta, 2018). The slower processing of the encryption or decryption of a larger data set of the sensor data issue can be addressed by developing a simplified architecture considering the supportability of critical applications, as shown below (Figure: 5).

Figure 5. Enhanced Architecture for IOT Device integration with Quantum Computing System with encryption and decryption of patient senor data

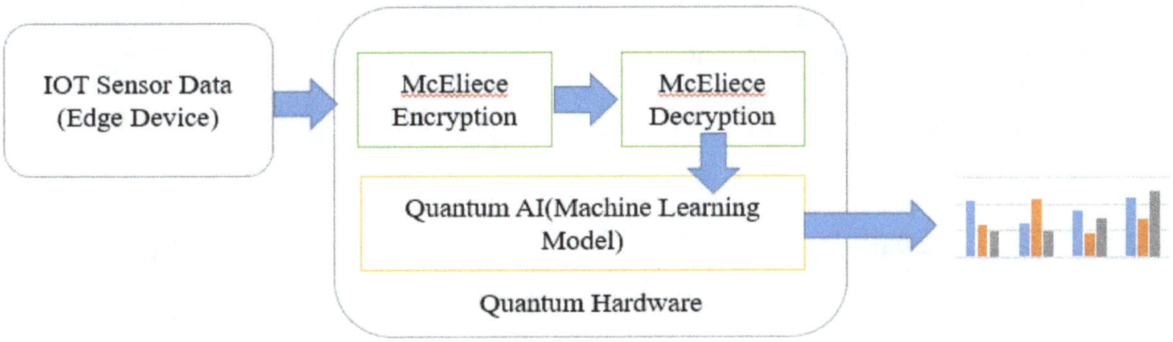

WHAT IS POST-QUANTUM MC-ELIECE CRYPTOSYSTEM PROCESS

The "McEliece" algorithm is an asymmetric encryption algorithm developed by Robert J. McEliece in 1978. The key benefit of the "McEliece" cryptosystem is to have a precise and faster encryption process and decryption. The McEliece encryption scheme, whose security breaks on the difficult problematic of decoding an unfamiliar error-correcting code value, must be described by a triple of procedures: key generation, encryption, and decryption procedure as shown in figure 2.

In the proposed research paperwork, the primary purpose usage of the "McEliece algorithm" is for encryption and decryption of the plain text information data values by introducing the complex error code while encrypting the data values, and finally, removing the errors while decrypting the data values. As shown in figure 6, the plain text from device "A" value is encapsulated into the blockchain, and hashing function is applied on the simple text data values once the processing is done. Then "McEliece algorithm" is used on the hash data values to generate the public key and encrypt the message. The message is securely transferred via an insecure channel to the destination. Then the data values are decrypted using the "McEliece algorithm" to generate the plain text in the human-readable form.

Figure 6. Schematic view of the McEliece a key generation, encryption and decryption process in the health care system

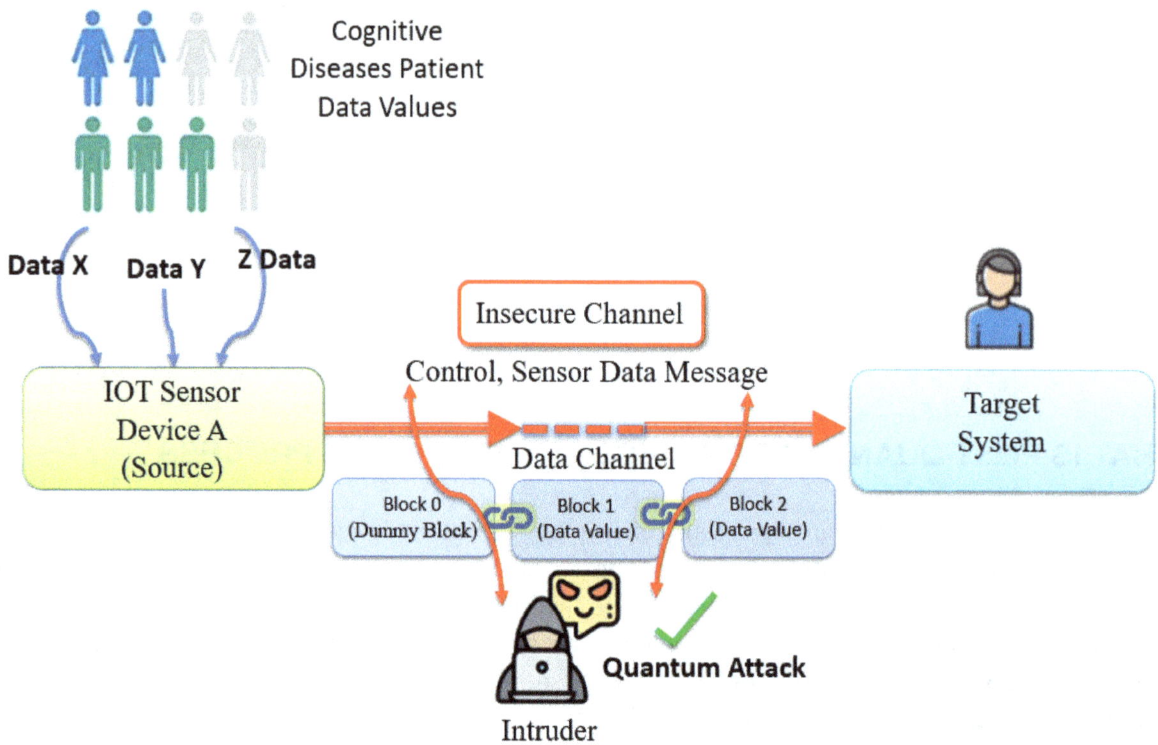

The encryption defining process, the below-mentioned four matrix needs to be considered for the calculation of the post-quantum McEliece-Cryptosystem calculation.

- The generator matrix (“G”), with the dimension value (“k,n”) having weight “d”
- The parity check matrix (“H”), with the dimension value (“k,n”)
- Invertible Binary matrix(“S”), with the dimension, is (“k,k”)
- Permutation matrix (“P”), with dimension, is (“n,n”) (that is, taking a single “one” in respective row and column and “0’s” everywhere else)

Note,

1. The Invertible Binary matrix will generate the random number, which will be in the range of ‘0’ (or) ‘1’.
2. Permutation matrix, P is selected such that P.PT= I
3. Parity check matrix is selected such that the dot product of the Generator matrix (G) and Parity check matrix (H) must be zero. H.G= 0
4. 4. The small word “t” is the number of errors that can be corrected.

$t = \left(\frac{d-1}{2}\right)$, where d is the weight of the generator matrix.

We can introduce more errors by using a bigger (higher k and n) generator matrix with more weight (higher 'd')

WHAT IS MC-ELIECE ENCRYPTION PROCESS

Where (S) is Invertible Binary matrix and (G) is Generator matrix and (P) is Permutation matrix
Message "m" will be encrypted as follows
Encryption Example:
Let us consider the Generator matrix *(G)*, with dimension (4,8) and weight 4. So n=4, k=8 and d=4.
This generator matrix can be used to correct only 1 error because

$$t = \left(\frac{d-1}{2}\right) = \left(\frac{4-1}{2}\right) = 1$$

Generator matrix, G is

$$\begin{bmatrix} 1 & 0 & 0 & 0 & 0 & 1 & 1 & 1 \\ 0 & 1 & 0 & 0 & 1 & 0 & 1 & 1 \\ 0 & 0 & 1 & 0 & 1 & 1 & 0 & 1 \\ 0 & 0 & 0 & 1 & 1 & 1 & 1 & 0 \end{bmatrix}$$

Parity check matrix, H is

$$\begin{bmatrix} 0 & 1 & 1 & 1 & 1 & 0 & 0 & 0 \\ 1 & 0 & 1 & 1 & 0 & 1 & 0 & 0 \\ 1 & 1 & 0 & 1 & 0 & 0 & 1 & 0 \\ 1 & 1 & 1 & 0 & 0 & 0 & 0 & 1 \end{bmatrix}$$

Binary Invertible matrix, S is

$$\begin{bmatrix} 0 & 1 & 1 & 0 \\ 0 & 1 & 0 & 1 \\ 1 & 1 & 1 & 1 \\ 1 & 0 & 0 & 0 \end{bmatrix}$$

Permutation matrix, P is

$$\begin{bmatrix} 1 & 0 & 0 & 0 & 0 & 0 & 0 & 0 \\ 0 & 1 & 0 & 0 & 0 & 0 & 0 & 0 \\ 0 & 0 & 1 & 0 & 0 & 0 & 0 & 0 \\ 0 & 0 & 0 & 1 & 0 & 0 & 0 & 0 \\ 0 & 0 & 0 & 0 & 1 & 0 & 0 & 0 \\ 0 & 0 & 0 & 0 & 0 & 1 & 0 & 0 \\ 0 & 0 & 0 & 0 & 0 & 0 & 1 & 0 \\ 0 & 0 & 0 & 0 & 0 & 0 & 0 & 1 \end{bmatrix}$$

If Message(m) to be transmitted is character "H", then the binary value for "H" is "0100 1000", that is 8 bits.

Take 1st part of binary value which is 0100 and take 2nd part of binary value which is 1000

Create public key Gprime ($G^{'}$), where $G' = S * G * P$ and error, "z" is a random number between 1 and 7. Let's say, z=5

$$\text{Public key Gprime } (G^{'}) = \begin{bmatrix} 0 & 1 & 1 & 0 & 0 & 1 & 1 & 0 \\ 0 & 1 & 0 & 1 & 0 & 1 & 0 & 1 \\ 1 & 1 & 1 & 1 & 1 & 1 & 1 & 1 \\ 1 & 0 & 0 & 0 & 0 & 1 & 1 & 1 \end{bmatrix}$$

Encryption is done on each part (first part and last part) of "m" separately as shown below

$$m^* \; G' \text{ for first part of m= } 0100 * \begin{bmatrix} 0 & 1 & 1 & 0 & 0 & 1 & 1 & 0 \\ 0 & 1 & 0 & 1 & 0 & 1 & 0 & 1 \\ 1 & 1 & 1 & 1 & 1 & 1 & 1 & 1 \\ 1 & 0 & 0 & 0 & 0 & 1 & 1 & 1 \end{bmatrix} = 01010101$$

$$m^* \; G' \text{ for second part of m= } 1000 * \begin{bmatrix} 0 & 1 & 1 & 0 & 0 & 1 & 1 & 0 \\ 0 & 1 & 0 & 1 & 0 & 1 & 0 & 1 \\ 1 & 1 & 1 & 1 & 1 & 1 & 1 & 1 \\ 1 & 0 & 0 & 0 & 0 & 1 & 1 & 1 \end{bmatrix} = 01100110$$

The outcome of result of X= 01010101(8bit) and Y=01100110(8bit)

Therefore the X= $0^{1Bit}\,1^{2Bit}\,0^{3Bit}\,1^{4Bit}\,0^{5Bit}\,1^{6Bit}\,0^{7Bit}\,1^{8Bit}$ and Y value is $0^{1Bit}\,1^{2Bit}\,1^{3Bit}\,0^{4Bit}\,0^{5Bit}\,1^{6Bit}\,1^{7Bit}\,0^{8Bit}$

As error, "z" = 5 (Random Number), we will flip the 5th bit value of X and Y, 5th bit value is 0 for X and Y. Flip it to 1.

After Flipping, the binary value of X will be, X= $0^{1Bit}\,1^{2Bit}\,0^{3Bit}\,1^{4Bit}\,1^{5Bit}\,1^{6Bit}\,0^{7Bit}\,1^{8Bit}$

After Flipping, the binary value of Y will be Y= $0^{1Bit}\,1^{2Bit}\,1^{3Bit}\,0^{4Bit}\,1^{5Bit}\,1^{6Bit}\,1^{7Bit}\,0^{8Bit}$

Convert binary values of X and Y to ASCII. Hence, X =] and Y= n

Note:- For each character to be encrypted, there will be 2 characters in encrypted file once encryption is done. Here, for character 'H', we got ']' and 'n' as the output after encryption.

Figure 7. Proposed framework of the Internet of Things (IoT) sensor encrypted data encapsulated into the classical block chain of the Patient data in the health care system

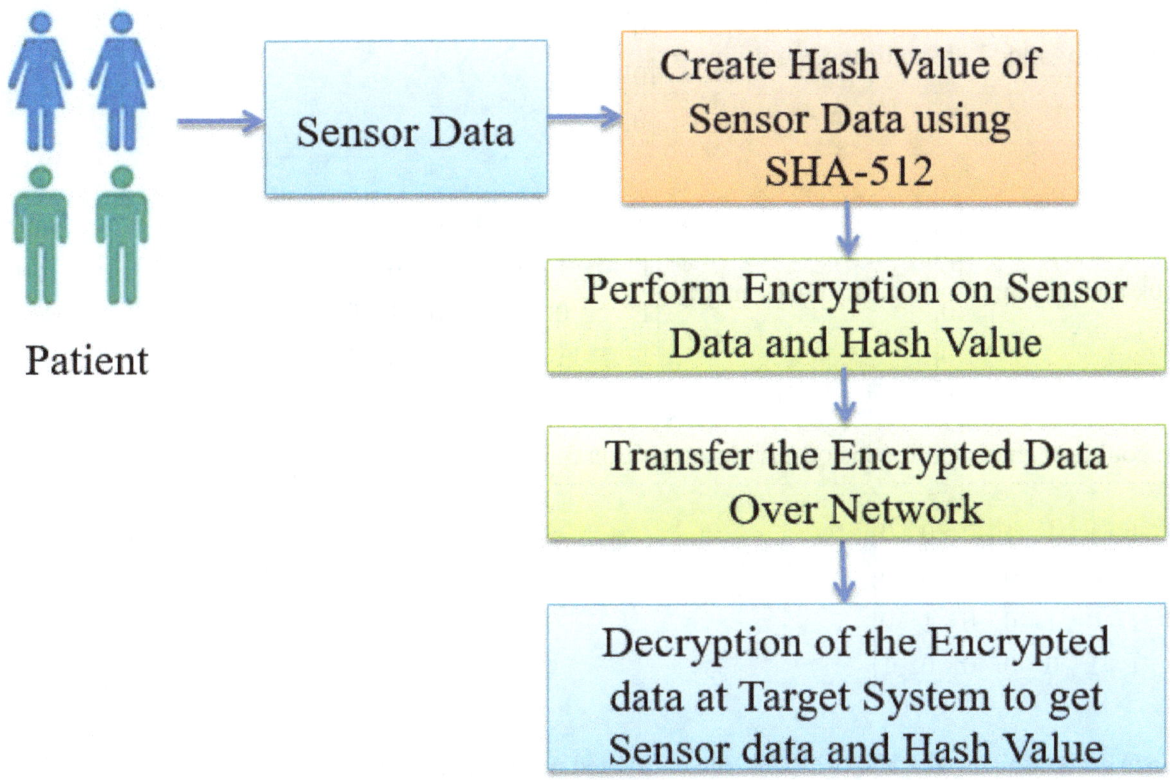

WHAT IS THE MC-ELIECE DECRYPTION PROCESS?

For the Decryption process, we are using the fast decryption process named as Syndrome Decoding method, and there is an efficient method for decoding binary linear codes.

If "c" is the encrypted message in binary, then syndrome is equal to dot product (mod2) of Parity check matrix (H) and the transpose of "C"

Lookup, this syndrome against each column of "H", and check-in which column position of "H" we are finding a match. That column position is the position where we have to correct/flip the bit of the encrypted binary message.

Decryption Example:

The encrypted message for the character 'H' is ']' and 'n'.

Binary form of ']' is 01010101(8bit). Let's call it c1.

Binary form of 'n' is 01100110(8bit). Let's call it c2.

$$\text{Syndrome= H.c}^T = \begin{bmatrix} 0 & 1 & 1 & 1 & 1 & 0 & 0 & 0 \\ 1 & 0 & 1 & 1 & 0 & 1 & 0 & 0 \\ 1 & 1 & 0 & 1 & 0 & 0 & 1 & 0 \\ 1 & 1 & 1 & 0 & 0 & 0 & 0 & 1 \end{bmatrix} * \begin{bmatrix} 0 \\ 1 \\ 1 \\ 0 \\ 1 \\ 1 \\ 1 \\ 0 \end{bmatrix} = \begin{bmatrix} 3 \\ 2 \\ 2 \\ 2 \end{bmatrix}$$

After taking mod2 of syndrome, syndrome = $\begin{bmatrix} 1 \\ 0 \\ 0 \\ 0 \end{bmatrix}$

Look up syndrome $\begin{bmatrix} 1 \\ 0 \\ 0 \\ 0 \end{bmatrix}$ in parity check matrix $\begin{bmatrix} 0 & 1 & 1 & 1 & 1 & 0 & 0 & 0 \\ 1 & 0 & 1 & 1 & 0 & 1 & 0 & 0 \\ 1 & 1 & 0 & 1 & 0 & 0 & 1 & 0 \\ 1 & 1 & 1 & 0 & 0 & 0 & 0 & 1 \end{bmatrix}$.

We could see that syndrome is occurring at position 5.

$$\begin{bmatrix} 0 & 1 & 1 & 1 & 1 & 0 & 0 & 0 \\ 1 & 0 & 1 & 1 & 0 & 1 & 0 & 0 \\ 1 & 1 & 0 & 1 & 0 & 0 & 1 & 0 \\ 1 & 1 & 1 & 0 & 0 & 0 & 0 & 1 \end{bmatrix}.$$

Hence correct/bitflip the 5th position of the encrypted message (in binary).
c1 after correction becomes 01011101
c2 after correction becomes 01100110
Take first four bits of c1 and take first four bits of c2
c1[0:4] = 0101
c2[0:4] = 0110.
First four bits of original message m will be c1*mod2(S^{-1})
m(message) = 0101
Last four bits of original message m will be c2*mod2(S^{-1})
m(message) = 0110

Here $S^{-1} = \begin{bmatrix} 0 & 0 & 0 & 1 \\ 1 & 1 & -1 & 1 \\ 0 & -1 & 1 & -1 \\ -1 & 0 & 1 & -1 \end{bmatrix}$ and $\text{mod2}(S^{-1}) = \begin{bmatrix} 0 & 0 & 0 & 1 \\ 1 & 1 & 1 & 1 \\ 0 & 1 & 1 & 1 \\ 1 & 0 & 1 & 1 \end{bmatrix}$

$$c1[0:4]^{*}\ \mathrm{mod2}(S^{-1}) = 0101^{*}\begin{bmatrix}0 & 0 & 0 & 1\\1 & 1 & 1 & 1\\0 & 1 & 1 & 1\\1 & 0 & 1 & 1\end{bmatrix} = [0100].\ \text{Lets call it U}$$

$$c2[0:4]^{*}\ \mathrm{mod2}(S^{-1}) = 0110^{*}\begin{bmatrix}0 & 0 & 0 & 1\\1 & 1 & 1 & 1\\0 & 1 & 1 & 1\\1 & 0 & 1 & 1\end{bmatrix} = [1000].\ \text{Let's call it V}$$

Concatenate U and V to get the binary value. In this case it is 0100 1000 which is equal to "H"

Figure 8. Tentative Architecture for IOT Device integration with Quantum Computing System

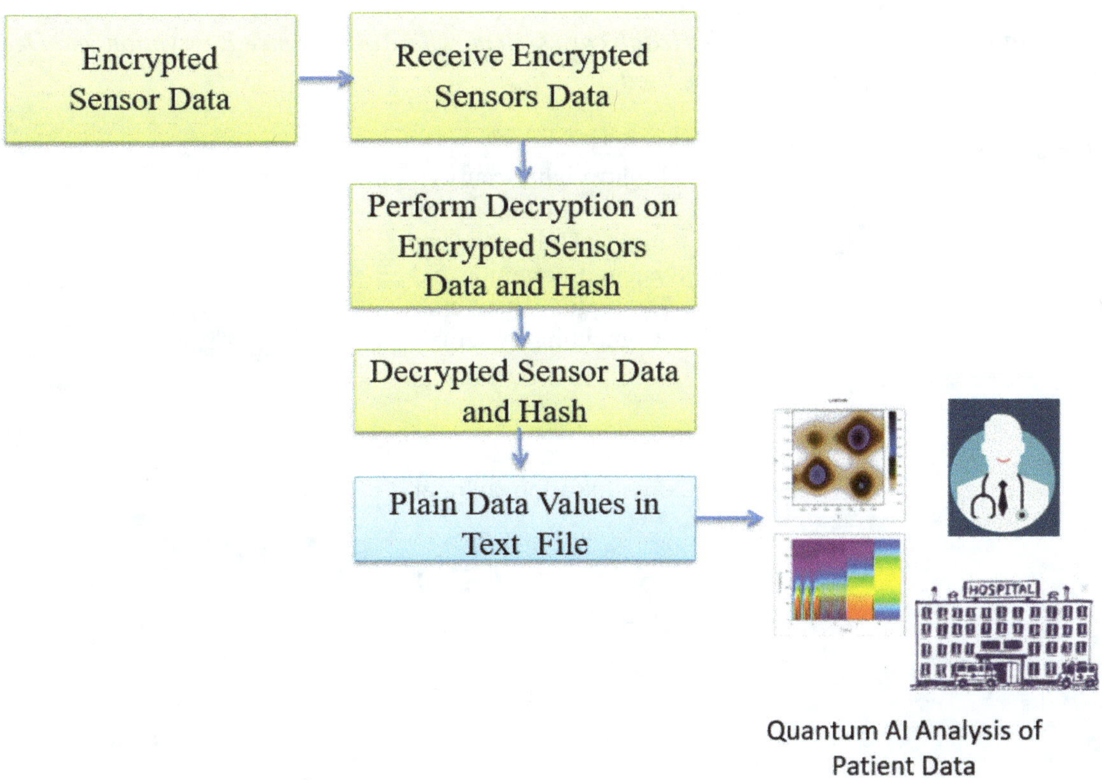

FUTURE RESEARCH DIRECTIONS

The core objective is to safeguard the end-to-end health care system from the current security vulnerability faced by the Internet of things (IoT) based health care communication system and the classical blockchain security attack. All when connected to the network is wide-open to more number of attacks. Thus security addition in the Internet of things (IoT) network will upsurge the trust level of users.

The number of security solutions is available in the literature for the Internet of things (IoT) as well as for the blockchain, and few newly developed security based on the traditional, outdated security solutions like AES, DES, RSA, and many more do not fit at all in resource-constrained Internet of things (IoT). The high risk of quantum computing attacks and other unknown future security risk factors. These traditional solutions take much power and resources from the Internet of things (IoT) use case devices. As a result, lightweight security algorithms are appropriate for Internet of things (IoT) devices due to their lower power requirements and optimum memory. The post-quantum algorithm "McEliece CryptoSystem" is an ideal lightweight algorithm and protects any future attacks.

The well-organized lightweight security solution of the Internet of things (IoT) is shown in figure 9. Can do real data collection using the Internet of things (IoT) sensor, achieves tasks such as data mining for judgment making, and is less susceptible to attacks. The future opportunity of this research work can be to propose a proficient method for sensing on securely collecting the data from in Internet of things (IoT) sensors and encrypting the blockchain data using post-quantum McEliece cryptosystem makes data more secure.

Figure 9. Future process model for IOT Health care system, where all advance Encryption and Decryption Quantum computing process can be used

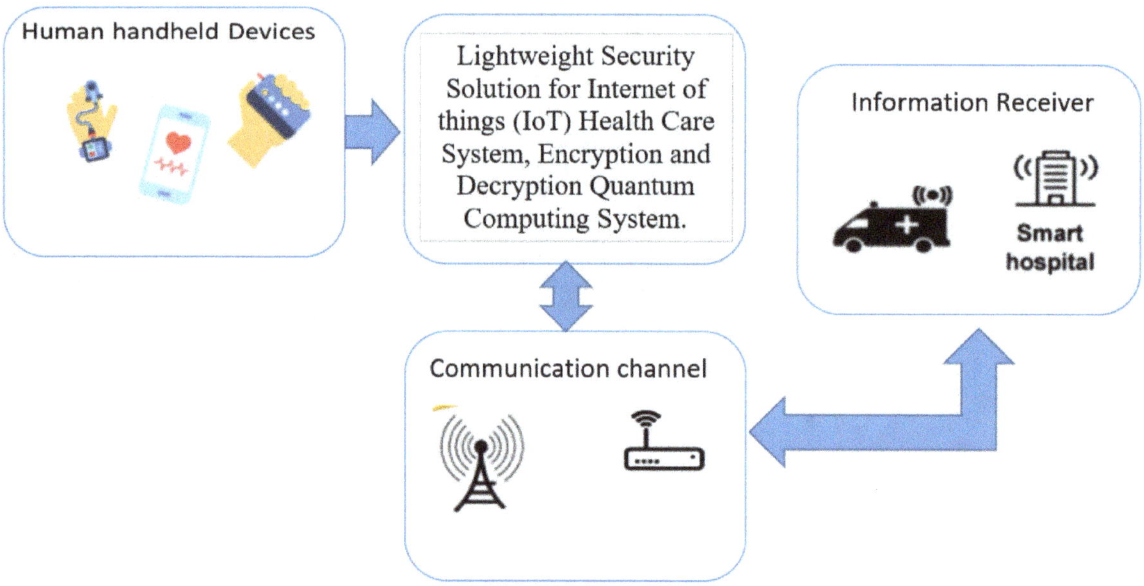

CONCLUSION

IoT health care environment is becoming more popular day by day, as the IoT allows remote location data to be collected more efficiently. The use of the IoT application, along with Quantum AI, in identifying cognitive diseases is becoming a vital part. The research papers focus on the extensive use of IoT sensors to collect the data from the remote location while transferring the data securely over the Internet and finally use Quantum AI to perform the data analytics. Advanced technologies in health care systems will enhance the prediction process faster and more accurately, and human error is removed. While transferring from the remote location, this work will ensure the data is securely transferred from source to destination without any alteration of the data values and transfer the data over the network layer. This research work can be extended further by integrating with the newer technologies.

ACKNOWLEDGMENT

First, I bow before the Lord Almighty with a grateful heart for his blessings, which have made me what I am. I show my respectful gratitude to Harish Sudarsanan, a second author contributing to this research work and his valuable time. I would like to start with my profound thanks to my Research Supervisor, Dr. Prof. Pritam Shah, Ph.D. Australia, Professor (Cyber Security Research Unit), Australia without his guidance, this would not have been possible, he has been a constant source of support, encouragement, guidance, motivation, and rationale thinking throughout my doctoral program. I express my special gratitude to Dr. Michael HM, Germany, for his encouragement, advice, and inspiration. I tell my appreciation to Dr. Mythili P. Rao, Dean - Languages, Research coordinator, Jain University, for making us ready to be part of the research. And I am very much thankful for Shweta Gupta, Editors, Jain University, and Bengaluru, India.

REFERENCES

Ablayev, Ablayev, Huang, Khadiev, Salikhova, & Wu. (2020). On quantum methods for machine learning problems part I: Quantum tools. *Big Data Mining and Analytics, 3*(1), 41-55. doi:10.26599/BDMA.9020016

Agrawal, R., Bu, L., & Kinsy, M. A. (2020). Quantum-Proof Lightweight McEliece Cryptosystem Co-processor Design. *IEEE 38th International Conference on Computer Design (ICCD),* 73-79. doi: 10.1109/ICCD50377.2020.00029

Akkaş, M., Sokullu, R., & Çetin, H. (2020). Healthcare and Patient Monitoring Using IoT. *Internet of Things., 11*, 100173. doi:10.1016/j.iot.2020.100173

Akshat. (2018). A Smart Healthcare Monitoring System Using Smartphone Interface. *2018 4th International Conference on Devices, Circuits and Systems (ICDCS)*, 228-231. doi: 10.1109/ICDCSyst.2018.8605142

Ara, A., & Ara, A. (2017). Case study: Integrating IoT, streaming analytics and machine learning to improve intelligent diabetes management system. *International Conference on Energy, Communication, Data Analytics and Soft Computing (ICECDS)*, 3179-3182. doi: 10.1109/ICECDS.2017.8390043

Arias, Wurm, Hoang, & Jin. (2015). Privacy and Security in Internet of Things and Wearable Devices. *IEEE Transactions on Multi-Scale Computing Systems, 1*(2), 99-109. doi:. doi:10.1109/TMSCS.2015.2498605

Bardis, N., Kharchenko, V., Potii, O., & Vambol, A. (2020). Post-Quantum Network Security: McEliece and Niederreiter Cryptosystems Analysis and Education Issues post-quantum cryptography. *WSEAS Transactions on Systems and Control, 15*, 627–634. doi:10.37394/23203.2020.15.62

Bektaş, M., & Görmüş, S. (2018). An energy efficient IoT protocol for healthcare at home. *26th Signal Processing and Communications Applications Conference (SIU)*, 1-4. doi: 10.1109/SIU.2018.8404663

Bhatt, V., & Chakraborty, S. (2020). Importance of Trust in IoT based Wearable Device Adoption by Patient: An Empirical Investigation. *Fourth International Conference on I-SMAC (IoT in Social, Mobile, Analytics and Cloud) (I-SMAC)*, 1226-1231. doi: 10.1109/I-SMAC49090.2020.9243533

Bisht, R. S., Jain, S., & Tewari, N. (2021). Study of Wearable IoT devices in 2021: Analysis & Future Prospects. *2nd International Conference on Intelligent Engineering and Management (ICIEM)*, 577-581. doi: 10.1109/ICIEM51511.2021.9445334

Bogdanov, S. I., Kudyshev, Z., Kildishev, A. V., Boltasseva, A., & Shalaev, V. M. (2019). *High-Speed Quantum Photonics with Plasmonic Metamaterials Empowered by Machine Learning. In IEEE Photonics Conference*. IPC. doi:10.1109/IPCon.2019.8908357

Budida, D. A. M., & Mangrulkar, R. S. (2017). Design and implementation of smart HealthCare system using IoT. *International Conference on Innovations in Embedded and Communication Systems (ICIIECS)*, 1-7. doi: 10.1109/ICIIECS.2017.8275903

Corchia, L. (2019). Radio-frequency Identification Based on Textile, Wearable, Chipless Tags for IoT Applications. *II Workshop on Metrology for Industry 4.0 and IoT (MetroInd4.0&IoT)*, 1-5. doi: 10.1109/METROI4.8792919

Gupta, HariPrasad, & Kumar. (2018). Bionics Based Emergency Contact for Treatment of Epilepsy. *Proceedings of the 2018 10th International Conference on Bioinformatics and Biomedical Technology*.

Gupta, S. (2020). Smartphone based Early Detection of Epileptic Seizures Using Machine Learning. *Proceedings of the 2020 12th International Conference on Bioinformatics and Biomedical Technology*.

Gupta, S., & Kumar, A. (2018). *Bionic Functionality of Prosthetic Hand. In Intelligent Communication, Control and Devices*. Springer.

Gupta, S., Mohanta, S., Chakraborty, M., & Ghosh, S. (2017). Quantum machine learning-using quantum computation in artificial intelligence and deep neural networks: Quantum computation and machine learning in artificial intelligence. *8th Annual Industrial Automation and Electromechanical Engineering Conference (IEMECON)*, 268-274. doi: 10.1109/IEMECON.2017.8079602

Hsu, C.-L., Chuang, T.-H., & Lin, T.-W. (2017). End-to-end authenticated key exchange agreement for wearable devices in IoT environments. *IEEE Great Lakes Biomedical Conference (GLBC)*, 1-1. doi: 10.1109/GLBC.2017.7928891

Jaiswal, K., Sobhanayak, S., Mohanta, B. K., & Jena, D. (2017). IoT-cloud based framework for patient's data collection in smart healthcare system using raspberry-pi. *2017 International Conference on Electrical and Computing Technologies and Applications (ICECTA)*, 1-4. doi: 10.1109/ICECTA.2017.8251967

Jangra, P., & Gupta, M. (2018). A Design of Real-Time Multilayered Smart Healthcare Monitoring Framework Using IoT. *International Conference on Intelligent and Advanced System (ICIAS)*, 1-5. doi: 10.1109/ICIAS.2018.8540606

John, C., Mueller, Z., Prayaga, L., & Devulapalli, K. (2020). *A Neural Network Model to Identify Relative Movements from Wearable Devices*. SoutheastCon. doi:10.1109/SoutheastCon44009.9368261

Kodali, R. K., Swamy, G., & Lakshmi, B. (2015). *An implementation of IoT for healthcare. In 2015 IEEE Recent Advances in Intelligent Computational Systems*. RAICS. doi:10.1109/RAICS.2015.7488451

Kudyshev, Z., Bogdanov, S., Isacsson, T., Kildishev, A. V., Boltasseva, A., & Shalaev, V. M. (2020). Merging Machine Learning with Quantum Photonics: Rapid Classification of Quantum Sources. *Conference on Lasers and Electro-Optics (CLEO)*, 1-2.

Lian, F., Wang, D., Chiu, R., Jiang, J., & Wang, Y.-P. (2019). Innovative Packaging Solutions of 3D Integration and System in Package for IoT/Wearable and 5G Application. *IEEE 21st Electronics Packaging Technology Conference (EPTC)*, 515-518. doi: 10.1109/EPTC47984.2019.9026573

Mehndiratta, N. (2020). A Yoking-Proof and PUF-based Mutual Authentication Scheme for Cloud-aided Wearable Devices. *IEEE International Conference for Innovation in Technology (INOCON)*, 1-4. doi: 10.1109/INOCON50539.2020.9298349

Odin Hashemi, S. H., & Hodtani, G. A. (2019). A Modified McEliece Public-Key Cryptosystem Based On Irregular Codes Of QC-LDPC and QC-MDPC. *27th Iranian Conference on Electrical Engineering (ICEE)*, 1373-1376. doi: 10.1109/IranianCEE.2019.8786376

P & Kumari. (2020). Quantum Algorithms for Machine Learning and Optimization. *2nd PhD Colloquium on Ethically Driven Innovation and Technology for Society (PhD EDITS)*, 1-2. doi: 10.1109/PhDEDITS51180.2020.9315301

Park, J., Kim, K., & Kwon, O. (2014). Comparison of machine learning algorithms to predict psychological wellness indices for ubiquitous healthcare system design. *Proceedings of the International Conference on Innovative Design and Manufacturing (ICIDM)*, 263-269. doi: 10.1109/IDAM.2014.6912705

Raj, C., Jain, C., & Arif, W. (2017). HEMAN: Health monitoring and nous: An IoT based e-health care system for remote telemedicine. *International Conference on Wireless Communications, Signal Processing and Networking (WiSPNET)*, 2115-2119, doi: 10.1109/WiSPNET.2017.8300134

Rashid, T., Hasan, M. N., & Mazumdar, P. S. (2021). An L-slot Compact Antenna for Medical, Wearable Device and IoT Applications. *International Conference on Information and Communication Technology for Sustainable Development (ICICT4SD)*, 100-104. doi: 10.1109/ICICT4SD50815.2021.9396832

Sarafrazi. (2019). Cracking the "Sepsis" Code: Assessing Time Series Nature of EHR Data,and Using Deep Learning for Early Sepsis Prediction. *2019 Computing in Cardiology (CinC)*, 1-4. doi:10.23919/CinC49843.2019.9005940

Sharma, V., & Vineeta, S. (2019). Future of Wearable Devices Using IoT Synergy in AI. *3rd International conference on Electronics, Communication and Aerospace Technology (ICECA)*, 138-142. doi: 10.1109/ICECA.2019.8821915

Sojuyigbe, S., & Daniel, K. (2015). Wearables/IOT devices: Challenges and solutions to integration of miniature antennas in close proximity to the human body. *2015 IEEE Symposium on Electromagnetic Compatibility and Signal Integrity*, 75-78. doi: 10.1109/EMCSI.2015.7107662

Tang, H. (2017). Integration benefits and challenges on Fan-Out to enable system in package for IoT/ Wearable Devices. *IEEE 19th Electronics Packaging Technology Conference (EPTC),* 1-4. doi: 10.1109/ EPTC.2017.8277425

Thompson, N., Steck, J., & Behrman, E. (2020). A non-algorithmic approach to "programming" quantum computers via machine learning. *IEEE International Conference on Quantum Computing and Engineering (QCE)*, 63-71. doi: 10.1109/QCE49297.2020.00019

Tripathi, V., & Shakeel, F. (2017). Monitoring Health Care System Using Internet of Things - An Immaculate Pairing. *2017 International Conference on Next Generation Computing and Information Systems (ICNGCIS)*, 153-158, 10.1109/ICNGCIS.2017.26

Worgan, P., Pappas, O., Omirou, T., & Collett, M. (2015). Flexible on-body coils for inductive power transfer to IoT garments and wearables. *IEEE 2nd World Forum on Internet of Things (WF-IoT),* 297-298, doi: 10.1109/WF-IoT.2015.7389069

Wu, F., Rüdiger, C., Redouté, J., & Yuce, M. R. (2018). WE-Safe: A wearable IoT sensor node for safety applications via LoRa. *IEEE 4th World Forum on Internet of Things (WF-IoT),* 144-148. doi: 10.1109/ WF-IoT.2018.8355234

Zhou, W., & Piramuthu, S. (2014). Security/privacy of wearable fitness tracking IoT devices. *9th Iberian Conference on Information Systems and Technologies (CISTI)*, 1-5. doi:10.1109/CISTI.2014.6877073

Zhou, Z., Yu, H., & Shi, H. (2015). Human Activity Recognition Based on Improved Bayesian Convolution Network to Analyze Health Care Data Using Wearable IoT Device. *IEEE Access: Practical Innovations, Open Solutions*, *8*, 86411–86418. doi:10.1109/ACCESS.2020.2992584

KEY TERMS AND DEFINITIONS

AI: Artificial intelligence.
BP: Blood pressure.
BT: Body temperature.
ECG: Electrocardiograph.
GLD: Glucose level detection.
GSR: Galvanic skin response.
HBR: Heartbeat rate.
ICU: Intensive care unit.
IoT: Internet of things.
ML: Machine learning.
QC: Quantum computation.

APPENDIX 1

Use Case Implementation, patients data trafered over IOT device to the Health care system

Result of McEliece Encrypted Data Values

Figure 10. Plain text of the IoT sensor data are encrypted

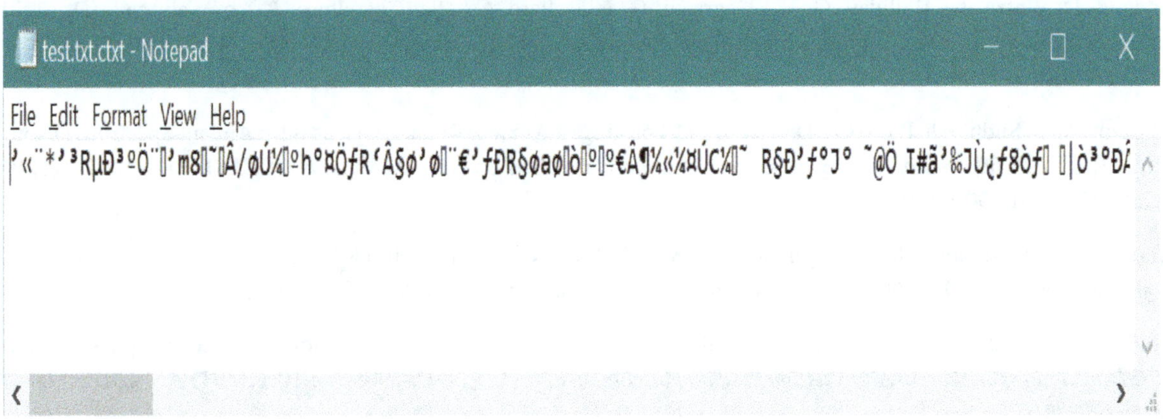

Result of McEliece DECRYPTED Data Values

Figure 11. Decrypted data values, at the target system

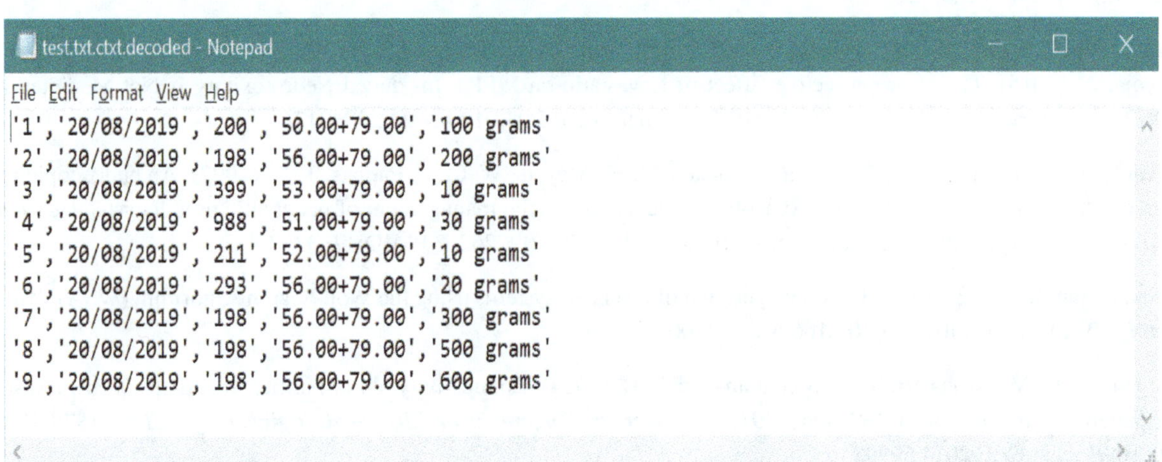

Compilation of References

Aarsland, D., Batzu, L., Halliday, G. M., Geurtsen, G. J., Ballard, C., Ray Chaudhuri, K., & Weintraub, D. (2021). Parkinson disease-associated cognitive impairment. *Nature Reviews. Disease Primers*, *7*(1), 47. doi:10.103841572-021-00280-3 PMID:34210995

Abhirami, A., & Sudheesh, P. (2019). Detection and Tracking of Anxiety Related Diseases for Autism Spectrum Disorder Using ECG. *2019 International Conference on Communication and Electronics Systems (ICCES)*, 1044-1052. 10.1109/ICCES45898.2019.9002160

Ablayev, Ablayev, Huang, Khadiev, Salikhova, & Wu. (2020). On quantum methods for machine learning problems part I: Quantum tools. *Big Data Mining and Analytics, 3*(1), 41-55. doi:10.26599/BDMA.9020016

Achille, A., & Soatto, S. (2018). Information dropout: Learning optimal representations through noisy computation. *IEEE Transactions on Pattern Analysis and Machine Intelligence*, *40*(12), 2897–2905. doi:10.1109/TPAMI.2017.2784440 PMID:29994167

Agrawal, R., Bu, L., & Kinsy, M. A. (2020). Quantum-Proof Lightweight McEliece Cryptosystem Co-processor Design. *IEEE 38th International Conference on Computer Design (ICCD),* 73-79. doi: 10.1109/ICCD50377.2020.00029

Agüero-Torres, H., Thomas, V. S., Winblad, B., & Fratiglioni, L. (2002). The impact of somatic and cognitive disorders on the functional status of the elderly. *Journal of Clinical Epidemiology*, *55*(10), 1007–1012. doi:10.1016/S0895-4356(02)00461-4 PMID:12464377

Aguirre-Vidal, Y., Montes, S., Tristan-López, L., Anaya-Ramos, L., Teiber, J., Ríos, C., Baron-Flores, V., & Monroy-Noyola, A. (2015). The Neuroprotective Effect of Lovastatin on MPP+-In- duced Neurotoxicity Is Not Mediated by PON2. *Neurotoxicology*, *48*, 166–170. doi:10.1016/j.neuro.2015.03.012 PMID:25842176

Ahearne, P. M., Baillie, J. M., Cotton, P. B., Baker, M. E., Meyers, W. C., & Pappas, T. N. (1992). An endoscopic retrograde cholangiopancreatography (ERCP)-based algorithm for the management of pancreatic pseudocysts. *American Journal of Surgery*, *163*(1), 111–116. doi:10.1016/0002-9610(92)90262-P PMID:1733357

Ahmadebrahimpour, E. (2019). Optimal operation of reservoir systems using the Wolf Search Algorithm (WSA). *Water Supply*, *19*(5), 1396–1404. doi:10.2166/ws.2019.005

Ahmadi, S. M. M., Mohajeri, N., & Soltanian-Zadeh, H. (2014). Connectivity abnormalities in autism spectrum disorder patients: A resting state fMRI study. *2014 22nd Iranian Conference on Electrical Engineering (ICEE),* 1878-1882. 10.1109/IranianCEE.2014.6999846

Air, T., Weightman, M. J., & Baune, B. T. (2015). Symptom severity of depressive symptoms impacts on social cognition performance in current but not remitted major depressive disorder. *Frontiers in Psychology*, *6*(AUG), 1–9. doi:10.3389/fpsyg.2015.01118 PMID:26300814

Akkaş, M., Sokullu, R., & Çetin, H. (2020). Healthcare and Patient Monitoring Using IoT. *Internet of Things., 11*, 100173. doi:10.1016/j.iot.2020.100173

Akshat. (2018). A Smart Healthcare Monitoring System Using Smartphone Interface. *2018 4th International Conference on Devices, Circuits and Systems (ICDCS)*, 228-231. doi: 10.1109/ICDCSyst.2018.8605142

Aladag, A., Muderrisoglu, S., Akbas, N., Zahmacioglu, O., & Bingol, H. (2018). Detecting Suicidal Ideation on Forums: Proof-of-Concept Study. *Journal of Medical Internet Research, 20*(6), e215. doi:10.2196/jmir.9840 PMID:29929945

Alam, S., Kwon, G.-R., & Initiative, A. D. (2017). Alzheimer disease classification using KPCA, LDA, and multi-kernel learning SVM. *International Journal of Imaging Systems and Technology, 27*(2), 133–143. doi:10.1002/ima.22217

Aldinger, K. A., & Doherty, D. (2016). *The genetics of cerebellar malformations.* Paper presented at the Seminars in Fetal and Neonatal Medicine.

Alexopoulos, G. S., Buckwalter, K., Olin, J., Martinez, R., Wainscott, C., & Krishnan, K. R. R. (2002). Comorbidity of late life depression: An opportunity for research on mechanisms and treatment. *Biological Psychiatry, 52*(6), 543–558. doi:10.1016/S0006-3223(02)01468-3 PMID:12361668

Aljarah, I., Al-Zoubi, A. M., Faris, H., Hassonah, M. A., Mirjalili, S., & Saadeh, H. (2018). Simultaneous feature selection and support vector machine optimization using the grasshopper optimization algorithm. *Cognitive Computation, 10*(3), 478–495. doi:10.100712559-017-9542-9

Álvarez, I., López, M., Górriz, J. M., Ramírez, J., Salas-Gonzalez, D., Puntonet, C. G., & Segovia, F. (2008). Automatic classification system for the diagnosis of alzheimer disease using Component-Based SVM aggregations. *International Conference on Neural Information Processing*, 402–409.

American Psychiatric Association & American Psychiatric Association. (2013). *Diagnostic and statistical manual of mental disorders: DSM-5*. Author.

American Psychiatric Association. (1980). Diagnostic and statistical manual of mental disorders (Vol. 3). Washington, DC: American Psychiatric Association.

Amukele, Ness, Tobian, Boyd, & Street. (2017). Drone transportation of blood products. *Transfusion, 57*(3), 582–588.

Anastasi, A. (1992). What counselors should know about the use and interpretation of psychological tests. *Journal of Counseling and Development, 70*(5), 610–615. doi:10.1002/j.1556-6676.1992.tb01670.x

Andersen, C. K., Wittrup-Jensen, K. U., Lolk, A., Andersen, K., & Kragh-Sørensen, P. (2004). Ability to perform activities of daily living is the main factor affecting quality of life in patients with dementia. *Health and Quality of Life Outcomes, 2*(1), 1–7. doi:10.1186/1477-7525-2-52 PMID:15383148

Andrzejak, R. G., Lehnertz, K., Mormann, F., Rieke, C., David, P., & Elger, C. E. (2001, November). Indications of Nonlinear Deterministic and Finite-dimensional Structures in Time Series of Brain Electrical Activity: Dependence on Recording Region and Brain State. *Physical Review E: Statistical, Nonlinear, and Soft Matter Physics, 64*(6), 061907. doi:10.1103/PhysRevE.64.061907 PMID:11736210

Anil Apak, R., Kose, G., Topaloglu, H., Anlar, B., Turanh, G., & Özdirim, E. (1999). Acute disseminated encephalomyelitis in childhood: Report of 10 cases. *Journal of Child Neurology, 14*(3), 198–201. doi:10.1177/088307389901400312 PMID:10190272

Anlar, B., Basaran, C., Kose, G., Guven, A., Haspolat, S., Yakut, A., ... Karaagaoglu, E. (2003). Acute disseminated encephalomyelitis in children: Outcome and prognosis. *Neuropediatrics, 34*(04), 194–199. doi:10.1055-2003-42208 PMID:12973660

Anurekha, G., & Geetha, P. (2018). Evidence Based Adaptive Neuro-Fuzzy Inference System for ASD Detection. *2018 3rd IEEE International Conference on Recent Trends in Electronics, Information & Communication Technology (RTEICT)*, 2188-2192. 10.1109/RTEICT42901.2018.9012400

Apak, R. A., Anlar, B., & Saatci, I. (1999). A case of relapsing acute disseminated encephalomyelitis with high dose corticosteroid treatment. *Brain & Development*, *21*(4), 279–282. doi:10.1016/S0387-7604(99)00011-X PMID:10392753

Ara, A., & Ara, A. (2017). Case study: Integrating IoT, streaming analytics and machine learning to improve intelligent diabetes management system. *International Conference on Energy, Communication, Data Analytics and Soft Computing (ICECDS)*, 3179-3182. doi: 10.1109/ICECDS.2017.8390043

Arias, Wurm, Hoang, & Jin. (2015). Privacy and Security in Internet of Things and Wearable Devices. *IEEE Transactions on Multi-Scale Computing Systems, 1*(2), 99-109. doi: . doi:10.1109/TMSCS.2015.2498605

Armstrong, M. J., & Okun, M. S. (2020). Diagnosis and treatment of Parkinson disease: A review. *Journal of the American Medical Association, 323*(6), 548–560. doi:10.1001/jama.2019.22360 PMID:32044947

Arns, M. (2012). EEG-based personalized medicine in ADHD: Individual alpha peak frequency as an endophenotype associated with nonresponse. *Journal of Neurotherapy*, *16*(2), 123–141. doi:10.1080/10874208.2012.677664

Arul Kumar, M. G. (2019). WCBAODV: An Efficacious approach to detect Wormhole attack in VANET using CBAODV Algorithm. *International Journal of Advanced Trends in Computer Science and Engineering*, 20-25.

Arulkumar, N. G. M. (2020). CPAODV: Classifying and Assigning 3 Level Preference to the Nodes in VANET Using AODV Based CBAODV Algorithm. In Intelligent Computing Paradigm and Cutting-edge Technologies. ICICCT 2019. Learning and Analytics in Intelligent Systems (pp. 432-445). Springer. doi:10.1007/978-3-030-38501-9_42

Ashour, A. S., El-Attar, A., Dey, N., Abd El-Kader, H., & Abd El-Naby, M. M. (2020). Long short term memory based patient-dependent model for FOG detection in Parkinson's disease. *Pattern Recognition Letters*, *131*, 23–29. doi:10.1016/j.patrec.2019.11.036

Askarzadeh, A. (2016). A novel metaheuristic method for solving constrained engineering optimization problems: Crow search algorithm. *Computers & Structures*, *169*, 1–12. doi:10.1016/j.compstruc.2016.03.001

Aslam, A. R., Hafeez, N., Heidari, H., & Altaf, M. A. B. (2021). An 8.62 μ W Processor for Autism Spectrum Disorder Classification using Shallow Neural Network. *2021 IEEE 3rd International Conference on Artificial Intelligence Circuits and Systems (AICAS),* 1-4. 10.1109/AICAS51828.2021.9458412

Association, A. (2015). 2015 Alzheimer's disease facts and figures. *Alzheimer's & Dementia*, *11*(3), 332–384. doi:10.1016/j.jalz.2015.02.003 PMID:25984581

Avants, B. B., Tustison, N., & Song, G. (2009). Advanced normalization tools (ANTS). *The Insight Journal*, *2*, 1–35.

Bader, M., Tannock, R., & Hadjikhani, N. (2018). The Zappel-Philipp a historical example of ADHD Clinics. *Attention Deficit and Hyperactivity Disorders, 10*(2), 119–127. doi:10.100712402-017-0239-4 PMID:28905267

Bailey, M. R., Pishchalnikov, Y. A., Sapozhnikov, O. A., Cleveland, R. O., McAteer, J. A., Miller, N. A., Pishchalnikova, I. V., Connors, B. A., Crum, L. A., & Evan, A. P. (2005). Cavitation detection during shock wave lithotripsy. *Ultrasound in Medicine & Biology*, *31*(9), 1245–1256. doi:10.1016/j.ultrasmedbio.2005.02.017 PMID:16176791

Bajwa, G., Dantu, R., Issadeen, M. F. M., & Joseph, R. M. (2013). Selftracking via brain-mobile-cloud interface. *Proceedings of the AAAI Spring Symposium Series.*

Balani, S., & De Choudhury, M. (2015). Detecting and Characterizing Mental Health Related Self-Disclosure in Social Media. *Proceedings of the 33Rd Annual ACM Conference Extended Abstracts on Human Factors in Computing Systems*. 10.1145/2702613.2732733

Balasingam. (2017). Drones in medicine—the rise of the machines. *International Journal of Clinical Practice*, *71*(9). doi:10.1111/ijcp.12989

Ball, N., Teo, W.-P., Chandra, S., & Chapman, J. (2019). Parkinson's disease and the environment. *Frontiers in Neurology*, *10*, 218. doi:10.3389/fneur.2019.00218 PMID:30941085

Banerjee, M., Hegde, S., Harish, T., Kulkarni, G. B., & Rao, N. (2021). In search of the 'self': Holistic rehabilitation in restoring cognition and recovering the 'self' following traumatic brain injury: A case report. *Neuro Rehabilitation*, 1-12.

Banerjee, M., & Kumar, K. (2020). Mood Induction Can Enhance Cognitive Remediation in Depression. *International Journal of Cognition and Behaviour*, *3*(1). Advance online publication. doi:10.23937/2690-3172/1710008

Barberger-Gateau, P., Fabrigoule, C., Helmer, C., Rouch, I., & Dartigues, J. F. (1999). Functional impairment in instrumental activities of daily living: An early clinical sign of dementia? *Journal of the American Geriatrics Society*, *47*(4), 456–462. doi:10.1111/j.1532-5415.1999.tb07239.x PMID:10203122

Bardis, N., Kharchenko, V., Potii, O., & Vambol, A. (2020). Post-Quantum Network Security: McEliece and Niederreiter Cryptosystems Analysis and Education Issues post-quantum cryptography. *WSEAS Transactions on Systems and Control*, *15*, 627–634. doi:10.37394/23203.2020.15.62

Barkley, R. A., & Edwards, G. H. (2006). *Attention-deficit*. Academic Press.

Barkley, R. A. (1997). *ADHD and the nature of self-control*. Guilford press.

Barkley, R. A. (1997). Behavioral inhibition, sustained attention, and executive functions: Constructing a unifying theory of ADHD. *Psychological Bulletin*, *121*(1), 65–94. doi:10.1037/0033-2909.121.1.65 PMID:9000892

Barkley, R. A. (2001). The executive functions and self-regulation: An evolutionary neuropsychological perspective. *Neuropsychology Review*, *11*(1), 1–29. doi:10.1023/A:1009085417776 PMID:11392560

Barlow, H. (2001). Redundancy reduction revisited. *Network (Bristol, England)*, *12*(3), 241–253. doi:10.1080/net.12.3.241.253 PMID:11563528

Barry, R. J., Clarke, A. R., & Johnstone, S. J. (2003). A review of electrophysiology in attention-deficit/hyperactivity disorder: I. Qualitative and quantitative electroencephalography. *Clinical Neurophysiology*, *114*(2), 171–183. doi:10.1016/S1388-2457(02)00362-0 PMID:12559224

Basaia, S., Agosta, F., Wagner, L., Canu, E., Magnani, G., Santangelo, R., & Filippi, M. (2019). Automated classification of Alzheimer's disease and mild cognitive impairment using a single MRI and deep neural networks. *NeuroImage. Clinical*, *21*, 101645. doi:10.1016/j.nicl.2018.101645 PMID:30584016

Bauman, M., & Kemper, T. L. (1985). Histoanatomic observations of the brain in early infantile autism. *Neurology*, *35*(6), 866–866. doi:10.1212/WNL.35.6.866 PMID:4000488

Baune, B. T., Miller, R., McAfoose, J., Johnson, M., Quirk, F., & Mitchell, D. (2010). The role of cognitive impairment in general functioning in major depression. *Psychiatry Research*, *176*(2–3), 183–189. doi:10.1016/j.psychres.2008.12.001 PMID:20138370

Bayindir, R., Yesilbudak, M., Colak, M., & Genc, N. (2017). A Novel Application of Naive Bayes Classifier in Photovoltaic Energy Prediction. *Proceedings of the 16th IEEE International Conference on Machine Learning and Applications*, 523–527. 10.1109/ICMLA.2017.0-108

Beach, T.G., Adler, C.H., Sue, L.I., Vedders, L., Lue, L., White, C.L. (2010). Multi-organ distribution of phosphorylated α-synuclein histopathology in subjects with Lewy body disorders. *Acta Neuropathol, 119*(6), 689–702. .95 doi:10.1007/s00401-010-0664-3

Beach, T. G., Carew, J., Serrano, G., Adler, C. H., Shill, H. A., Sue, L. I., Sabbagh, M. N., Akiyama, H., & Cuenca, N. (2014). Phosphorylated α-synuclein-immunoreactive retinal neuronal elements in Parkinson's disease subjects. *Neuroscience Letters, 571*, 34–38. doi:10.1016/j.neulet.2014.04.027 PMID:24785101

Beck, J. S., & Beck, A. T. (1995). Cognitive therapy: Basics and beyond (No. Sirsi). New York: Guilford Press.

Bee, H. (2000). The developing child (9th ed.). Academic Press.

Bega, D., Gonzalez-Latapi, P., Zadikoff, C., Spies, W., & Simuni, T. (2015). Is there a role for DAT-SPECT imaging in a specialty movement disorders practice? *Neurodegenerative Diseases, 15*(2), 81–86. doi:10.1159/000370116 PMID:25592727

Bektaş, M., & Görmüş, S. (2018). An energy efficient IoT protocol for healthcare at home. *26th Signal Processing and Communications Applications Conference (SIU)*, 1-4. doi: 10.1109/SIU.2018.8404663

Benes, F. M. (2006). *The development of the prefrontal cortex: The maturation of neurotransmitter systems and their interactions*. Academic Press.

Beniczky, S., Polster, T., Kjaer, T. W., & Hjalgrim, H. (2013). Detection of generalized tonic-clonic seizures by a wireless wrist accelerometer: A prospective, multicenter study. *Epilepsia, 54*(4), e58–e61. doi:10.1111/epi.12120 PMID:23398578

Berg, D., Postuma, R. B., Bloem, B., Chan, P., Dubois, B., Gasser, T., Goetz, C. G., Halliday, G. M., Hardy, J., Lang, A. E., Litvan, I., Marek, K., Obeso, J., Oertel, W., Olanow, C. W., Poewe, W., Stern, M., & Deuschl, G. (2014). Time to redefine PD? Introductory statement of the MDS Task Force on the definition of Parkinson's disease. *Movement Disorders, 29*(4), 454–462. doi:10.1002/mds.25844 PMID:24619848

Bharanidharan, N., & Rajaguru, H. (2020). Performance enhancement of swarm intelligence techniques in dementia classification using dragonfly-based hybrid algorithms. *International Journal of Imaging Systems and Technology, 30*, 57–74.

Bhatt, V., & Chakraborty, S. (2020). Importance of Trust in IoT based Wearable Device Adoption by Patient: An Empirical Investigation. *Fourth International Conference on I-SMAC (IoT in Social, Mobile, Analytics and Cloud) (I-SMAC)*, 1226-1231. doi: 10.1109/I-SMAC49090.2020.9243533

Bianchi, F. M., Maiorino, E., Kampffmeyer, M. C., Rizzi, A., & Jenssen, R. (2017). *An overview and comparative analysis of recurrent neural networks for short term load forecasting*. arXiv:1705.04378

Biscetti, L., Salvadori, N., Farotti, L., Cataldi, S., Eusebi, P., Paciotti, S., & Parnetti, L. (2019). The added value of Aβ42/Aβ40 in the CSF signature for routine diagnostics of Alzheimer's disease. *Clinica Chimica Acta, 494*, 71–73. doi:10.1016/j.cca.2019.03.001 PMID:30844364

Bisgin, H., Bera, T., Ding, H., Semey, H. G., Wu, L., Liu, Z., Barnes, A. E., Langley, D. A., Pava-Ripoll, M., Vyas, H. J., Tong, W., & Xu, J. (2018). Comparing SVM and ANN-based machine learning methods for species identification of food contaminating beetles. *Scientific Reports, 8*(1), 1–12. doi:10.103841598-018-24926-7 PMID:29695741

Bisht, R. S., Jain, S., & Tewari, N. (2021). Study of Wearable IoT devices in 2021: Analysis & Future Prospects. *2nd International Conference on Intelligent Engineering and Management (ICIEM)*, 577-581. doi: 10.1109/ICIEM51511.2021.9445334

Blair, C., & Diamond, A. (2008). The promotion of self regulation as a means of preventing school failure. *Development and Psychopathology*, *20*(3), 899–911. doi:10.1017/S0954579408000436 PMID:18606037

Bogdanov, S. I., Kudyshev, Z., Kildishev, A. V., Boltasseva, A., & Shalaev, V. M. (2019). *High-Speed Quantum Photonics with Plasmonic Metamaterials Empowered by Machine Learning. In IEEE Photonics Conference*. IPC. doi:10.1109/IPCon.2019.8908357

Bogle, Rosamond, Snyder, & Zègre-Hemsey. (2019). The case for droneassisted emergency response to cardiac arrest: An optimized statewide deployment approach. *North Carolina Medical Journal*, *80*(4), 204–212.

Borcea, C., Ding, X., Gehani, N., Curtmola, R., Khan, M. A., & Debnath, H. (2015). Avatar: mobile distributed computing in the cloud. *Proceedings of the 3rd IEEE International Conference on Mobile Cloud Computing, Services, and Engineering, Mobile-Cloud 2015*, 151–156. 10.1109/MobileCloud.2015.22

Botvinick, M., Nystrom, L. E., Fissell, K., Carter, C. S., & Cohen, J. D. (1999). Conflict monitoring versus selection-for-action in anterior cingulate cortex. *Nature*, *402*(6758), 179–181. doi:10.1038/46035 PMID:10647008

Boutros, N., Fraenkel, L., & Feingold, A. (2005). A four-step approach for developing diagnostic tests in psychiatry: EEG in ADHD as a test case. *The Journal of Neuropsychiatry and Clinical Neurosciences*, *17*(4), 455–464. doi:10.1176/jnp.17.4.455 PMID:16387983

Braak, H., Del Tredici, K., Rüb, U., de Vos, R. A., Steur, E. N. J., & Braak, E. (2003). Staging of brain pathology related to sporadic Parkinson's disease. *Neurobiology of Aging*, *24*(2), 197–211. doi:10.1016/S0197-4580(02)00065-9 PMID:12498954

Brain Anatomy and How the Brain Works. (2021). Retrieved 9 October 2021, from https://www.hopkinsmedicine.org/health/conditions-and-diseases/anatomy-of-the-brain

Braun, Gertz, & Furer. (2019). The promising future of drones in prehospital medical care and its application to battlefield medicine. *The Journal of Trauma and Acute Care Surgery*, *87*, S28–S34.

Brownlee, J. (2011). *Clever algorithms: Nature-inspired programming recipes*. Jason Brownlee.

Budida, D. A. M., & Mangrulkar, R. S. (2017). Design and implementation of smart HealthCare system using IoT. *International Conference on Innovations in Embedded and Communication Systems (ICIIECS)*, 1-7. doi: 10.1109/ICIIECS.2017.8275903

Burks, H. F. (1960). The hyperkinetic child. *Exceptional Children*, *27*(1), 18–26. doi:10.1177/001440296002700105

Buschert, V., Bokde, A. L., & Hampel, H. (2010). Cognitive intervention in Alzheimer disease. *Nature Reviews. Neurology*, *6*(9), 508–517. doi:10.1038/nrneurol.2010.113 PMID:20717104

Cai, X., Gao, X., & Xue, Y. (2016). Improved bat algorithm with optimal forage strategy and random disturbance strategy. *International Journal of Bio-inspired Computation*, *8*(4), 205–214. doi:10.1504/IJBIC.2016.078666

Callaway, E., Halliday, R., & Naylor, H. (1983). Hyperactive children's event-related potentials fail to support underarousal and maturational-lag theories. *Archives of General Psychiatry*, *40*(11), 1243–1248. doi:10.1001/archpsyc.1983.01790100089012 PMID:6639294

Callegari, D., Conte, E., & Ferreto, T. (2014). EpiCare - a home care platform based on mobile cloud computing to assist epilepsy diagnosis. *Proceedings of the 4th International Conference on Wireless Mobile Communication and Healthcare, MOBIHEALTH 2014*, 148–151. 10.4108/icst.mobihealth.2014.257379

Cameron, I., Cardy, A., Crawford, J., du Toit, S., Hay, S., Lawton, K., Mitchell, K., Sharma, S., Shivaprasad, S., Winning, S., & Reid, I. C. (2011). Measuring depression severity in general practice: Discriminatory performance of the PHQ-9, HADS-D, and BDI-II. *The British Journal of General Practice*, *61*(588), e419–e426. doi:10.3399/bjgp11X583209 PMID:21722450

Casanova, M. F., van Kooten, I. A., Switala, A. E., van Engeland, H., Heinsen, H., Steinbusch, H. W., Hof, P. R., Trippe, J., Stone, J., & Schmitz, C. (2006). Minicolumnar abnormalities in autism. *Acta Neuropathologica*, *112*(3), 287–303. doi:10.100700401-006-0085-5 PMID:16819561

Caseras, X., Garner, M., Bradley, B. P., & Mogg, K. (2007). Biases in Visual Orienting to Negative and Positive Scenes in Dysphoria: An Eye Movement Study. *Journal of Abnormal Psychology*, *116*(3), 491–497. doi:10.1037/0021-843X.116.3.491 PMID:17696705

Casey, B. J., Castellanos, F. X., Giedd, J. N., Marsh, W. L., Hamburger, S. D., Schubert, A. B., Vauss, Y. C., Vaituzis, A. C., Dickstein, D. P., Sarfatti, S., & Rapoport, J. L. (1997). Implication of right frontostriatal circuitry in response inhibition and attention-deficit/hyperactivity disorder. *Journal of the American Academy of Child and Adolescent Psychiatry*, *36*(3), 374–383. doi:10.1097/00004583-199703000-00016 PMID:9055518

Castellanos, F. X. (2001). Neuroimaging studies of ADHD. *Stimulant drugs and ADHD, Basic and Clinical Neuroscience*, 243–258.

Chabot, R. J., & Serfontein, G. (1996). Quantitative electroencephalographic profiles of children with attention deficit disorder. *Biological Psychiatry*, *40*(10), 951–963. doi:10.1016/0006-3223(95)00576-5 PMID:8915554

Chakravarty, A. (2001). Neurologic illness following post-exposure prophylaxis with purifiled chick embryo cell antirabies vaccine. *The Journal of the Association of Physicians of India*, *49*, 927–928. PMID:11837768

Charletta, D., Gorelick, P. B., Dollear, T., Freels, S., & Harris, Y. (1995). CT and MRI fndings among African-Americans with Alzheimer's disease, vascular dementia, and stroke without dementia. *Neurology*, *45*(8), 1456–1461. doi:10.1212/WNL.45.8.1456 PMID:7644040

Chaudhuri, K. R., Healy, D. G., & Schapira, A. H. (2006). Non-motor symptoms of Parkinson's disease: Diagnosis and management. *Lancet Neurology*, *5*(3), 235–245. doi:10.1016/S1474-4422(06)70373-8 PMID:16488379

Chaudhuri, K. R., & Schapira, A. H. (2009). Non-motor symptoms of Parkinson's disease: Dopaminergic pathophysiology and treatment. *Lancet Neurology*, *8*(5), 464–474. doi:10.1016/S1474-4422(09)70068-7 PMID:19375664

Chen, T., & Guestrin, C. (2016). XGBoost: A scalable tree boosting system. In *Proceedings of the 22Nd ACM SIGKDD International Conference on Knowledge Discovery and Data Mining, KDD '16*. ACM. 10.1145/2939672.2939785

Chen, A. C., Oathes, D. J., Chang, C., Bradley, T., Zhou, Z. W., Williamsa, L. M., Glover, G. H., Deisseroth, K., & Etkin, A. (2013). Causal interactions between fronto-parietal central executive and default-mode networks in humans. *Proceedings of the National Academy of Sciences of the United States of America*, *110*(49), 19944–19949. doi:10.1073/pnas.1311772110 PMID:24248372

Cheng, Y., Luo, S., & Lin, H. (2016). Investigating the Performance on Comprehending 3D Social Emotion through a Mobile Learning System for Individuals with Autistic Spectrum Disorder. *2016 5th IIAI International Congress on Advanced Applied Informatics (IIAI-AAI)*, 414-417. 10.1109/IIAI-AAI.2016.138

Cherdal, S., & Mouline, S. (2016). A Petri Net model to simulate and analyse cerebral folate deficiency and hyperhomocysteinemia effects in Autism Spectrum Disorder. *2016 7th International Conference on Sciences of Electronics, Technologies of Information and Telecommunications (SETIT)*, 279-284. 10.1109/SETIT.2016.7939880

Chess, S. (1960). Diagnosis and treatment of the hyperactive child. *New York State Journal of Medicine*, *60*, 2379–2385. PMID:13809736

Chiang, H.-S., Sangaiah, A. K., Chen, M.-Y., & Liu, J.-Y. (2020). A novel artificial bee colony optimization algorithm with SVM for bio-inspired software-defined networking. *International Journal of Parallel Programming*, *48*(2), 310–328. doi:10.100710766-018-0594-6

Chrisman, B. (2018). Analysis of Sex and Recurrence Ratios in Simplex and Multiplex Autism Spectrum Disorder Implicates Sex-Specific Alleles as Inheritance Mechanism. *2018 IEEE International Conference on Bioinformatics and Biomedicine (BIBM)*, 1470-1477. 10.1109/BIBM.2018.8621554

Claesson, Svensson, & Nordberg. (2017). Drones may be used to save lives in out of hospital cardiac arrest due to drowning. *Resuscitation*, *114*, 152–156.

Cohen, N., Mor, N., & Henik, A. (2015). Linking executive control and emotional response: A training procedure to reduce rumination. *Clinical Psychological Science*, *3*(1), 15–25. doi:10.1177/2167702614530114

Contaldo, C., Högger, D. C., Khorrami Borozadi, M., Stotz, M., Platz, U., Forster, N., Lindenblatt, N., & Giovanoli, P. (2012). Radial pressure waves mediate apoptosis and functional angiogenesis during wound repair in ApoE deficient mice. *Microvascular Research*, *84*(1), 24–33. doi:10.1016/j.mvr.2012.03.006 PMID:22504489

Corbetta, M., & Shulman, G. L. (2002). Control of goal-directed and stimulus-driven attention in the brain. *Nature Reviews. Neuroscience*, *3*(3), 201–215. doi:10.1038/nrn755 PMID:11994752

Corchia, L. (2019). Radio-frequency Identification Based on Textile, Wearable, Chipless Tags for IoT Applications. *II Workshop on Metrology for Industry 4.0 and IoT (MetroInd4.0&IoT)*, 1-5. doi: 10.1109/METROI4.8792919

Corne, D. W., & Lones, M. A. (2018). *Evolutionary algorithms.* arXiv preprint arXiv:1805.11014.

Costafreda, S. G., Dinov, I. D., Tu, Z., Shi, Y., Liu, C. Y., Kloszewska, I., Mecocci, P., Soininen, H., Tsolaki, M., Vellas, B., Wahlund, L.-O., Spenger, C., Toga, A. W., Lovestone, S., & Simmons, A. (2011). Automated hippocampal shape analysis predicts the onset of dementia in mild cognitive impairment. *NeuroImage*, *56*(1), 212–219. doi:10.1016/j.neuroimage.2011.01.050 PMID:21272654

Coune, P. G., Schneider, B. L., & Aebischer, P. (2012). Parkinson's Disease: Gene Therapies. *Cold Spring Harbor Perspectives in Medicine*, *4*(4), a009431. Advance online publication. doi:10.1101/cshperspect.a009431 PMID:22474617

Courchesne, E., Mouton, P. R., Calhoun, M. E., Semendeferi, K., Ahrens-Barbeau, C., Hallet, M. J., Barnes, C. C., & Pierce, K. (2011). Neuron number and size in prefrontal cortex of children with autism. *Journal of the American Medical Association*, *306*(18), 2001–2010. doi:10.1001/jama.2011.1638 PMID:22068992

Crichton, A. (1798). *An inquiry into the nature and origin of mental derangement: comprehending a concise system of the physiology and pathology of the human mind. and a history of the passions and their effects* (Vol. 2). Academic Press.

Daches, S., & Mor, N. (2014). Training ruminators to inhibit negative information: A preliminary report. *Cognitive Therapy and Research*, *38*(2), 160–171. doi:10.100710608-013-9585-5

Dale, R., De Sousa, C., Chong, W., Cox, T., Harding, B., & Neville, B. (2000). Acute disseminated encephalomyelitis, multiphasic disseminated encephalomyelitis and multiple sclerosis in children. *Brain*, *123*(12), 2407–2422. doi:10.1093/brain/123.12.2407 PMID:11099444

Daoud, H. G., Abdelhameed, A. M., & Bayoumi, M. (2018). Automatic Epileptic Seizure Detection Based on Empirical Mode Decomposition An Deep Neural Network. *Proceedings of the IEEE 14th International Colloquium on Signal Processing Its Applications*, 182–186. 10.1109/CSPA.2018.8368709

Darwish, A. (2018). Bio-inspired computing: Algorithms review, deep analysis, and the scope of applications. *Future Computing and Informatics Journal*, *3*(2), 231–246. doi:10.1016/j.fcij.2018.06.001

Das, R. (2010). A comparison of multiple classification methods for diagnosis of Parkinson disease. *Expert Systems with Applications*, *37*(2), 1568–1572. doi:10.1016/j.eswa.2009.06.040

Dauer, W., & Przedborski, S. (2003). Parkinson's disease: Mechanisms and models. *Neuron*, *39*(6), 889–909. doi:10.1016/S0896-6273(03)00568-3 PMID:12971891

Davie, C. A. (2008). A review of Parkinson's disease. *British Medical Bulletin*, *86*(1), 109–127. doi:10.1093/bmb/ldn013 PMID:18398010

De Lau, L. M., & Breteler, M. M. (2006). Epidemiology of Parkinson's disease. *Lancet Neurology*, *5*(6), 525–535. doi:10.1016/S1474-4422(06)70471-9 PMID:16713924

De Lissnyder, E., Koster, E. H. W., Everaert, J., Schacht, R., Van den Abeele, D., & De Raedt, R. (2012). Internal cognitive control in clinical depression: General but no emotion-specific impairments. *Psychiatry Research*, *199*(2), 124–130. doi:10.1016/j.psychres.2012.04.019 PMID:22578821

De Raedt, R., & Koster, E. H. W. (2010). Understanding vulnerability for depression from a cognitive neuroscience perspective: A reappraisal of attentional factors and a new conceptual framework. *Cognitive, Affective & Behavioral Neuroscience*, *10*(1), 50–70. doi:10.3758/CABN.10.1.50 PMID:20233955

DeLong, E. R., DeLong, D. M., & Clarke-Pearson, D. L. (1988). Comparing the areas under two or more correlated receiver operating characteristic curves: A nonparametric approach ". *Biometrics*, *44*(3), 837–845. doi:10.2307/2531595 PMID:3203132

Demeyer, I., De Lissnyder, E., Koster, E. H. W., & De Raedt, R. (2012). Rumination mediates the relationship between impaired cognitive control for emotional information and depressive symptoms: A prospective study in remitted depressed adults. *Behaviour Research and Therapy*, *50*(5), 292–297. doi:10.1016/j.brat.2012.02.012 PMID:22449892

Dempster, T. (2012). *An investigation into the optimum training paradigm for alpha electroencephalographic biofeedback*. Canterbury Christ Church University.

Deng, L., & Dong, Y. (2014). Deep learning: Methods and applications. *Found. Trends® Signal Process, 7*(3–4), 197–387. doi:10.1007/978-981-13-3459-7_3

Deng, H., Wang, P., & Jankovic, J. (2018). The genetics of Parkinson disease. *Ageing Research Reviews*, *42*, 72–85. doi:10.1016/j.arr.2017.12.007 PMID:29288112

Deshmukh, S., & Shah, R. (2016). Computation offloading frameworks in mobile cloud computing: a survey. *Proceedings of the 2016 IEEE International Conference on Current Trends in Advanced Computing, ICCTAC 2016*, 1–5. 10.1109/ICCTAC.2016.7567332

Diamond, A. (2000). Close interrelation of motor development and cognitive development and of the cerebellum and prefrontal cortex. *Child Development*, *71*(1), 44–56. doi:10.1111/1467-8624.00117 PMID:10836557

Dickson, D. W. (2012). Parkinson's disease and parkinsonism: Neuropathology. *Cold Spring Harbor Perspectives in Medicine*, *2*(8), a009258. doi:10.1101/cshperspect.a009258 PMID:22908195

Direito, B., Teixeira, C., Ribeiro, B., Castelo-Branco, M., Sales, F., & Dourado, A. (2012). Modeling epileptic brain states using EEG spectral analysis and topographic mapping. *Journal of Neuroscience Methods*, *210*(2), 220–229. doi:10.1016/j.jneumeth.2012.07.006 PMID:22850556

Dolgin, E. (2018). *This Seizure-Detecting Smartwatch Could Save Your Life*. https://spectrum.ieee.org/the-human-os/biomedical/diagnostics/this-seizuredetecting-smartwatch-could-save-your-life

Dorigo, M., Maniezzo, V., & Colorni, A. (1996). Ant system: Optimization by a colony of cooperating agents. *IEEE Transactions on Systems, Man, and Cybernetics. Part B, Cybernetics*, *26*(1), 29–41. doi:10.1109/3477.484436 PMID:18263004

Douglas, V. I. (1983). Attention and cognitive problems. *Developmental Neuropsychiatry*, 280-329.

Douglas, V. I. (1999). Cognitive control processes in attention deficit/hyperactivity disorder. In *Handbook of disruptive behavior disorders* (pp. 105–138). Springer. doi:10.1007/978-1-4615-4881-2_5

Douglas, V. I., & Parry, P. A. (1983). Effects of reward on delayed reaction time task performance of hyperactive children. *Journal of Abnormal Child Psychology*, *11*(2), 313–326. doi:10.1007/BF00912094 PMID:6619440

Doukas, C., & Maglogiannis, I. (2011). Managing wearable sensor data through Cloud Computing. *Proceedings of the 2011 3rd IEEE International Conference on Cloud Computing Technology and Science, CloudCom 2011*, 440–445. 10.1109/CloudCom.2011.65

Dris, A. B., Alsalman, A., Al-Wabil, A., & Aldosari, M. (2019). Intelligent Gaze-Based Screening System for Autism. *2nd International Conference on Computer Applications & Information Security (ICCAIS)*, 1-5. 10.1109/CAIS.2019.8769452

Dukart, J., Mueller, K., Barthel, H., Villringer, A., Sabri, O., & Schroeter, M. L. (2013). Meta-analysis based SVM classification enables accurate detection of Alzheimer's disease across different clinical centers using FDG-PET and MRI. *Psychiatry Research: Neuroimaging*, *212*(3), 230–236. doi:10.1016/j.pscychresns.2012.04.007 PMID:23149027

Dykman, R. A., Holcomb, P. J., Oglesby, D. M., & Ackerman, P. T. (1982). Electrocortical frequencies in hyperactive, learning-disabled, mixed, and normal children. *Biological Psychiatry*. PMID:7104419

Ebaugh, F. G. (1923). Neuropsychiatric sequelae of acute epidemic encephalitis in children. *American Journal of Diseases of Children*, *25*(2), 89–97.

Eberhart, R., & Kennedy, J. (1995). A new optimizer using particle swarm theory. *MHS'95. Proceedings of the Sixth International Symposium on Micro Machine and Human Science*, 39–43. 10.1109/MHS.1995.494215

Edwards, T. J., Sherr, E. H., Barkovich, A. J., & Richards, L. J. (2014). Clinical, genetic and imaging findings identify new causes for corpus callosum development syndromes. *Brain*, *137*(6), 1579–1613. doi:10.1093/brain/awt358 PMID:24477430

Eesa, A. S., Brifcani, A. M., & Orman, Z. (2013). Cuttlefish algorithm-a novel bio-inspired optimization algorithm. *International Journal of Scientific and Engineering Research*, *4*, 1978–1986.

Eesa, A. S., Brifcani, A. M., & Orman, Z. (2014). A new tool for global optimization problems-cuttlefish algorithm. *International Journal of Mathematical, Computational. Natural and Physical Engineering*, *8*, 1208–1211.

Eesa, A. S., Orman, Z., & Brifcani, A. M. (2015). A novel feature-selection approach based on the cuttlefish optimization algorithm for intrusion detection systems. *Expert Systems with Applications*, *42*(5), 2670–2679. doi:10.1016/j.eswa.2014.11.009

Elobeid, A., Libard, S., Leino, M., Popova, S. N., & Alafuzoff, I. (2016, April). Altered proteins in the aging brain. *Journal of Neuropathology and Experimental Neurology*, *75*(4), 316–325. doi:10.1093/jnen/nlw002 PMID:26979082

Engel, J. Jr. (2001). A proposed diagnostic scheme for people with epileptic seizures and with epilepsy: Report of the ILAE task force on classification and terminology. *Epilepsia*, *42*(6), 796–803. doi:10.1046/j.1528-1157.2001.10401.x PMID:11422340

Eremina, G., & Smolin, A. (2021). Numerical modeling of shockwave treatment of knee joint. *Materials (Basel)*, *14*(24), 7678. doi:10.3390/ma14247678 PMID:34947273

Erhan, D., Bengio, Y., Courville, A., Manzagol, P.-A., Vincent, P., & Bengio, S. (2010). Why does unsupervised pre-training help deep learning? *Journal of Machine Learning Research*, *11*, 625–660.

Erickson, B. J., Korfiatis, P., Akkus, Z., & Kline, T. L. (2017). Machine learning for medical imaging. *Radiographics*, *37*(2), 505–515. doi:10.1148/rg.2017160130 PMID:28212054

Esteva, A. (2019). A deep learning model for early prediction of Alzheimer's disease dementia based on hippocampal magnetic resonance imaging data. *Alzheimer's & Dementia*, *15*(8), 1059–1070. doi:10.1016/j.jalz.2019.02.007 PMID:31201098

Evans, C. (2007). Cognitive–behavioural therapy with older people. *Advances in Psychiatric Treatment*, *13*(2), 111–118. doi:10.1192/apt.bp.106.003020

Evans, N. R., Tarkin, J. M., Buscombe, J. R., Markus, H. S., Rudd, J. H., & Warburton, E. A. (2018). Erratum: PET imaging of the neurovascular interface in cerebrovascular disease. *Nature Reviews. Neurology*, *14*(5), 313–313. doi:10.1038/nrneurol.2018.42 PMID:29611539

Ewees, A. A., Abd Elaziz, M., & Houssein, E. H. (2018). Improved grasshopper optimization algorithm using opposition-based learning. *Expert Systems with Applications*, *112*, 156–172. doi:10.1016/j.eswa.2018.06.023

Fabre, M., & Buser, P. (1980). Structures involved in acquisition and performance of visually guided movements in the cat. *Acta Neurobiologiae Experimentalis*, *40*, 95–116. PMID:7424596

Fadhil, T. Z., & Mandeel, A. R. (2018). Live Monitoring System for Recognizing Varied Emotions of Autistic Children. *2018 International Conference on Advanced Science and Engineering (ICOASE)*, 151-155. 10.1109/ICOASE.2018.8548931

Fadi, A., Carette, R., Elbattah, M., Dequen, G., Guérin, J.-L., & Cilia, F. (2018). Visualization of Eye-Tracking Patterns in Autism Spectrum Disorder: Method and Dataset. *2018 Thirteenth International Conference on Digital Information Management (ICDIM)*, 248-253. 10.1109/ICDIM.2018.8846967

Falkensammer, F., Rausch-Fan, X., Schaden, W., Kivaranovic, D., & Freudenthaler, J. (2015). Impact of extracorporeal shockwave therapy on tooth mobility in adult orthodontic patients: A randomized single-center placebo-controlled clinical trial. *Journal of Clinical Periodontology*, *42*(3), 294–301. doi:10.1111/jcpe.12373 PMID:25640577

Fang, P., Zeng, L. L., Shen, H., Wang, L., Li, B., Liu, L., & Hu, D. (2012). Increased Cortical-Limbic Anatomical Network Connectivity in Major Depression Revealed by Diffusion Tensor Imaging. *PLoS One*, *7*(9), e45972. Advance online publication. doi:10.1371/journal.pone.0045972 PMID:23049910

Fan, Y., Resnick, S. M., Wu, X., & Davatzikos, C. (2008). Structural and functional biomarkers of prodromal Alzheimer's disease: A high-dimensional pattern classification study. *NeuroImage*, *41*(2), 277–285. doi:10.1016/j.neuroimage.2008.02.043 PMID:18400519

Fareed & Al-Atroshi. (2021). *Australia Patent No. 2020103911*. Australian Government.

Feero, W. G., Guttmacher, A. E., & Collins, F. S. (2010). Genomic medicine—An updated primer. *The New England Journal of Medicine*, *362*(21), 2001–2011. doi:10.1056/NEJMra0907175 PMID:20505179

Feng, T., Xie, L., Yao, J., & Xu, J. (in press). UAV-Enabled Data Collection for Wireless Sensor Networks with Distributed Beamforming. *IEEE Transactions on Wireless Communications*. Advance online publication. doi:10.1109/TWC.2021.3103739

Fernando, N., Loke, S. W., & Rahayu, W. (2013). Mobile cloud computing: A survey. *Future Generation Computer Systems*, *29*(1), 84–106. doi:10.1016/j.future.2012.05.023

Fischl, B. (2012). FreeSurfer. *NeuroImage*, *62*(2), 774–781. doi:10.1016/j.neuroimage.2012.01.021 PMID:22248573

Fisher, R. S., Van Emde Boas, W., & Blume, W. (2005). Epileptic seizures and epilepsy: Definitions proposed by the International League Against Epilepsy (ILAE) and the International Bureau for Epilepsy (IBE). *Epilepsia*, *46*(4), 470–472. doi:10.1111/j.0013-9580.2005.66104.x PMID:15816939

Foland-Ross, L. C., Hamilton, J. P., Joormann, J., Berman, M. G., Jonides, J., & Gotlib, I. H. (2013). The Neural Basis of Difficulties Disengaging From Negative Irrelevant Material in Major Depression. *Psychological Science*, *24*(3), 334–344. doi:10.1177/0956797612457380 PMID:23334445

Forkan, A., Khalil, I., & Tari, Z. (2014). CoCaMAAL: A cloud-oriented context-aware middleware in ambient assisted living. *Future Generation Computer Systems*, *35*, 114–127. doi:10.1016/j.future.2013.07.009

Fortino, M. P., & di Fatta, G. (2012). BodyCloud: integration of cloud computing and body sensor networks. *Proceedings of the 4th IEEE International Conference on Cloud Computing Technology and Science (CloudCom '12)*, 851–856. 10.1109/CloudCom.2012.6427537

Frankle, W. G., Slifstein, M., Talbot, P. S., & Laruelle, M. (2005). Neuroreceptor imaging in psychiatry: Theory and applications. *International Review of Neurobiology*, *67*, 385–440. doi:10.1016/S0074-7742(05)67011-0 PMID:16291028

Frisoni, G. B., Bocchetta, M., Chételat, G., Rabinovici, G. D., De Leon, M. J., Kaye, J., Reiman, E. M., Scheltens, P., Barkhof, F., Black, S. E., Brooks, D. J., Carrillo, M. C., Fox, N. C., Herholz, K., Nordberg, A., Jack, C. R., Jagust, W. J., Johnson, K. A., Rowe, C. C., ... DeCarli, C. (2013). Imaging markers for Alzheimer disease: Which vs how. *Neurology*, *81*(5), 487–500. doi:10.1212/WNL.0b013e31829d86e8 PMID:23897875

Fujinami, R. S., & Oldstone, M. (1985). Amino acid homology between the encephalitogenic site of myelin basic protein and virus: Mechanism for autoimmunity. *Science*, *230*(4729), 1043–1045. doi:10.1126cience.2414848 PMID:2414848

Furia, J. P., Rompe, J. D., Cacchio, A., Del Buono, A., & Maffulli, N. (2013). A single application of low energy radial extracorporeal shock wave therapy is effective for the management of chronic patellar tendinopathy. *Knee Surgery, Sports Traumatology, Arthroscopy*, *21*(2), 346–350. doi:10.100700167-012-2057-8 PMID:22627667

Fuster, J. M. (1997). Network memory. *Trends in Neurosciences*, *20*(10), 451–459. doi:10.1016/S0166-2236(97)01128-4 PMID:9347612

Gabbard, C. (1989). Foot lateralization and psychomotor control in four-year-olds. *Perceptual and Motor Skills*, *68*(2), 675–678. doi:10.2466/pms.1989.68.2.675 PMID:2717370

Galasko, D., Hansen, L. A., Katzman, R., Wiederholt, W., Masliah, E., Terry, R., Hill, L. R., Lessin, P., & Thal, L. J. (1994). Clinical-neuropathological correlations in Alzheimer's disease and related dementias. *Archives of Neurology*, *51*(9), 888–895. doi:10.1001/archneur.1994.00540210060013 PMID:8080388

Galety, M. G. (2019). OSSR-P: Ontological service searching and ranking system for PaaS services. *Int. J. Adv. Trends Comput. Sci. Eng*, 271-276.

Galety, M. G. A. A. (2020). Improved Crypto Algorithm for High-Speed Internet of Things (IoT) Applications. Springer. doi:10.1007/978-3-030-38501-9_28

Gamaethige, C., Gunathilake, U., Jayasena, D., Manike, H., Samarasinghe, P., & Yatanwala, T. (2017). "SenseA"-Autism Early Signs and Pre-Aggressive Detector through Image Processing. *2017 Asia Modelling Symposium (AMS)*, 125-130. 10.1109/AMS.2017.28

Gardner, H. (1993). *Multiple intelligences: The theory in practice*. Basic Books.

Garg, R. K. (2003). Acute disseminated encephalomyelitis. *Postgraduate Medical Journal*, *79*(927), 11–17. doi:10.1136/pmj.79.927.11 PMID:12566545

Garnefski, N., & Kraaij, V. (2006). Relationships between cognitive emotion regulation strategies and depressive symptoms: A comparative study of five specific samples. *Personality and Individual Differences*, *40*(8), 1659–1669. doi:10.1016/j.paid.2005.12.009

Garnefski, N., Teerds, J., Kraaij, V., Legerstee, J., & van den Kommer, T. (2004). Cognitive emotion regulation strategies and depressive symptoms: Differences between males and females. *Personality and Individual Differences*, *36*(2), 267–276. doi:10.1016/S0191-8869(03)00083-7

Gates, N. J., Valenzuela, M., Sachdev, P. S., Singh, N. A., Baune, B. T., Brodaty, H., ... Singh, M. A. F. (2011). Study of Mental Activity and Regular Training (SMART) in at risk individuals: A randomised double blind, sham controlled, longitudinal trial. *BMC Geriatrics*, *11*(1), 1–15. doi:10.1186/1471-2318-11-19 PMID:21510896

Gerdesmeyer, L., & Krath, A. (2014). ESWT and knee arthroplasty: radial shock wave therapy in ligament pain after total knee arthroplasty. Multidisciplinary medical applications, 84–96.

Gevensleben, H., Holl, B., Albrecht, B., Vogel, C., Schlamp, D., Kratz, O., Studer, P., Rothenberger, A., Moll, G. H., & Heinrich, H. (2009). Is neurofeedback an efficacious treatment for ADHD? A randomised controlled clinical trial. *Journal of Child Psychology and Psychiatry, and Allied Disciplines*, *50*(7), 780–789. doi:10.1111/j.1469-7610.2008.02033.x PMID:19207632

Ghazi, M., Nielsen, M., Pai, A., Cardoso, M. J., Modat, M., Ourselin, S., & Sørensen, L. (2019). Training recurrent neural networks robust to incomplete data: Application to Alzheimer's disease progression modeling. *Medical Image Analysis*, *53*, 39–46. doi:10.1016/j.media.2019.01.004 PMID:30682584

Glauser. (2018). Blood-delivering drones saving lives in Africa and maybe soon in Canada. Canadian Medical Association Journal, 190(3), E88–E89.

Goedert, M., Spillantini, M. G., Del Tredici, K., & Braak, H. (2012). 100 years of Lewy pathology. *Nature Reviews. Neurology*, *9*(1), 13–24. doi:10.1038/nrneurol.2012.242 PMID:23183883

Goldman, J., & Patel, R. (2015). Diagnosis of Parkinson's disease: Progress and future prospects. *Journal of Parkinsonism and Restless Legs Syndrome*, *19*, 19. Advance online publication. doi:10.2147/JPRLS.S62065

Gold, P. W., Drevets, W. C., Charney, D. S., & Drevets, W. C. (2002). New insights into the role of cortisol and the glucocorticoid receptor in severe depression. *Biological Psychiatry*, *52*(5), 381–385. doi:10.1016/S0006-3223(02)01480-4 PMID:12242053

Gonzalez, C., Bonilla, S., Flores, A. I., Cano, E., & Liste, I. (2016). An Update on Human Stem Cell-Based Therapy in Parkinson's Disease. *Current Stem Cell Research & Therapy*, *11*(7), 561–568. Advance online publication. doi:10.2174/1574888X10666150531172612 PMID:26027681

Goodfellow, I., Pouget-Abadie, J., Mirza, M., Xu, B., Warde-Farley, D., Ozair, S., Courville, A., & Bengio, Y. (2014). Generative adversarial nets. Advances in Neural Information Processing Systems, 2672–2680.

Gottfredson, G. D., Jones, E. M., & Holland, J. L. (1993). Personality and vocational interests: The relation of Holland's six interest dimensions to five robust dimensions of personality. *Journal of Counseling Psychology*, *40*(4), 518–524. doi:10.1037/0022-0167.40.4.518

Gouse, D. G. (2018). Improved Reconfigurable based Lightweight Crypto Algorithms for IoT based Applications. *Journal of Advanced Research in Dynamical & Control Systems*, 186-193.

Goyal, P., Pandey, S., & Jain, K. (2018). Introduction to natural language processing and deep learning. In Deep Learning for Natural Language Processing (pp. 1–74). Springer. doi:10.1007/978-1-4842-3685-7_1

Grillner, S., Markram, H., De Schutter, E., Silberberg, G., & LeBeau, F. E. (2005). Microcircuits in action–from CPGs to neocortex. *Trends in Neurosciences*, *28*(10), 525–533. doi:10.1016/j.tins.2005.08.003 PMID:16118022

Gulshan, V., Peng, L., Coram, M., Stumpe, M. C., Wu, D., Narayanaswamy, A., Venugopalan, S., Widner, K., Madams, T., Cuadros, J., Kim, R., Raman, R., Nelson, P. C., Mega, J. L., & Webster, D. R. (2016). Development and validation of a deep learning algorithm for detection of diabetic retinopathy in retinal fundus photograph. *Journal of the American Medical Association*, *316*(22), 2402–2410. doi:10.1001/jama.2016.17216 PMID:27898976

Gunduz, H. (2019). Deep learning-based Parkinson's disease classification using vocal feature sets. *IEEE Access: Practical Innovations, Open Solutions*, *7*, 115540–115551. doi:10.1109/ACCESS.2019.2936564

Gupta, HariPrasad, & Kumar. (2018). Bionics Based Emergency Contact for Treatment of Epilepsy. *Proceedings of the 2018 10th International Conference on Bioinformatics and Biomedical Technology.*

Gupta, S., & Kant, V. (2020). A Comparative Analysis of Genetic Programming and Genetic Algorithm on Multi-Criteria Recommender Systems. *2020 5th International Conference on Communication and Electronics Systems (ICCES).*

Gupta, S., HariPrasad, S. A., & Kumar, A. (2018). Bionics Based Emergency Contact for Treatment of Epilepsy. *Proceedings of the 2018 10th International Conference on Bioinformatics and Biomedical Technology*, 46–50. 10.1145/3232059.3232064

Gupta, A., Ayhan, M., & Maida, A. (2013). Natural image bases to represent neuroimaging data. *International conference on machine learning*, 987–994.

Gupta, D., & Ahlawat, A. K. (2017). Usability feature selection via MBBAT: A novel approach. *Journal of Computational Science*, *23*, 195–203. doi:10.1016/j.jocs.2017.06.005

Gupta, D., Julka, A., Jain, S., Aggarwal, T., Khanna, A., Arunkumar, N., & de Albuquerque, V. H. (2018). Optimized cuttlefish algorithm for diagnosis of Parkinson's disease. *Cognitive Systems Research*, *52*, 36–48. doi:10.1016/j.cogsys.2018.06.006

Gupta, D., Sundaram, S., Khanna, A., Hassanien, A. E., & De Albuquerque, V. H. (2018). Improved diagnosis of Parkinson's disease using optimized crow search algorithm. *Computers & Electrical Engineering*, *68*, 412–424. doi:10.1016/j.compeleceng.2018.04.014

Gupta, S. (2014). *Repetitive Transcranial Magnetic Stimulation (RTMS) for the Treatment of Depression*. Migraine and Parkinson's Disease.

Gupta, S. (2020). Smartphone based Early Detection of Epileptic Seizures Using Machine Learning. *Proceedings of the 2020 12th International Conference on Bioinformatics and Biomedical Technology*, 38–42. 10.1145/3405758.3405763

Gupta, S. (2020). Smartphone based Early Detection of Epileptic Seizures Using Machine Learning. *Proceedings of the 2020 12th International Conference on Bioinformatics and Biomedical Technology.*

Gupta, S., & Kumar, A. (2018). *Bionic Functionality of Prosthetic Hand. In Intelligent Communication, Control and Devices*. Springer.

Gupta, S., Mohanta, S., Chakraborty, M., & Ghosh, S. (2017). Quantum machine learning-using quantum computation in artificial intelligence and deep neural networks: Quantum computation and machine learning in artificial intelligence. *8th Annual Industrial Automation and Electromechanical Engineering Conference (IEMECON)*, 268-274. doi: 10.1109/IEMECON.2017.8079602

Gupta, S., Singh, V. K., & ... (2015). Bionics Based Solar Powered Clothing for Treating Parkinson's Disease and Epilepsy. *International Journal of Life Sciences Biotechnology and Pharma Research*, *4*, 132.

Gupta, Y., Lama, R. K., Lee, S.-W., & Kwon, G.-R. (2020). An MRI brain disease classification system using PDFB-CT and GLCM with kernel-SVM for medical decision support. *Multimedia Tools and Applications*, *79*(43-44), 32195–32224. doi:10.100711042-020-09676-x

Halfin, A. (2007, November). Depression: The benefits of early and appropriate treatment. *The American Journal of Managed Care*, *13*(4, Suppl), S92–S97. PMID:18041868

Halvorsen, M., Hagen, R., Hjemdal, O., Eriksen, M. S., Sørli, Å. J., Waterloo, K., Eisemann, M., & Wang, C. E. A. (2014). Metacognitions and Thought Control Strategies in Unipolar Major Depression: A Comparison of Currently Depressed, Previously Depressed, and Never-Depressed Individuals. *Cognitive Therapy and Research*, *39*(1), 31–40. doi:10.100710608-014-9638-4

Hand, D. J., & Till, R. J. (2001). A simple generalization of the area under the ROC curve for multiple class classification problems. *Machine Learning*, *45*(2), 171–186. doi:10.1023/A:1010920819831

Happ, C., & Greven, S. (2018). Multivariate functional principal component analysis for data observed on different (dimensional) domains. *Journal of the American Statistical Association*, *113*(522), 649–659. doi:10.1080/01621459.2016.1273115

Hartman-Maeir, A., Harel, H., & Katz, N. (2009). Kettle Test—A brief measure of cognitive functional performance: Reliability and validity in stroke rehabilitation. *The American Journal of Occupational Therapy*, *63*(5), 592–599. doi:10.5014/ajot.63.5.592 PMID:19785258

Hasan, R., Hossain, M. M., & Khan, R. (2015). Aura: An IoT based cloud infrastructure for localized mobile computation outsourcing. *Proceedings of the 3rd IEEE International Conference on Mobile Cloud Computing, Services, and Engineering, MobileCloud 2015*, 183–188. 10.1109/MobileCloud.2015.37

Hastie, T., Tibshirani, R., & Friedman, J. H. (2009). Statistics The Elements of Statistical Learning. *The Mathematical Intelligencer*, *27*, 83–85.

Hawkes, C. H., Tredici, K. D., & Braak, H. (2007). Parkinson's disease: A dual-hit hypothesis. *Neuropathology and Applied Neurobiology*, *33*(6), 599–614. doi:10.1111/j.1365-2990.2007.00874.x PMID:17961138

Healy, D. G., Falchi, M., O'Sullivan, S. S., Bonifati, V., Durr, A., Bressman, S., Brice, A., Aasly, J., Zabetian, C. P., Goldwurm, S., Ferreira, J. J., Tolosa, E., Kay, D. M., Klein, C., Williams, D. R., Marras, C., Lang, A. E., Wszolek, Z. K., Berciano, J., ... Wood, N. W. (2008). Phenotype, genotype, and worldwide genetic penetrance of LRRK2-associated Parkinson's disease: A case-control study. *Lancet Neurology*, *7*(7), 583–590. doi:10.1016/S1474-4422(08)70117-0 PMID:18539534

Hegarty, S. V., O'Keeffe, G. W., & Sullivan, A. M. (2014). Neurotrophic Factors: From Neurodevelopmental Regulators to Novel Therapies for Parkinson's Disease. *Neural Regeneration Research*, *9*, 1708–1711. doi:10.4103/1673-5374.143410 PMID:25422631

Heidari, A. A., Faris, H., Aljarah, I., & Mirjalili, S. (2019). An efficient hybrid multilayer perceptron neural network with grasshopper optimization. *Soft Computing*, *23*(17), 7941–7958. doi:10.100700500-018-3424-2

Helm, K., Viol, K., Weiger, T. M., Tass, P. A., Grefkes, C., Del Monte, D., & Schiepek, G. (2018). *Neuropsychiatric Disease and Treatment Dovepress Neuronal connectivity in major depressive disorder: A systematic review*. doi:10.2147/NDT.S170989

Hemachudha, T., Griffin, D. E., Giffels, J. J., Johnson, R. T., Moser, A. B., & Phanuphak, P. (1987). Myelin basic protein as an encephalitogen in encephalomyelitis and polyneuritis following rabies vaccination. *The New England Journal of Medicine*, *316*(7), 369–374. doi:10.1056/NEJM198702123160703 PMID:2433582

Hertel, P. T., & Hardin, T. S. (1990). Remembering With and Without Awareness in a Depressed Mood: Evidence of Deficits in Initiative. *Journal of Experimental Psychology. General*, *119*(1), 45–59. doi:10.1037/0096-3445.119.1.45 PMID:2141063

Hesse, A., Brändle, E., Wilbert, D., Köhrmann, K. U., & Alken, P. (2003). Study on the prevalence and incidence of urolithiasis in Germany comparing the years 1979 vs. 2000. *European Urology*, *44*(6), 709–713. doi:10.1016/S0302-2838(03)00415-9 PMID:14644124

Hichem, H., Elkamel, M., Rafik, M., Mesaaoud, M. T., & Ouahiba, C. (2019). A new binary grasshopper optimization algorithm for feature selection problem. *Journal of King Saud University-Computer and Information Sciences*.

Hojjati, S. H., Ebrahimzadeh, A., Khazaee, A., Babajani-Feremi, A., & Initiative, A. D. (2017). Predicting conversion from MCI to AD using resting-state fMRI, graph theoretical approach and SVM. *Journal of Neuroscience Methods*, *282*, 69–80. doi:10.1016/j.jneumeth.2017.03.006 PMID:28286064

Honton, B., & Laperche, C. (2021). Why and how do I use Shockwave? [Pourquoi et comment j'utilise le Shockwave?]. *Annales de Cardiologie et d'Angeiologie*, *70*(6), 425–431. doi:10.1016/j.ancard.2021.10.016 PMID:34740397

Hoorelbeke, K., Koster, E. H. W., Demeyer, I., Loeys, T., & Vanderhasselt, M.-A. (2016). Effects of Cognitive Control Training on the Dynamics of (Mal). *Adaptive Emotion Regulation in Daily Life.*, *16*(August), 945–956. Advance online publication. doi:10.1037/emo0000169 PMID:27177250

Hopfner, F., Künstner, A., Müller, S. H., Künzel, S., Zeuner, K. E., Margraf, N. G., Deuschl, G., Baines, J. F., & Kuhlenbäumer, G. (2017). Gut microbiota in Parkinson disease in a northern German cohort. *Brain Research*, *1667*, 41–45. doi:10.1016/j.brainres.2017.04.019 PMID:28506555

Hosseini-Asl, E., Gimel'farb, G., & El-Baz, A. (2016). *Alzheimer's disease diagnostics by a deeply supervised adaptable 3D convolutional network*. arXiv preprint arXiv:1607.00556.

Hosseini, M. P., Pompili, D., Elisevich, K., & Soltanian-Zadeh, H. (2017, December). Optimized Deep Learning for EEG Big Data and Seizure Prediction BCI via Internet of Things. *IEEE Transactions on Big Data*, *3*(4), 392–404. doi:10.1109/TBDATA.2017.2769670

Hosseini, S. H. R., Kohno, Y., & Takayama, K. (2005). Micro-explosives induced underwater shock waves for medical applications. *Science and Technology of Energetic Materials*, *6*, 411–415.

Hosseini, S. H. R., Menezes, V., Moosavi-Nejad, S., Ohki, T., Nakagawa, A., Tominaga, T., & Takayama, K. (2006). Development of shock wave assisted therapeutic devices and establishment of shock wave therapy. *Minimally Invasive Therapy & Allied Technologies*, *15*(4), 230–240. doi:10.1080/13645700600836315 PMID:16966137

Hsu, C.-L., Chuang, T.-H., & Lin, T.-W. (2017). End-to-end authenticated key exchange agreement for wearable devices in IoT environments. *IEEE Great Lakes Biomedical Conference (GLBC)*, 1-1. doi: 10.1109/GLBC.2017.7928891

Hua, M., Yang, L., Wu, Q., Li, C., & Swindlehurst, A. L. (2021). UAV-Assisted Intelligent Reflecting Surface Symbiotic Radio System. *IEEE Transactions on Wireless Communications*, *20*(9), 5769–5785.

Huang, F., Elazab, A., OuYang, L., Tan, J., Wang, T., & Lei, B. (2019). Sparse Low-rank Constrained Adaptive Structure Learning using Multi-template for Autism Spectrum Disorder Diagnosis. *2019 IEEE 16th International Symposium on Biomedical Imaging (ISBI 2019),* 1555-1558. 10.1109/ISBI.2019.8759487

Huang, D., Zhang, X., Kang, M., & Luo, J. (2010). MobiCloud: building secure cloud framework for mobile computing and communication. *Proceedings of the 5th IEEE International Symposium on Service-Oriented SystemEngineering, SOSE 2010*, 27–34. 10.1109/SOSE.2010.20

Hubens, N. (2018). *Deep inside: autoencoders—towards data science*. Google Scholar.

Hueber, W., Sands, B. E., Lewitzky, S., Vandemeulebroecke, M., Reinisch, W., Higgins, P. D., ... Karczewski, M. (2012). Secukinumab, a human anti-IL-17A monoclonal antibody, for moderate to severe Crohn's disease: Unexpected results of a randomised, double-blind placebo-controlled trial. *Gut*, *61*(12), 1693–1700. doi:10.1136/gutjnl-2011-301668 PMID:22595313

Huerta-Canepa, G., & Lee, D. (2010). A virtual cloud computing provider for mobile devices. In *Proceedings of the 1st ACM Workshop on Mobile Cloud Computing and Services: Social Networks and Beyond (MCS '10)*. ACM. 10.1145/1810931.1810937

Hu, Z., Wang, J., Zhang, C., Luo, Z., Luo, X., Xiao, L., & Shi, J. (2021). Uncertainty Modeling for Multi center Autism Spectrum Disorder Classification Using Takagi-Sugeno-Kang Fuzzy Systems. *IEEE Transactions on Cognitive and Developmental Systems*, 1. Advance online publication. doi:10.1109/TCDS.2021.3073368

Hwang, E. J., Park, S., Jin, K.-N., Kim, J. I., Choi, S. Y., Lee, J. H., Goo, J. M., Aum, J., Yim, J.-J., Cohen, J. G., Ferretti, G. R., & Park, C. M. (2019). Development and validation of a deep learning-based automated detection algorithm for major thoracic diseases on chest radiographs. *JAMA Network Open*, *2*(3), e191095. doi:10.1001/jamanetworkopen.2019.1095 PMID:30901052

Hynson, J., Kornberg, A., Coleman, L., Shield, L., Harvey, A., & Kean, M. (2001). Clinical and neuroradiologic features of acute disseminated encephalomyelitis in children. *Neurology*, *56*(10), 1308–1312. doi:10.1212/WNL.56.10.1308 PMID:11376179

Ibrahim, H. T., Mazher, W. J., Ucan, O. N., & Bayat, O. (2019). A grasshopper optimizer approach for feature selection and optimizing SVM parameters utilizing real biomedical data sets. *Neural Computing & Applications*, *31*(10), 5965–5974. doi:10.100700521-018-3414-4

Islam, J., & Zhang, Y. (2017). A novel deep learning based multiclass classification method for Alzheimer's disease detection using brain MRI data. *International conference on brain informatics*, 213–222. 10.1007/978-3-319-70772-3_20

Islam, S., Akter, T., Zakir, S., Sabreen, S., & Hossain, M. I. (2020). Autism Spectrum Disorder Detection in Toddlers for Early Diagnosis Using Machine Learning. *2020 IEEE Asia-Pacific Conference on Computer Science and Data Engineering (CSDE)*, 1-6. 10.1109/CSDE50874.2020.9411531

Ivry, R. (1997). Cerebellar timing systems. *International Review of Neurobiology*, *41*, 555–573. doi:10.1016/S0074-7742(08)60370-0 PMID:9378608

Jadhav, R. S., Gavasane, A., & Agrawal, A. (2020). Improved theory for shock waves using the OBurnett equations. *Journal of Fluid Mechanics*, 929.

Jaiswal, K., Sobhanayak, S., Mohanta, B. K., & Jena, D. (2017). IoT-cloud based framework for patient's data collection in smart healthcare system using raspberry-pi. *2017 International Conference on Electrical and Computing Technologies and Applications (ICECTA)*, 1-4. doi: 10.1109/ICECTA.2017.8251967

Jangra, P., & Gupta, M. (2018). A Design of Real-Time Multilayered Smart Healthcare Monitoring Framework Using IoT. *International Conference on Intelligent and Advanced System (ICIAS)*, 1-5. doi: 10.1109/ICIAS.2018.8540606

Jankovic, J. (2008). Parkinson's disease: Clinical features and diagnosis. *Journal of Neurology, Neurosurgery, and Psychiatry*, *79*(4), 368–376. doi:10.1136/jnnp.2007.131045 PMID:18344392

Jankovic, J., McDermott, M., Carter, J., Gauthier, S., Goetz, C., Golbe, L., Huber, S., Koller, W., Olanow, C., Shoulson, I., Stern, M., Tanner, C., & Weiner, W. (1990). Variable expression of Parkinson's disease: A base-line analysis of the DATATOP cohort. The Parkinson Study Group. *Neurology*, *40*(10), 1529–1534. doi:10.1212/WNL.40.10.1529 PMID:2215943

Jansen, W. J., Ossenkoppele, R., Knol, D. L., Tijms, B. M., Scheltens, P., Verhey, F. R. J., Visser, P. J., Aalten, P., Aarsland, D., Alcolea, D., Alexander, M., Almdahl, I. S., Arnold, S. E., Baldeiras, I., Barthel, H., van Berckel, B. N. M., Bibeau, K., Blennow, K., Brooks, D. J., ... Zetterberg, H. (2015). Prevalence of cerebral amyloid pathology in persons without dementia: A meta-analysis. *Journal of the American Medical Association*, *313*(19), 1924–1938. doi:10.1001/jama.2015.4668 PMID:25988462

Jebran. (2020). Detection of Lesions for Diabetic Retinopathy By using Machine Learning Algorithms. *International Journal of Recent Technology and Engineering*, *8*, 1160–1166.

Jebran, P. M., & Gupta, S. (2021). Pre-Diabetic Retinopathy identification using hybridGenetic Algorithm-Neural Network classifier. *Journal of Physics: Conference Series*.

Jia, X., Shi, L., Qian, T., Li, Y., Wang, D., Liang, P., & Li, K. (2018). Improved gray matter atrophy detection in Alzheimer disease in Chinese populations using Chinese brain template ". *Alzheimer Disease and Associated Disorders*, *32*(4), 309–313. doi:10.1097/WAD.0000000000000264 PMID:30024411

John, C., Mueller, Z., Prayaga, L., & Devulapalli, K. (2020). *A Neural Network Model to Identify Relative Movements from Wearable Devices*. SoutheastCon. doi:10.1109/SoutheastCon44009.9368261

John, H. (1979). Metacognition and cognitive monitoring: A new area of cognitive-developmental inquiry. *The American Psychologist*, *34*(10), 906–911. doi:10.1037/0003-066X.34.10.906

Johnson, K. A., Fox, N. C., Sperling, R. A., & Klunk, W. E. (2012). Brain imaging in Alzheimer disease. *Cold Spring Harbor Perspectives in Medicine*, *2*(4), a006213. doi:10.1101/cshperspect.a006213 PMID:22474610

Joormann, J., & Gotlib, I. H. (2008). Updating the Contents of Working Memory in Depression: Interference From Irrelevant Negative Material. *Journal of Abnormal Psychology*, *117*(1), 182–192. doi:10.1037/0021-843X.117.1.182 PMID:18266496

Joshi, D. M., Rana, N. K., & Misra, V. (2010). Classification of brain cancer using artificial neural network. *2010 2nd international conference on electronic computer technology*, 112–116.

Jo, T., Nho, K., & Saykin, A. J. (2019). Deep learning in Alzheimer's disease: Diagnostic classification and prognostic prediction using neuroimaging data. *Frontiers in Aging Neuroscience*, *11*, 220. doi:10.3389/fnagi.2019.00220 PMID:31481890

Judd, L. L., Akiskal, H. S., Maser, J. D., Zeller, P. J., Endicott, J., Coryell, W., Paulus, M. P., Kunovac, J. L., Leon, A. C., Mueller, T. I., Rice, J. A., & Keller, M. B. (1998). Major depressive disorder: A prospective study of residual subthreshold depressive symptoms as predictor of rapid relapse. *Journal of Affective Disorders*, *50*(2–3), 97–108. doi:10.1016/S0165-0327(98)00138-4 PMID:9858069

Junninen, H., Niska, H., Tuppurainen, K., Ruuskanen, J., & Kolehmainen, M. (2004). Methods for imputation of missing values in air quality data sets. *Atmospheric Environment*, *38*(18), 2895–2907. doi:10.1016/j.atmosenv.2004.02.026

K. & Jaganathan. (2021). Graph Convolutional Model to Diagnose Autism Spectrum Disorder Using Rs-Fmri Data. *2021 5th International Conference on Computer, Communication and Signal Processing (ICCCSP),* 1-5. 10.1109/ICCCSP52374.2021.9465490

Kägi, G., Bhatia, K. P., & Tolosa, E. (2010). The role of DAT-SPECT in movement disorders. *Journal of Neurology, Neurosurgery, and Psychiatry*, *81*(1), 5–12. doi:10.1136/jnnp.2008.157370 PMID:20019219

Kalia LV, Lang AE. (2015), Parkinson's disease. *Lancet*, *386*(9996), 896–912. . doi:10.1016/S0140-6736(14)61393-3

Kalia, L. V., Brotchie, J. M., & Fox, S. H. (2013). Novel nondopaminergic targets for motor features of Parkinson's disease: Review of recent trials. *Movement Disorders*, *28*(2), 131–144. doi:10.1002/mds.25273 PMID:23225267

Kamathe, R. S., & Joshi, K. R. (2018). A novel method based on independent component analysis for brain MR image tissue classification into CSF, WM and GM for atrophy detection in Alzheimer's disease. *Biomedical Signal Processing and Control*, *40*, 41–48. doi:10.1016/j.bspc.2017.09.005

Kanter, D., Horensky, D., Sperling, R., Kaplan, J., Malachowski, M., & Churchill, W. (1995). Plasmapheresis in fulminant acute disseminated encephalomyelitis. *Neurology*, *45*(4), 824–827. doi:10.1212/WNL.45.4.824 PMID:7723979

Karno, M., Golding, J. M., Sorenson, S. B., & Burnam, M. A. (1988). The epidemiology of obsessive-compulsive disorder in five US communities. *Archives of General Psychiatry*, *45*(12), 1094–1099. doi:10.1001/archpsyc.1988.01800360042006 PMID:3264144

Katzenschlager, R. (2014). Parkinson's disease: Recent advances. *Journal of Neurology*.

Katzenschlager, R., Head, J., Schrag, A., Ben-Shlomo, Y., Evans, A., & Lees, A. J. (2008). Fourteen-year final report of the randomized PDRG-UK trial comparing three initial treatments in PD. *Neurology*, *71*(7), 474–480. doi:10.1212/01.wnl.0000310812.43352.66 PMID:18579806

Keegan, M., Pineda, A., McClelland, R., Darby, C., Rodriguez, M., & Weinshenker, B. (2002). Plasma exchange for severe attacks of CNS demyelination: Predictors of response. *Neurology*, *58*(1), 143–146. doi:10.1212/WNL.58.1.143 PMID:11781423

Kehoe, E. G., McNulty, J. P., Mullins, P. G., & Bokde, A. L. (2014). Advances in MRI biomarkers for the diagnosis of Alzheimer's disease. *Biomarkers in Medicine*, *8*(9), 1151–1169. doi:10.2217/bmm.14.42 PMID:25402585

Kerestes, R., Ladouceur, C. D., Meda, S., Nathan, P. J., Blumberg, H. P., Maloney, K., Ruf, B., Saricicek, A., Pearlson, G. D., Bhagwagar, Z., & Phillips, M. L. (2012). Abnormal prefrontal activity subserving attentional control of emotion in remitted depressed patients during a working memory task with emotional distracters. *Psychological Medicine*, *42*(1), 29–40. doi:10.1017/S0033291711001097 PMID:21733287

Khagi, B., Lee, K. H., Choi, K. Y., Lee, J. J., Kwon, G.-R., & Yang, H.-D. (2021). VBM-Based Alzheimer's Disease Detection from the Region of Interest of T1 MRI with Supportive Gaussian Smoothing and a Bayesian Regularized Neural Network. *Applied Sciences (Basel, Switzerland)*, *11*(13), 6175. doi:10.3390/app11136175

Khanna, T. (1990). *Foundations of neural networks*. Addison-Wesley Longman Publishing Co., Inc.

Khelil, A., Shaikh, F. K., Sheikh, A. A., Felemban, E., & Bojan, H. (2014). DigiAID: A wearable health platform for automated self-tagging in emergency cases. *Proceedings of the 4th International Conference on Wireless Mobile Communication and Healthcare, MOBIHEALTH2014*, 296–299. 10.4108/icst.mobihealth.2014.257541

Kiernan, R. J., Mueller, J., Langston, J. W., & Van Dyke, C. R. A. I. G. (1987). The Neurobehavioral Cognitive Status Examination: A brief but differentiated approach to cognitive assessment. *Annals of Internal Medicine*, *107*(4), 481–485. doi:10.7326/0003-4819-107-4-481 PMID:3631786

Kim, D. H., Wit, H., & Thurston, M. (2018). Artificial intelligence in the diagnosis of Parkinson's disease from ioflupane-123 single-photon emission computed tomography dopamine transporter scans using transfer learning. *Nuclear Medicine Communications*, *39*(10), 887–893. doi:10.1097/MNM.0000000000000890 PMID:30080748

Kleanthi, G., & Maria, G. (2021). Alexithymia, Stress and Depression in Infertile Women: A Case Control Study. *Materia Socio-Medica*, *33*(1), 70–74. doi:10.5455/msm.2021.33.70-74 PMID:34012355

Knight, M. J., & Baune, B. T. (2018). Executive Function and Spatial Cognition Mediate Psychosocial Dysfunction in Major Depressive Disorder. *Frontiers in Psychiatry*, *9*(October), 3–6. doi:10.3389/fpsyt.2018.00539 PMID:30420817

Knobel, M., Wolman, M. B., & Mason, E. (1959). Hyperkinesis and organicity in children. *A.M.A. Archives of General Psychiatry*, *1*(3), 310–321. doi:10.1001/archpsyc.1959.03590030094011 PMID:14410146

Kobilecki, C. (2020). Update on the diagnosis and management of Parkinson's disease. *Clinical Medicine*, *20*(4), 393–398. doi:10.7861/clinmed.2020-0220 PMID:32675145

Kodali, R. K., Swamy, G., & Lakshmi, B. (2015). *An implementation of IoT for healthcare. In 2015 IEEE Recent Advances in Intelligent Computational Systems*. RAICS. doi:10.1109/RAICS.2015.7488451

Kordower, J. H., Olanow, C. W., Dodiya, H. B., Chu, Y., Beach, T. G., Adler, C. H., Halliday, G. M., & Bartus, R. T. (2013). Disease duration and the integrity of the nigrostriatal system in Parkinson's disease. *Brain*, *136*(8), 2419–2431. doi:10.1093/brain/awt192 PMID:23884810

Koster, E. (2011). Understanding depressive rumination. *Dissertation*, *32*(0), 1–32.

Koster, E. H. W., Hoorelbeke, K., Onraedt, T., Owens, M., & Derakshan, N. (2017). Cognitive control interventions for depression: A systematic review of findings from training studies. *Clinical Psychology Review*, *53*, 79–92. doi:10.1016/j.cpr.2017.02.002 PMID:28273486

Kouli, A., Torsney, K. M., & Kuan, W. L. (2018). Parkinson's Disease: Etiology, Neuropathology, and Pathogenesis. In *Parkinson's Disease: Pathogenesis and Clinical Aspects*. doi:10.15586/codonpublications.parkinsonsdisease.2018.ch1

Kowalski, P. A., Łukasik, S., Charytanowicz, M., & Kulczycki, P. (2018). Optimizing clustering with cuttlefish algorithm. *Conference on Information Technology, Systems Research and Computational Physics*, 34–43.

Kraaij, V., Garnefski, N., De Wilde, E. J., Dijkstra, A., Gebhardt, W., Maes, S., & Ter Doest, L. (2003). Negative Life Events and Depressive Symptoms in Late Adolescence: Bonding and Cognitive Coping as Vulnerability Factors? *Journal of Youth and Adolescence*, *32*(3), 185–193. doi:10.1023/A:1022543419747

Kraft, B., Jonassen, R., Stiles, T. C., & Landrø, N. I. (2017). Dysfunctional metacognitive beliefs are associated with decreased executive control. *Frontiers in Psychology*, *8*(APR), 1–6. doi:10.3389/fpsyg.2017.00593 PMID:28469590

Krupski, A., Raskin, D. C., & Bakan, P. (1971). Physiological and personality correlates of commission errors in an auditory vigilance task. *Psychophysiology*, *8*(3), 304–311. doi:10.1111/j.1469-8986.1971.tb00460.x PMID:5093973

Kudyshev, Z., Bogdanov, S., Isacsson, T., Kildishev, A. V., Boltasseva, A., & Shalaev, V. M. (2020). Merging Machine Learning with Quantum Photonics: Rapid Classification of Quantum Sources. *Conference on Lasers and Electro-Optics (CLEO)*, 1-2.

Kumar, Y., Dewal, M., & Anand, R. (2014, October). Epileptic Seizures Detection in EEG Using DWT-based ApEn and Artificial Neural Network. *Signal, Image and Video Processing*, *8*(7), 1323–1334. doi:10.100711760-012-0362-9

Kurth, F., Gaser, C., & Luders, E. (2015). A 12-step user guide for analysing voxel-wise gray matter asymmetries in statistical parametric mapping (SPM). *Nature Protocols*, *10*(2), 293–304. doi:10.1038/nprot.2015.014 PMID:25591011

Lacor, P. N. (2004). Synaptic targeting by Alzheimer's-related amyloid β oligomers. *The Journal of Neuroscience: The Official Journal of the Society for Neuroscience, 24*(45), 10191–10200. doi:10.1523/JNEUROSCI.3432-04.2004 PMID:15537891

Lahmiri, S., & Boukadoum, M. (2014). New approach for automatic classification of Alzheimer's disease, mild cognitive impairment and healthy brain magnetic resonance images. *Healthcare Technology Letters, 1*(1), 32–36. doi:10.1049/htl.2013.0022 PMID:26609373

LaMantia, A., & Rakic, P. (1990). Axon overproduction and elimination in the corpus callosum of the developing rhesus monkey. *The Journal of Neuroscience: The Official Journal of the Society for Neuroscience, 10*(7), 2156–2175. doi:10.1523/JNEUROSCI.10-07-02156.1990 PMID:2376772

Latif, G., Butt, M. M., Khan, A. H., Butt, M. O., & Al-Asad, J. F. (2017). Automatic multimodal brain image classification using MLP and 3D glioma tumor reconstruction. *2017 9th IEEE-GCC Conference and Exhibition (GCCCE)*, 1–9.

Laufer, M. W., Denhoff, E., & Solomons, G. (2011). Hyperkinetic impulse disorder in children's behavior problems. *Journal of Attention Disorders, 15*(8), 620–625. doi:10.1177/1087054711413043 PMID:22131306

Lazar, M., Weinstein, D. M., Tsuruda, J. S., Hasan, K. M., Arfanakis, K., Meyerand, M. E., Badie, B., Rowley, H. A., Haughton, V., Field, A., & Alexander, A. L. (2003). White matter tractography using diffusion tensor deflection. *Human Brain Mapping, 18*(4), 306–321. doi:10.1002/hbm.10102 PMID:12632468

Le, G.V. (2015). A tutorial on deep learning part 2: autoencoders, convolutional neural networks and recurrent neural networks. *Google Brain*, 1–20.

Leake, J. A., Albani, S., Kao, A. S., Senac, M. O., Billman, G. F., Nespeca, M. P., Paulino, A. D., Quintela, E. R., Sawyer, M. H., & Bradley, J. S. (2004). Acute disseminated encephalomyelitis in childhood: Epidemiologic, clinical and laboratory features. *The Pediatric Infectious Disease Journal, 23*(8), 756–764. doi:10.1097/01.inf.0000133048.75452.dd PMID:15295226

Leech, R., & Sharp, D. J. (2014). The role of the posterior cingulate cortex in cognition and disease. *Brain, 137*(1), 12–32. doi:10.1093/brain/awt162 PMID:23869106

Lee, D., & Lozano, A. (2018). The Future of Surgical Treatments for Parkinson's Disease. *Journal of Parkinson's Disease, 8*(s1), S79–S83. doi:10.3233/JPD-181467 PMID:30584156

Lee, H., Perry, G., Moreira, P. I., Garrett, M. R., Liu, Q., Zhu, X., Takeda, A., Nunomura, A., & Smith, M. A. (2005). Tau phosphorylation in Alzheimer's disease: Pathogen or protector? *Trends in Molecular Medicine, 11*(4), 164–169. doi:10.1016/j.molmed.2005.02.008 PMID:15823754

Lees, A. J., Hardy, J., & Revesz, T. (2009). Parkinson's disease. *Lancet, 373*(9680), 2055–2066. doi:10.1016/S0140-6736(09)60492-X PMID:19524782

Le, H. N., & Boyd, R. C. (2006). Prevention of major depression: Early detection and early intervention in the general population. *Clin Neuropsychiatry, 3*(1), 6–22.

Levine, G. N., Gomes, A. S., Arai, A. E., Bluemke, D. A., Flamm, S. D., Kanal, E., Manning, W. J., Martin, E. T., Smith, J. M., Wilke, N., & Shellock, F. S. (2007). Safety of magnetic resonance imaging in patients with cardiovascular devices: an American Heart Association scientific statement from the Committee on Diagnostic and Interventional Cardiac Catheterization, Council on Clinical Cardiology, and the Council on Cardiovascular Radiology and Intervention: endorsed by the American College of Cardiology Foundation, the North American Society for Cardiac Imaging, and the Society for Cardiovascular Magnetic Resonance. *Circulation, 116*(24), 2878–2891. doi:10.1161/CIRCULATIONAHA.107.187256 PMID:18025533

Levin, J., Hasan, A., & Höglinger, G. U. (2015). Psychosis in Parkinson's disease: Identification, prevention and treatment. *Journal of Neural Transmission (Vienna, Austria)*. Advance online publication. doi:10.100700702-015-1400-x PMID:25894288

Li, F. & Liu, M. (2018). *Alzheimer's disease diagnosis based on multiple cluster dense convolutional network*. doi:10.1016/j.compmedimag.2018.09.009

Lian, F., Wang, D., Chiu, R., Jiang, J., & Wang, Y.-P. (2019). Innovative Packaging Solutions of 3D Integration and System in Package for IoT/Wearable and 5G Application. *IEEE 21st Electronics Packaging Technology Conference (EPTC)*, 515-518. doi: 10.1109/EPTC47984.2019.9026573

Li, H., Li, J., Liu, M., Ding, Z., & Gong, F. (2021). Energy Harvesting and Resource Allocation for Cache-Enabled UAV Based IoT NOMA Networks. *IEEE Transactions on Vehicular Technology*, *70*(9), 9625–9630.

Li, J., Fong, S., Wong, R. K., Millham, R., & Wong, K. K. (2017). Elitist binary wolf search algorithm for heuristic feature selection in high-dimensional bioinformatics datasets. *Scientific Reports*, *7*(1), 1–14. doi:10.103841598-017-04037-5 PMID:28659577

Lin, W., Lin, W., Chen, G., Zhang, H., Gao, Q., Huang, Y., Tong, T., & Du, M. (2021). Bidirectional Mapping of Brain MRI and PET With 3D Reversible GAN for the Diagnosis of Alzheimer's Disease. *Frontiers in Neuroscience*, *15*, 357. doi:10.3389/fnins.2021.646013 PMID:33935634

Lipton, H. L. (1975). Theiler's virus infection in mice: An unusual biphasic disease process leading to demyelination. *Infection and Immunity*, *11*(5), 1147–1155. doi:10.1128/iai.11.5.1147-1155.1975 PMID:164412

Lipton, Z. C., Kale, D. C., Elkan, C., & Wetzel, R. (2016a). Learning to diagnose with LSTM recurrent neural networks. *Proceedings of the International Conference on Learning Representations (ICLR)*.

Little, M., McSharry, P., Hunter, E., Spielman, J., & Ramig, L. (2008). Suitability of dysphonia measurements for telemonitoring of Parkinson's disease. *Nature Proceedings*, 1–1. doi:10.1038/npre.2008.2298.1

Litvak, A. M. (1943). Encephalitis complicating measles: Report of fifty-six cases with follow-up studies in thirty-two. *American Journal of Diseases of Children*, *65*(2), 265–295. doi:10.1001/archpedi.1943.02010140073006

Liu, S., Liu, S., Cai, W., Pujol, S., Kikinis, R., & Feng, D. (2014). Early diagnosis of Alzheimer's disease with deep learning. *2014 IEEE 11th international symposium on biomedical imaging (ISBI)*, 1015–1018.

Liu, F., Shu, P., & Jin, H. (2013). Gearing resource-poor mobile devices with powerful clouds: Architectures, challenges, and applications. *IEEE Wireless Communications*, *20*(3), 14–21. doi:10.1109/MWC.2013.6549279

Liu, M., An, Y., Hu, X., Langer, D., Newschaffer, C., & Shea, L. (2013). An evaluation of identification of suspected autism spectrum disorder (ASD) cases in early intervention (EI) records. *2013 IEEE International Conference on Bioinformatics and Biomedicine*, 566-571. 10.1109/BIBM.2013.6732559

Liu, M., Zhang, D., Shen, D., & Initiative, A. D. (2012). Ensemble sparse classification of Alzheimer's disease. *NeuroImage*, *60*(2), 1106–1116. doi:10.1016/j.neuroimage.2012.01.055 PMID:22270352

Liu, M., Zhang, J., Adeli, E., & Shen, D. (2018). Landmark-based deep multi-instance learning for brain disease diagnosis. *Medical Image Analysis*, *43*, 157–168. doi:10.1016/j.media.2017.10.005 PMID:29107865

Liu, S., Liu, S., Cai, W., Che, H., Pujol, S., Kikinis, R., Feng, D., Fulham, M. J., & Adni. (2014). Multimodal neuroimaging feature learning for multiclass diagnosis of Alzheimer's disease. *IEEE Transactions on Biomedical Engineering*, *62*(4), 1132–1140. doi:10.1109/TBME.2014.2372011 PMID:25423647

Liu, Y., Julkunen, V., Paajanen, T., Westman, E., Wahlund, L.-O., Aitken, A., Sobow, T., Mecocci, P., Tsolaki, M., Vellas, B., Muehlboeck, S., Spenger, C., Lovestone, S., Simmons, A., & Soininen, H. (2012). Education increases reserve against Alzheimer's disease-evidence from structural MRI analysis. *Neuroradiology*, *54*(9), 929–938. doi:10.100700234-012-1005-0 PMID:22246242

Losada, D., Crestani, F., & Parapar, J. (2017). eRISK 2017: CLEF Lab on Early Risk Prediction on the Internet: Experimental Foundations. *Lecture Notes in Computer Science*, *10456*, 346–360. doi:10.1007/978-3-319-65813-1_30

Loske, A. M. (2017). *Medical and biomedical applications of shock waves*. Academic Press.

Loske, A. M., Campos-Guillen, J., de Icaza, M., Fernández, F., & Castaño-Tostado, E. (2012) Improved shock-wave-assisted bacteria transformation. In Shock waves. Springer.

Lubar, J. F., & Shouse, M. N. (1976). EEG and behavioral changes in a hyperkinetic child concurrent with training of the sensorimotor rhythm (SMR). *Biofeedback and Self-Regulation*, *1*(3), 293–306. doi:10.1007/BF01001170 PMID:990355

Lu, D., Popuri, K., Ding, G. W., Balachandar, R., & Beg, M. F. (2018). Multimodal and multiscale deep neural networks for the early diagnosis of Alzheimer's disease using structural MR and FDG-PET images. *Scientific Reports*, *8*(1), 5697. doi:10.103841598-018-22871-z PMID:29632364

Luo, S., Li, X., & Li, J. (2017). Automatic Alzheimer's disease recognition from MRI data using deep learning method. *Zeitschrift für Angewandte Mathematik und Physik*, *05*(09), 1892–1898. doi:10.4236/jamp.2017.59159

Madhoo, M., & Levine, S. Z. (2015). Initial Severity Effects on Residual Symptoms in Response and Remission: A STAR*D Study during and after Failed Citalopram Treatment. *Journal of Clinical Psychopharmacology*, *35*(4), 450–453. doi:10.1097/JCP.0000000000000354 PMID:26066336

Manser, R., Cooper, M., & Trefusis, J. (2012). Beliefs about Emotions as a Metacognitive Construct: Initial Development of a Self-Report Questionnaire Measure and Preliminary Investigation in Relation to Emotion Regulation. *Clinical Psychology & Psychotherapy*, *19*(3), 235–246. doi:10.1002/cpp.745 PMID:21374759

Marchetti, I., Koster, E. H. W., Sonuga-Barke, E. J., & De Raedt, R. (2012). The Default Mode Network and recurrent depression: A neurobiological model of cognitive risk factors. *Neuropsychology Review*, *22*(3), 229–251. doi:10.100711065-012-9199-9 PMID:22569771

Márquez, F., & Yassa, M. A. (2019). Neuroimaging biomarkers for Alzheimer's disease. *Molecular Neurodegeneration*, *14*(1), 1–14. doi:10.118613024-019-0325-5 PMID:31174557

Martínez-Álvarez, F., Asencio-Cortés, G., Torres, J. F., Gutiérrez-Avilés, D., Melgar-García, L., Pérez-Chacón, R., Rubio-Escudero, C., Riquelme, J. C., & Troncoso, A. (2020). Coronavirus optimization algorithm: A bioinspired metaheuristic based on the COVID-19 propagation model. *Big Data*, *8*(4), 308–322. doi:10.1089/big.2020.0051 PMID:32716641

Martinez-Martin, P., Rodriguez-Blazquez, C., Kurtis, M.M., & Chaudhuri, K.R. (2011). The impact of non-motor symptoms on health-related quality of life of patients with Parkinson's disease. *Mov Disord*, *26*(3), 399–406. . doi:10.1002/mds.23462

Marwan, Y., Husain, W., Alhajii, W., & Mogawer, M. (2014). Extracorporeal shock wave therapy relieved pain in patients with coccydynia: A report of two cases. *The Spine Journal*, *14*(1), e1–e4. doi:10.1016/j.spinee.2013.07.438 PMID:24094989

Marzbani, H., Marateb, H. R., & Mansourian, M. (2016). Neurofeedback: A comprehensive review on system design, methodology and clinical applications. *Basic and Clinical Neuroscience*, *7*(2), 143. doi:10.15412/J.BCN.03070208 PMID:27303609

Marzuki, N. A., Husain, W., & Shahiri, A. M. (2016). Myepipal, Mobile application for managing, monitoring and predicting epilepsy patient. In *Proceedings of the International Conferenceon Advances in Information and Communication Technology*, (pp. 383–392). Springer.

Masse, Bussel, Serteyn, Arends, & Penders. (2013). Miniaturized wireless ECG monitor for real-time detection of epileptic seizures. *Transactions on Embedded Computing Systems, 12*(4).

Mäthger, L. M., Denton, E. J., Marshall, N. J., & Hanlon, R. T. (2009). Mechanisms and behavioural functions of structural coloration in cephalopods. *Journal of the Royal Society, Interface*, *6*(suppl_2), S149–S163. doi:10.1098/rsif.2008.0366.focus PMID:19091688

Matsumoto, S., Horiguchi, S., Shigeno, H., & Okada, K. (2016). Visual Effect on the Odor Identification Ability of Children with Autism Spectrum Disorder. *2016 IEEE International Conference on Healthcare Informatics (ICHI)*, 349-355. 10.1109/ICHI.2016.63

Matthew, Yang, Islam, & Khaled. (2019). Functional connectivity magnetic resonance imaging classification of autism spectrum disorder using the multisite ABIDE dataset. *2019 IEEE EMBS International Conference on Biomedical & Health Informatics (BHI)*, 1-4. 10.1109/BHI.2019.8834653

Mayberg, S. (1997). Limbic-Cortical Dysregulation : Depression. *Journal of Neuropsychiatry*, *9*(4), 471–481. PMID:9276848

McCollough, C. H., & Leng, S. (2020). Use of artificial intelligence in computed tomography dose optimisation. *Annals of the ICRP*, *49*(1_suppl), 113–125. doi:10.1177/0146645320940827 PMID:32870019

McIntyre, R. S., Cha, D. S., Soczynska, J. K., Woldeyohannes, H. O., Gallaugher, L. A., Kudlow, P., Alsuwaidan, M., & Baskaran, A. (2013). Cognitive deficits and functional outcomes in major depressive disorder: Determinants, substrates, and treatment interventions. *Depression and Anxiety*, *30*(6), 515–527. doi:10.1002/da.22063 PMID:23468126

McKhann, G., Drachman, D., Folstein, M., Katzman, R., Price, D., & Stadlan, E. M. (1984). Clinical diagnosis of Alzheimer's disease Report of the NINCDS-ADRDA Work Group under the auspices of Department of Health and Human Services Task Force on Alzheimer's Disease. *Neurology*, *34*(7), 939–939. doi:10.1212/WNL.34.7.939 PMID:6610841

Md, G., & Gouse, D. K. (2009). Web Mining: A Review of Present Research Techniques, and Its Software. *Journal of Computer Information Systems*, 75–83.

Mehndiratta, N. (2020). A Yoking-Proof and PUF-based Mutual Authentication Scheme for Cloud-aided Wearable Devices. *IEEE International Conference for Innovation in Technology (INOCON)*, 1-4. doi: 10.1109/INOCON50539.2020.9298349

Menezes, V., Mathew, Y., Takayama, K., Kanno, A., & Hosseini, H. (2012). Laser plasma jet driven microparticles for DNA/drug delivery. *PLoS One*, *7*(11), e50823. doi:10.1371/journal.pone.0050823 PMID:23226394

Meraihi, Y., Gabis, A. B., Mirjalili, S., & Ramdane-Cherif, A. (2021). Grasshopper optimization algorithm: Theory, variants, and applications. *IEEE Access: Practical Innovations, Open Solutions*, *9*, 50001–50024. doi:10.1109/ACCESS.2021.3067597

Metcalfe, J., & Mischel, W. (1999). A hot/cool-system analysis of delay of gratification: Dynamics of willpower. *Psychological Review*, *106*(1), 3–19. doi:10.1037/0033-295X.106.1.3 PMID:10197361

Mirjalili, S. (2015). Moth-flame optimization algorithm: A novel nature-inspired heuristic paradigm. *Knowledge-Based Systems*, *89*, 228–249. doi:10.1016/j.knosys.2015.07.006

Mirjalili, S. (2015). The ant lion optimizer. *Advances in Engineering Software*, *83*, 80–98. doi:10.1016/j.advengsoft.2015.01.010

Mirjalili, S. (2016). Dragonfly algorithm: A new meta-heuristic optimization technique for solving single-objective, discrete, and multi-objective problems. *Neural Computing & Applications*, *27*(4), 1053–1073. doi:10.100700521-015-1920-1

Mirjalili, S., & Lewis, A. (2016). The whale optimization algorithm. *Advances in Engineering Software*, *95*, 51–67. doi:10.1016/j.advengsoft.2016.01.008

Mirjalili, S., Mirjalili, S. M., & Lewis, A. (2014). Grey wolf optimizer. *Advances in Engineering Software*, *69*, 46–61. doi:10.1016/j.advengsoft.2013.12.007

Misman, M. F. (2019). Classification of Adults with Autism Spectrum Disorder using Deep Neural Network. *2019 1st International Conference on Artificial Intelligence and Data Sciences (AiDAS)*, 29-34. 10.1109/AiDAS47888.2019.8970823

Mitragotri, S. (2013). Devices for overcoming biological barriers: The use of physical forces to disrupt the barriers. *Advanced Drug Delivery Reviews*, *65*(1), 100–103. doi:10.1016/j.addr.2012.07.016 PMID:22960787

Miyake, A., Friedman, N. P., Emerson, M. J., Witzki, A. H., Howerter, A., & Wager, T. D. (2000). The Unity and Diversity of Executive Functions and Their Contributions to Complex "Frontal Lobe" Tasks: A Latent Variable Analysis. *Cognitive Psychology*, *41*(1), 49–100. doi:10.1006/cogp.1999.0734 PMID:10945922

Mohammad Galety, F. H. (2021). Deep Neural Network Concepts for Classification using Convolutional Neural Network: A Systematic Review and Evaluation. *Technium: Romanian Journal of Applied Sciences and Technology*, 58-70. doi:10.47577/technium.v3i8.4554

Mohd, M. S., Aimie-Salleh, N., Wahab, A. H. A., Sahalan, M., & Ashari, U. M. M. (2020). Heart Rate Variability Response on Autism Spectrum Disorder and Typical Development Children. *2020 4th International Symposium on Multidisciplinary Studies and Innovative Technologies (ISMSIT)*, 1-3. 10.1109/ISMSIT50672.2020.9255015

Monastra, V. J., Lubar, J. F., Linden, M., VanDeusen, P., Green, G., Wing, W., Phillips, A., & Fenger, T. N. (1999). Assessing attention deficit hyperactivity disorder via quantitative electroencephalography: An initial validation study. *Neuropsychology*, *13*(3), 424–433. doi:10.1037/0894-4105.13.3.424 PMID:10447303

Moon, H. E., & Paek, S. H. (2015). Mitochondrial dysfunction in Parkinson's disease. *Experimental Neurobiology*, *24*(2), 103–116. doi:10.5607/en.2015.24.2.103 PMID:26113789

Morgan, J. P. M., Hamm, M., Schmitz, C., & Brem, M. H. (2021). Return to play after treating acute muscle injuries in elite football players with radial extracorporeal shock wave therapy. *Journal of Orthopaedic Surgery and Research*, *16*(1), 708. doi:10.118613018-021-02853-0 PMID:34876172

Mulders, P. C., van Eijndhoven, P. F., Schene, A. H., Beckmann, C. F., & Tendolkar, I. (2015). Resting-state functional connectivity in major depressive disorder: A review. *Neuroscience and Biobehavioral Reviews*, *56*, 330–344. doi:10.1016/j.neubiorev.2015.07.014 PMID:26234819

Mulero-Pázmány, Jenni-Eiermann, & Strebel, Sattler, Negro, & Tablado. (2017). Unmanned aircraft systems as a new source of disturbance for wildlife: A systematic review. *PLoS One*, *12*(6).

Murphy, F. C., Michael, A., & Sahakian, B. J. (2012). Emotion modulates cognitive flexibility in patients with major depression. *Psychological Medicine*, *42*(7), 1373–1382. doi:10.1017/S0033291711002418 PMID:22067530

Murray, E. A., Wise, S. P., & Drevets, W. C. (2011). Localization of dysfunction in major depressive disorder: Prefrontal cortex and amygdala. *Biological Psychiatry*, *69*(12), e43–e54. doi:10.1016/j.biopsych.2010.09.041 PMID:21111403

Murthy, J., Yangala, R., Meena, A., & Reddy, J. J. (1999). Acute disseminated encephalomyelitis: Clinical and MRI study from South India. *Journal of the Neurological Sciences*, *165*(2), 133–138. doi:10.1016/S0022-510X(99)00094-5 PMID:10450798

Murthy, S. K., Faden, H. S., Cohen, M. E., & Bakshi, R. (2002). Acute disseminated encephalomyelitis in children. *Pediatrics, 110*(2), e21–e21. doi:10.1542/peds.110.2.e21 PMID:12165620

Musallam, S., Andersen, R. A., Corneil, B. D., Greger, B., & Scherberger, H. (2010). *U.S. Patent No. 7,826,894*. Washington, DC: U.S. Patent and Trademark Office.

Muty, N., & Azizul, Z. (2016). Detecting arm flapping in children with Autism Spectrum Disorder using human pose estimation and skeletal representation algorithms. *2016 International Conference On Advanced Informatics: Concepts, Theory And Application (ICAICTA)*, 1-6. 10.1109/ICAICTA.2016.7803118

Nauck, T., Lohrer, H., & Schöll, J. (2014). Paradigm shift: ESWT applied to growth plates: radial shock wave therapy in patients with apophysitis calcanei. Multidisciplinary medical applications, 70–82.

Neisius, A., Lipkin, M. E., Rassweiler, J. J., Zhong, P., Preminger, G. M., & Knoll, T. (2015). Shock wave lithotripsy: The new phoenix? *World Journal of Urology, 33*(2), 213–221. doi:10.100700345-014-1369-3 PMID:25081010

Nichols, W. C., Pankratz, N., Marek, D. K., Pauciulo, M. W., Elsaesser, V. E., Halter, C. A., Rudolph, A., Wojcieszek, J., Pfeiffer, R. F., & Foroud, T. (2009). Mutations in GBA are associated with familial Parkinson disease susceptibility and age at onset. *Neurology, 72*(4), 310–316. doi:10.1212/01.wnl.0000327823.81237.d1 PMID:18987351

Nigg, J. T., & Casey, B. J. (2005). An integrative theory of attention-deficit/hyperactivity disorder based on the cognitive and affective neurosciences. *Development and Psychopathology, 17*(3), 785–806. doi:10.1017/S0954579405050376 PMID:16262992

Niranjan, R. (2014). The Role of Inflammatory and Oxidative Stress Mechanisms in the Pathogenesis of Parkinson's Disease: Focus on Astrocytes. *Molecular Neurobiology, 49*(1), 28–38. doi:10.100712035-013-8483-x PMID:23783559

Nishikawa, M., Ichiyama, T., Hayashi, T., Ouchi, K., & Furukawa, S. (1999). Intravenous immunoglobulin therapy in acute disseminated encephalomyelitis. *Pediatric Neurology, 21*(2), 583–586. doi:10.1016/S0887-8994(99)00042-9 PMID:10465150

Nolen Hoeksema, S., & Davis, R. N. (2000). Cognitive inflexibility among ruminators and nonruminators. *Cognitive Therapy and Research, 24*(6), 699–711. doi:10.1023/A:1005591412406

Norman, D. A., & Shallice, T. (1986). Attention to action: willed and automatic control of behaviour. In Consciousness and self-regulation (4th ed.). Plenum Press. doi:10.1007/978-1-4757-0629-1_1

Northoff, G., Wiebking, C., Feinberg, T., & Panksepp, J. (2011). The "resting-state hypothesis" of major depressive disorder-A translational subcortical-cortical framework for a system disorder. *Neuroscience and Biobehavioral Reviews, 35*(9), 1929–1945. doi:10.1016/j.neubiorev.2010.12.007 PMID:21192971

Obsessive-Compulsive Disorder. (2021). Retrieved 9 October 2021, from https://www.helpguide.org/articles/anxiety/obssessive-compulsive-disorder-ocd.htm

Odin Hashemi, S. H., & Hodtani, G. A. (2019). A Modified McEliece Public-Key Cryptosystem Based On Irregular Codes Of QC-LDPC and QC-MDPC. *27th Iranian Conference on Electrical Engineering (ICEE)*, 1373-1376. doi: 10.1109/IranianCEE.2019.8786376

Okamura, N., Harada, R., Furumoto, S., Arai, H., Yanai, K., & Kudo, Y. (2014). Tau PET imaging in Alzheimer's disease. *Current Neurology and Neuroscience Reports, 14*(11), 500. doi:10.100711910-014-0500-6 PMID:25239654

Omar, Mishra, & Bajpai. (2018). Machine Learning Techniques to Predict Autism Spectrum Disorder. *2018 IEEE Punecon*, 1-5. . doi:10.1109/PUNECON.2018.8745405

Orlandi, S., Manfredi, C., Bocchi, L., & Scattoni, M. L. (2012). Automatic newborn cry analysis: A Non-invasive tool to help autism early diagnosis. *Annual International Conference of the IEEE Engineering in Medicine and Biology Society*, 2953-2956. 10.1109/EMBC.2012.6346583

Othman, M., & Wahab, A. (2010). Affective face processing analysis in autism using electroencephalogram. *Proceeding of the 3rd International Conference on Information and Communication Technology for the Moslem World (ICT4M)*, E23-E27. 10.1109/ICT4M.2010.5971907

Othman, M., Madani, S. A., & Khan, S. U. (2014). A survey of mobile cloud computing application models. *IEEE Communications Surveys and Tutorials*, *16*(1), 393–413. doi:10.1109/SURV.2013.062613.00160

Ou, Y.-N., Xu, W., Li, J.-Q., Guo, Y., Cui, M., Chen, K.-L., Huang, Y.-Y., Dong, Q., Tan, L., & Yu, J.-T. (2019). FDG-PET as an independent biomarker for Alzheimer's biological diagnosis: A longitudinal study. *Alzheimer's Research & Therapy*, *11*(1), 1–11. doi:10.118613195-019-0512-1 PMID:31253185

P & Kumari. (2020). Quantum Algorithms for Machine Learning and Optimization. *2nd PhD Colloquium on Ethically Driven Innovation and Technology for Society (PhD EDITS)*, 1-2. doi: 10.1109/PhDEDITS51180.2020.9315301

Pacific, A. S. (2006). *Dementia in the Asia Pacific Region: The Epidemic Is Here*. Academic Press.

Palaniappan, P., Seshadri, S., Girimaji, S. C., & Srinath, S. (2013). Pattern of comorbidities in Indian children and adolescents with attention deficit hyperactivity disorder. *European Psychiatry*, *28*, 1. doi:10.1016/S0924-9338(13)77398-X

Palmer, K., Fratiglioni, L., & Winblad, B. (2003). What is mild cognitive impairment? Variations in definitions and evolution of nondemented persons with cognitive impairment. *Acta Neurologica Scandinavica*, *107*, 14–20. doi:10.1034/j.1600-0404.107.s179.2.x PMID:12603245

Papageorgiou, C., & Wells, A. (2009). A prospective test of the clinical metacognitive model of rumination and depression. *International Journal of Cognitive Therapy*, 2(2), 123–131. doi:10.1521/ijct.2009.2.2.123

Park, M., McDonald, D., & Cha, M. (2013) Perception differences between the depressed and nondepressed users in Twitter. In *International AAAI Conference on Web and Social Media (ICWSM)*. The AAAI Press.

Park, R. J., Goodyer, I. M., & Teasdale, J. D. (2004). *Effects of induced rumination and distraction on mood and overgeneral autobiographical memory in adolescent*. Academic Press.

Park, J., Kim, K., & Kwon, O. (2014). Comparison of machine learning algorithms to predict psychological wellness indices for ubiquitous healthcare system design. *Proceedings of the International Conference on Innovative Design and Manufacturing (ICIDM)*, 263-269. doi: 10.1109/IDAM.2014.6912705

Parlar, T. (2021). A heuristic approach with artificial neural network for Parkinson's disease. *International Journal of Applied Mathematics Electronics and Computers*, *9*(1), 1–6. doi:10.18100/ijamec.802599

Paul, L. K., Corsello, C., Kennedy, D. P., & Adolphs, R. (2014). Agenesis of the corpus callosum and autism: A comprehensive comparison. *Brain*, *137*(6), 1813–1829. doi:10.1093/brain/awu070 PMID:24771497

Payan, A., & Montana, G. (2015). *Predicting Alzheimer's disease: a neuroimaging study with 3D convolutional neural networks*. arXiv preprint arXiv:1502.02506.

Pedregosa, F., Varoquaux, G., Gramfort, A., Michel, V., Thirion, B., Grisel, O., Blondel, M., Prettenhofer, P., Weiss, R., & Dubourg, V. (2011). Scikit-learn: Machine learning in Python. *Journal of Machine Learning Research*, *12*, 2825–2830.

Pelvig, D. P., Pakkenberg, H., Stark, A. K., & Pakkenberg, B. (2008). Neocortical glial cell numbers in human brains. *Neurobiology of Aging*, *29*(11), 1754–1762. doi:10.1016/j.neurobiolaging.2007.04.013 PMID:17544173

Pennequin, V., Questel, F., Delaville, E., Delugre, M., & Maintenant, C. (2019). Metacognition and emotional regulation in children from 8 to 12 years old. *The British Journal of Educational Psychology*, *90*(S1), 1–16. doi:10.1111/bjep.12305 PMID:31292954

Perera, T., Lee, W.-L., Jones, M., Tan, J. L., Proud, E. L., Begg, A., Sinclair, N. C., Peppard, R., & McDermott, H. J. (2019). A palm-worn device to quantify rigidity in Parkinson's disease. *Journal of Neuroscience Methods*, *317*, 113–120. doi:10.1016/j.jneumeth.2019.02.006 PMID:30776378

Perneczky, R., Wagenpfeil, S., Komossa, K., Grimmer, T., Diehl, J., & Kurz, A. (2006). Mapping scores onto stages: Mini-mental state examination and clinical dementia rating. *The American Journal of Geriatric Psychiatry*, *14*(2), 139–144. doi:10.1097/01.JGP.0000192478.82189.a8 PMID:16473978

Petersen, R. C. (2004). Mild cognitive impairment as a diagnostic entity. *Journal of Internal Medicine*, *256*(3), 183–194. doi:10.1111/j.1365-2796.2004.01388.x PMID:15324362

Petersen, R. C., Aisen, P. S., Beckett, L. A., Donohue, M. C., Gamst, A. C., Harvey, D. J., Jack, C. R., Jagust, W. J., Shaw, L. M., Toga, A. W., Trojanowski, J. Q., & Weiner, M. W. (2010). Alzheimer's disease neuroimaging initiative (ADNI): Clinical characterization. *Neurology*, *74*(3), 201–209. doi:10.1212/WNL.0b013e3181cb3e25 PMID:20042704

Petersen, R. C., Caracciolo, B., Brayne, C., Gauthier, S., Jelic, V., & Fratiglioni, L. (2014). Mild cognitive impairment: A concept in evolution. *Journal of Internal Medicine*, *275*(3), 214–228. doi:10.1111/joim.12190 PMID:24605806

Picardi, A., Lega, I., Tarsitani, L., Caredda, M., Matteucci, G., Zerella, M., Miglio, R., Gigantesco, A., Cerbo, M., Gaddini, A., Spandonaro, F., & Biondi, M.The SET-DEP Group. (2016). A randomised controlled trial of the effectiveness of a program for early detection and treatment of depression in primary care. *Journal of Affective Disorders*, *198*, 96–101. doi:10.1016/j.jad.2016.03.025 PMID:27015158

Pickett, J., Xiu, E., Tuchman, R., Dawson, G., & Lajonchere, C. (2011). Mortality in individuals with autism, with and without epilepsy. *Journal of Child Neurology*, *26*(8), 932–939. doi:10.1177/0883073811402203 PMID:21471551

Pingali, S. (2014). Sunderajan J. A study of comorbidities in attention deficit hyperactivity disorder: A retrospective analysis of case records. *AP J Psychol Med*, *15*(2), 206–210.

Pisner, D. A., Shumake, J., Beevers, C. G., & Schnyer, D. M. (2018). A Reproducible Neurobiology of Depressive Rumination. *bioRxiv*.

Plant, C., Teipel, S. J., Oswald, A., Böhm, C., Meindl, T., Mourao-Miranda, J., Bokde, A. W., Hampel, H., & Ewers, M. (2010). Automated detection of brain atrophy patterns based on MRI for the prediction of Alzheimer's disease. *NeuroImage*, *50*(1), 162–174. doi:10.1016/j.neuroimage.2009.11.046 PMID:19961938

Plesner, A. M., Arlien-Søborg, P., & Herning, M. (1998). Neurological complications to vaccination against Japanese encephalitis. *European Journal of Neurology*, *5*(5), 479–485. doi:10.1046/j.1468-1331.1998.550479.x PMID:10210877

Poewe, W., Seppi, K., Tanner, C. M., Halliday, G. M., Brundin, P., Volkmann, J., Schrag, A.-E., & Lang, A. E. (2017). Parkinson disease. *Nature Reviews. Disease Primers*, *3*(1), 1–21. doi:10.1038/nrdp.2017.13 PMID:28332488

Prasad, G., Abhishek, P., & Karthick, R. (2018). Influence of Unmanned Aerial Vehicle in Medical Product Transport. *International Journal of Intelligent Unmanned Systems*, *7*(2), 88–94.

Preminger, G., Badlani, G., & Kavoussi, L. (Eds.). (2012). *Smith's textbook on endourology*. John Wiley and Sons.

Puelles, L. (2001). Thoughts on the development, structure and evolution of the mammalian and avian telencephalic pallium. *Philosophical Transactions of the Royal Society of London. Series B, Biological Sciences*, *356*(1414), 1583–1598. doi:10.1098/rstb.2001.0973 PMID:11604125

Puthal, D., Obaidat, M. S., Nanda, P., Prasad, M., Mohanty, S. P., & Zomaya, A. Y. (2018, May). Secure and Sustainable Load Balancing of Edge Data Centers in Fog Computing. *IEEE Communications Magazine*, *56*(5), 60–65. doi:10.1109/MCOM.2018.1700795

Qian, N. (1999). On the momentum term in gradient descent learning algorithms. *Neural Networks*, *12*(1), 145–151. doi:10.1016/S0893-6080(98)00116-6 PMID:12662723

Qidwai, U., & Connor, O. (2018). A General Purpose Game Module for Children with Autism Spectrum Disorder. *2018 IEEE-EMBS Conference on Biomedical Engineering and Sciences (IECBES)*, 426-431. 10.1109/IECBES.2018.8626699

Quay, H. C. (1997). Inhibition and attention deficit hyperactivity disorder. *Journal of Abnormal Child Psychology*, *25*(1), 7–13. doi:10.1023/A:1025799122529 PMID:9093895

Raj, C., Jain, C., & Arif, W. (2017). HEMAN: Health monitoring and nous: An IoT based e-health care system for remote telemedicine. *International Conference on Wireless Communications, Signal Processing and Networking (WiSPNET)*, 2115-2119, doi: 10.1109/WiSPNET.2017.8300134

Ramirez-Duque, A. A., Frizera-Neto, A., & Bastos, T. F. (2018). Robot-Assisted Diagnosis for Children with Autism Spectrum Disorder Based on Automated Analysis of Nonverbal Cues. *2018 7th IEEE International Conference on Biomedical Robotics and Biomechatronics (Biorob),* 456-461. 10.1109/BIOROB.2018.8487909

Rashid, T., Hasan, M. N., & Mazumdar, P. S. (2021). An L-slot Compact Antenna for Medical, Wearable Device and IoT Applications. *International Conference on Information and Communication Technology for Sustainable Development (ICICT4SD),* 100-104. doi: 10.1109/ICICT4SD50815.2021.9396832

Rassweiler, J., Rassweiler, M. C., Frede, T., & Alken, P. (2014). Extracorporeal shock wave lithotripsy: An opinion on its future. *Indian Journal of Urology*, *30*(1), 73–79. doi:10.4103/0970-1591.124211 PMID:24497687

Rassweiler, J., Rassweiler, M. C., Kenngott, H., Frede, T., Michel, M. S., Alken, P., & Clayman, R. (2013). The past, present and future of minimally invasive therapy in urology: A review and speculative outlook. *Minimally Invasive Therapy & Allied Technologies*, *22*(4), 200–209. doi:10.3109/13645706.2013.816323 PMID:23808367

Reginold, W., Lang, A. E., Marras, C., Heyn, C., Alharbi, M., & Mikulis, D. J. (2014). Longitudinal quantitative MRI in multiple system atrophy and progressive supranuclear palsy. *Parkinsonism & Related Disorders*, *20*(2), 222–225. doi:10.1016/j.parkreldis.2013.10.002 PMID:24239142

Rehman, F. U. (2020). Impact of bioinspired nanotechnology on brain diseases amelioration. *Biometrical Letters*, *6*, 17–22.

Rice, S., Goodall, J., Hetrick, S., Parker, A., Gilbertson, T., Amminger, G., Davey, C. G., McGorry, P. D., Gleeson, J., & Alvarez-Jimenez, M. (2014). Online and Social Networking Interventions for the Treatment of Depression in Young People: A Systematic Review. *Journal of Medical Internet Research*, *16*(9), e206. doi:10.2196/jmir.3304 PMID:25226790

Rive, M. M., Van Rooijen, G., Veltman, D. J., Phillips, M. L., Schene, A. H., & Ruhé, H. G. (2013). Neuroscience and Biobehavioral Reviews Neural correlates of dysfunctional emotion regulation in major depressive disorder. A systematic review of neuroimaging studies. *Neuroscience and Biobehavioral Reviews*, *37*(10), 2529–2553. doi:10.1016/j.neubiorev.2013.07.018 PMID:23928089

Rivers, T. M., Sprunt, D., & Berry, G. (1933). Observations on attempts to produce acute disseminated encephalomyelitis in monkeys. *The Journal of Experimental Medicine*, *58*(1), 39–53. doi:10.1084/jem.58.1.39 PMID:19870180

Robakowska, Ślęzak, & Tyrańska-Fobke. (2019). Operational and financial considerations of using drones for medical support of mass events in Poland. *Disaster Medicine and Public Health Preparedness*, *13*(3), 527–532.

Rock, P. L., Roiser, J. P., Riedel, W. J., & Blackwell, A. D. (2014). Cognitive impairment in depression: A systematic review and meta-analysis. *Psychological Medicine*, *44*(10), 2029–2040. doi:10.1017/S0033291713002535 PMID:24168753

Rockwood, K., Howard, K., MacKnight, C., & Darvesh, S. (1999). Spectrum of disease in vascular cognitive impairment. *Neuroepidemiology*, *18*(5), 248–254. doi:10.1159/000026219 PMID:10461050

Roebers, C. M. (2017). Executive function and metacognition: Towards a unifying framework of cognitive self-regulation. *Developmental Review*, *45*, 31–51. doi:10.1016/j.dr.2017.04.001

Roman, U. K. D., & Lausen, H. (2005). *The Web Service Modeling Ontology Wsmo*. Final Version. http://www.wsmo.org/TR/d2/v1.1/

Rompe, J. D., Furia, J., Cacchio, A., Schmitz, C., & Maffulli, N. (2015). Radial shock wave treatment alone is less efficient than radial shock wave treatment combined with tissue-specific plantar fasciastretching in patients with chronic plantar heel pain. *International Journal of Surgery*, *24*, 135–142. doi:10.1016/j.ijsu.2015.04.082 PMID:25940060

Ronald, T. (1998). Consensus report of the working group on: "Molecular and biochemical markers of Alzheimer's disease. *Neurobiology of Aging*, *19*, 109–116. PMID:9558143

Roopa, B. S., & Manjunatha Prasad, R. (2019). Concatenating framework in ASD analysis towards research progress. *2019 1st International Conference on Advanced Technologies in Intelligent Control, Environment, Computing & Communication Engineering (ICATIECE)*, 269-271. 10.1109/ICATIECE45860.2019.9063816

Rosenberger, A. L., Halenar, L., & Cooke, S. B. (2011). The making of platyrrhine semifolivores: Models for the evolution of folivory in primates. *Anatomical Record (Hoboken, N.J.)*, *294*(12), 2112–2130. doi:10.1002/ar.21510 PMID:22042497

Rosser Jr., Parker, & Vignesh. (2018). Medical applications of drones for disaster relief: A review of the literature. *Surgical Technology International*, *33*, 17–22.

Rozenthal, M., Laks, J., & Engelhardt, E. (2004). Aspectos neuropsicológicos da depressão. *Revista de Psiquiatria Do Rio Grande Do Sul*, *26*(2), 204–212. doi:10.15900101-81082004000200010

Rubia, K., Overmeyer, S., Taylor, E., Brammer, M., Williams, S. C., Simmons, A., & Bullmore, E. T. (1999). Hypofrontality in attention deficit hyperactivity disorder during higher-order motor control: A study with functional MRI. *The American Journal of Psychiatry*, *156*(6), 891–896. doi:10.1176/ajp.156.6.891 PMID:10360128

Russo, S. (2014). Avascular osteonecrosis of the femoral head. Multidisciplinary medical applications, 144–161.

Sachan, D. (2016). The age of drones: What might it mean for health? *Lancet*, *387*, 1803–1804.

Sadato, N., & Tanabe, H. C. (2012). Neural substrates and inter-individual functional connectivity during mutual gaze and joint attention using dual functional MRI. *2012 ICME International Conference on Complex Medical Engineering (CME)*, 527-530. 10.1109/ICCME.2012.6275596

Sahlas, D., Miller, S., Guerin, M., Veilleux, M., & Francis, G. (2000). Treatment of acute disseminated encephalomyelitis with intravenous immunoglobulin. *Neurology*, *54*(6), 1370–1372. doi:10.1212/WNL.54.6.1370 PMID:10746613

Sahu, B., Gouse, M., Ranjan Pattnaik, C., & Nandan Mohanty, S. (2021, February). MMFA-SVM: New bio-marker gene discovery algorithms for cancer gene expression. *Materials Today: Proceedings*. Advance online publication. doi:10.1016/j.matpr.2020.11.617

Saitoh, K., Ménard, A., & Grillner, S. (2007). Tectal control of locomotion, steering, and eye movements in lamprey. *Journal of Neurophysiology*, *97*(4), 3093–3108. doi:10.1152/jn.00639.2006 PMID:17303814

Salas, C., Broglio, C., & Rodríguez, F. (2003). Evolution of forebrain and spatial cognition in vertebrates: Conservation across diversity. *Brain, Behavior and Evolution*, *62*(2), 72–82. doi:10.1159/000072438 PMID:12937346

Salem, O., Naseem, A., & Mehaoua, A. (2014). Epileptic Seizure Detection from EEG Signal Using Discrete Wavelet Transform and Ant Colony Classifier. *Proceedings of the IEEE International Conference on Communications*, 3529–3534. 10.1109/ICC.2014.6883868

Samad, M. D., Diawara, N., Bobzien, J. L., Harrington, J. W., Witherow, M. A., & Iftekharuddin, K. M. (2018, February). A Feasibility Study of Autism Behavioral Markers in Spontaneous Facial, Visual, and Hand Movement Response Data. *IEEE Transactions on Neural Systems and Rehabilitation Engineering*, *26*(2), 353–361. doi:10.1109/TNSRE.2017.2768482 PMID:29432106

Samanta, D. D. S. (2021). *A Novel Approach for Web Mining Taxonomy for High-Performance Computing. Kolkata, India*. Springer., doi:10.1007/978-981-16-4284-5_37

Samie, F., Paul, S., Bauer, L., & Henkel, J. (2018). Highly Efficient And Accurate Seizure Prediction on Constrained IoT Devices. *Proceedings of the Design, Automation Test in Europe Conference Exhibition*, 955–960. 10.23919/DATE.2018.8342147

Sarafrazi. (2019). Cracking the "Sepsis" Code: Assessing Time Series Nature of EHR Data,and Using Deep Learning for Early Sepsis Prediction. *2019 Computing in Cardiology (CinC),* 1-4. doi:10.23919/CinC49843.2019.9005940

Saranya & Anandan. (2021). Autism Spectrum Prognosis using Worm Optimized Extreme Learning Machine (WOEM) Technique. *2021 International Conference on Advance Computing and Innovative Technologies in Engineering (ICACITE)*, 636-641. 10.1109/ICACITE51222.2021.9404729

Sareen, S., Sood, S. K., & Gupta, S. K. (2016). An automatic prediction of epileptic seizures using cloud computing and wireless sensor networks. Journal of Medical Systems, 40(11). doi:10.100710916-016-0579-1

Sareen, S., Sood, S. K., & Gupta, S. K. (2016). A cloud-based seizure alert system for epileptic patients that uses higher-order statistics. *Computing in Science & Engineering*, *18*(5), 56–67. doi:10.1109/MCSE.2016.82

Saremi, S., Mirjalili, S., & Lewis, A. (2017). Grasshopper optimisation algorithm: Theory and application. *Advances in Engineering Software*, *105*, 30–47. doi:10.1016/j.advengsoft.2017.01.004

Satyanarayanan, M., Bahl, P., C'aceres, R., & Davies, N. (2009). The case for VM-based cloudlets in mobile computing. *IEEE Pervasive Computing*, *8*(4), 14–23. doi:10.1109/MPRV.2009.82

Sayeed, M. A., Mohanty, S. P., Kougianos, E., & Zaveri, H. (2018). A Fast and Accurate Approach for Real-Time Seizure Detection in the IoMT. *Proceedings of the IEEE International Smart Cities Conference (ISC2).* 10.1109/ISC2.2018.8656713

Sayeed, M. A., Mohanty, S. P., Kougianos, E., & Zaveri, H. (2018). An Energy Efficient Epileptic Seizure Detector. *Proceedings of the IEEE International Conference on Consumer Electronics (ICCE)*, 1–4.

Scales, C. D. Jr, Smith, A. C., Hanley, J. M., & Saigal, C. S. (2012). Prevalence of kidney stones in the United States. *European Urology*, *62*(1), 160–165. doi:10.1016/j.eururo.2012.03.052 PMID:22498635

Scharoun, S. M., & Bryden, P. J. (2014). Hand preference, performance abilities, and hand selection in children. *Frontiers in Psychology*, *5*, 82. doi:10.3389/fpsyg.2014.00082 PMID:24600414

Schattenfroh, C. (2004). Acute disseminated encephalomyelitis after active immunization against early summer encephalitis. *Der Nervenarzt*, *75*(8), 776–779. PMID:15309308

Scheltens, P., Leys, D., Barkhof, F., Huglo, D., Weinstein, H. C., Vermersch, P., Kuiper, M., Steinling, M., Wolters, E. C., & Valk, J. (1992). Atrophy of medial temporal lobes on MRI in "probable" Alzheimer's disease and normal ageing: Diagnostic value and neuropsychological correlates. *Journal of Neurology, Neurosurgery, and Psychiatry*, *55*(10), 967–972. doi:10.1136/jnnp.55.10.967 PMID:1431963

Schmitz, C., Császár, N. B. M., Rompe, J. D., Chaves, H., & Furia, J. P. (2013). Treatment of chronic plantar fasciopathy with extracorporeal shock waves [review]. *Journal of Orthopaedic Surgery and Research*, *8*(1), 31–42. doi:10.1186/1749-799X-8-31 PMID:24004715

Schrag, A., Horsfall, L., Walters, K., Noyce, A., & Petersen, I. (2015). Prediagnostic presentations of Parkinson's disease in primary care: A case-control study. *Lancet Neurology*, *14*(1), 57–64. doi:10.1016/S1474-4422(14)70287-X PMID:25435387

Schulte, C., & Gasser, T. (2011). Genetic basis of Parkinson's disease: Inheritance, penetrance, and expression. *The Application of Clinical Genetics*, *1*(4), 67–80. PMID:23776368

Schwarz, S., Mohr, A., Knauth, M., Wildemann, B., & Storch–Hagenlocher, B. (2001). Acute disseminated encephalomyelitis: A follow-up study of 40 adult patients. *Neurology*, *56*(10), 1313–1318. doi:10.1212/WNL.56.10.1313 PMID:11376180

Segovia, F., Górriz, J. M., Ramírez, J., Salas-González, D., Álvarez, I., López, M., Chaves, R., & Padilla, P. (2010). Classification of functional brain images using a GMM-based multi-variate approach. *Neuroscience Letters*, *474*(1), 58–62. doi:10.1016/j.neulet.2010.03.010 PMID:20227464

Sehgal, S., Agarwal, M., Gupta, D., Sundaram, S., & Bashambu, A. (2020). Optimized grass hopper algorithm for diagnosis of Parkinson's disease. *SN Applied Sciences*, *2*(6), 1–18. doi:10.100742452-020-2826-9

Shafto, M. A., & Tyler, L. K. (2014). Language in the aging brain: The network dynamics of cognitive decline and preservation. *Science*, *346*(6209), 583–587. doi:10.1126cience.1254404 PMID:25359966

Shahar, E., Andraus, J., Savitzki, D., Pilar, G., & Zelnik, N. (2002). Outcome of severe encephalomyelitis in children: Effect of high-dose methylprednisolone and immunoglobulins. *Journal of Child Neurology*, *17*(11), 810–814. doi:10.1177/08830738020170111001 PMID:12585719

Sharma, V., & Vineeta, S. (2019). Future of Wearable Devices Using IoT Synergy in AI. *3rd International conference on Electronics, Communication and Aerospace Technology (ICECA)*, 138-142. doi: 10.1109/ICECA.2019.8821915

Sharma, P., Jain, R., Sharma, M., & Gupta, D. (2019). Parkinson's diagnosis using ant-lion optimisation algorithm. *International Journal of Innovative Computing and Applications*, *10*(3/4), 138–146. doi:10.1504/IJICA.2019.103370

Sheng, J., Wang, B., Zhang, Q., Liu, Q., Ma, Y., Liu, W., Shao, M., & Chen, B. (2019). A novel joint HCPMMP method for automatically classifying Alzheimer's and different stage MCI patients. *Behavioural Brain Research*, *365*, 210–221. doi:10.1016/j.bbr.2019.03.004 PMID:30836158

Shin, H.-W., & Chung, S. J. (2012). Drug-induced parkinsonism. *Journal of Clinical Neurology (Seoul, Korea)*, *8*(1), 15–21. doi:10.3988/jcn.2012.8.1.15 PMID:22523509

Shi, Z., He, L., Suzuki, K., Nakamura, T., & Itoh, H. (2009). Survey on neural networks used for medical image processing. *International Journal of Computational Science*, *3*, 86. PMID:26740861

Shukla, P., Shen, X., Allott, R., Swanson, P., & Fitzpatrick, M. E. (2021). Response of silicon nitride ceramics subject to laser shock treatment. *Ceramics International*, *47*(24), 34538–34553. doi:10.1016/j.ceramint.2021.08.369

Siegel, D. J. (2010). *The Mindful Therapist: A Clinician's Guide to Mindsight and Neural Integration (Norton Series on Interpersonal Neurobiology)*. WW Norton & Company.

Simms, M. L., Kemper, T. L., Timbie, C. M., Bauman, M. L., & Blatt, G. J. (2009). The anterior cingulate cortex in autism: Heterogeneity of qualitative and quantitative cytoarchitectonic features suggests possible subgroups. *Acta Neuropathologica, 118*(5), 673–684. doi:10.100700401-009-0568-2 PMID:19590881

Simon, D. K., Tanner, C. M., & Brundin, P. (2020). Parkinson disease epidemiology, pathology, genetics, and pathophysiology. *Clinics in Geriatric Medicine, 36*(1), 1–12. doi:10.1016/j.cger.2019.08.002 PMID:31733690

Simon-Sanchez, J., Schulte, C., Bras, J. M., Sharma, M., Gibbs, J. R., Berg, D., Paisan-Ruiz, C., Lichtner, P., Scholz, S. W., Hernandez, D. G., Krüger, R., Federoff, M., Klein, C., Goate, A., Perlmutter, J., Bonin, M., Nalls, M. A., Illig, T., Gieger, C., ... Gasser, T. (2009). Genome-wide association study reveals genetic risk underlying Parkinson's disease. *Nature Genetics, 41*(12), 1308–1312. doi:10.1038/ng.487 PMID:19915575

Simonsen, A. H., Herukka, S.-K., Andreasen, N., Baldeiras, I., Bjerke, M., Blennow, K., Engelborghs, S., Frisoni, G. B., Gabryelewicz, T., Galluzzi, S., Handels, R., Kramberger, M. G., Kulczyńska, A., Molinuevo, J. L., Mroczko, B., Nordberg, A., Oliveira, C. R., Otto, M., Rinne, J. O., ... Waldemar, G. (2017). Recommendations for CSF AD biomarkers in the diagnostic evaluation of dementia. *Alzheimer's & Dementia, 13*(3), 274–284. doi:10.1016/j.jalz.2016.09.008 PMID:28341065

Sin, D. S., Kim, M. H., Park, S.-A., Joo, M. C., & Kim, M. S. (2018). Crossed cerebellar diaschisis: Risk factors and correlation to functional recovery in intracerebral hemorrhage. *Annals of Rehabilitation Medicine, 42*(1), 8. doi:10.5535/arm.2018.42.1.8 PMID:29560319

Singh, A. K., Kumar, A., Mahmud, M., Kaiser, M. S., & Kishore, A. (2021). COVID-19 Infection detection from chest X-ray images using hybrid social group optimization and support vector classifier. *Cognitive Computation*, 1–13. doi:10.100712559-021-09848-3 PMID:33688379

Smarr, K., & Keefer, A. (2011). Measures of depression and depressive symptoms: Beck Depression Inventory-II (BDI-II), Center for Epidemiologic Studies Depression Scale (CES-D), Geriatric Depression Scale (GDS), Hospital Anxiety and Depression Scale (HADS), and Patient Health Questionna. *Arthritis Care and Research, 63*(S11), S454–S466. doi:10.1002/acr.20556 PMID:22588766

Smith, S. M. (2000). *BET: Brain extraction tool. Oxford Centre for Functional Magnetic Resonance Imaging of the Brain, Department of Clinical Neurology, Oxford University, John Radclife Hospital.*

Snyder, H. R. (2014). Major Depressive Disorder is Associated with Broad Impairments on Neuropsychological Measures of Executive Function: A Meta-Analysis and Review. *Psychological Bulletin, 139*(1), 81–132. doi:10.1037/a0028727 PMID:22642228

Sojuyigbe, S., & Daniel, K. (2015). Wearables/IOT devices: Challenges and solutions to integration of miniature antennas in close proximity to the human body. *2015 IEEE Symposium on Electromagnetic Compatibility and Signal Integrity*, 75-78. doi: 10.1109/EMCSI.2015.7107662

Solem, S., Hagen, R., Hoksnes, J. J., & Hjemdal, O. (2016). The metacognitive model of depression: An empirical test in a large Norwegian sample. *Psychiatry Research, 242*, 171–173. doi:10.1016/j.psychres.2016.05.056 PMID:27285952

Song, J., Zheng, J., Li, P., Lu, X., Zhu, G., & Shen, P. (2021). An Effective Multimodal Image Fusion Method Using MRI and PET for Alzheimer's Disease Diagnosis. *Frontiers in Digital Health, 3*, 19. doi:10.3389/fdgth.2021.637386 PMID:34713109

Spada, M. M., Georgiou, G. A., & Wells, A. (2010). The relationship among metacognitions, attentional control, and state anxiety. *Cognitive Behaviour Therapy, 39*(1), 64–71. doi:10.1080/16506070902991791 PMID:19735025

Spada, M. M., Mohiyeddini, C., & Wells, A. (2008). Measuring metacognitions associated with emotional distress: Factor structure and predictive validity of the metacognitions questionnaire 30. *Personality and Individual Differences*, *45*(3), 238–242. doi:10.1016/j.paid.2008.04.005

Spillantini, M. G., Crowther, R. A., Jakes, R., Hasegawa, M., & Goedert, M. (1998). α-Synuclein in filamentous inclusions of Lewy bodies from Parkinson's disease and dementia with Lewy bodies. *Proceedings of the National Academy of Sciences of the United States of America*, *95*(11), 6469–6473. doi:10.1073/pnas.95.11.6469 PMID:9600990

Spillantini, M. G., Schmidt, M. L., Lee, V. M., Trojanowski, J. Q., Jakes, R., & Goedert, M. (1997). Alpha-synuclein in Lewy bodies. *Nature*, *388*(6645), 839–840. doi:10.1038/42166 PMID:9278044

Sprich, S., Biederman, J., Crawford, M. H., Mundy, E., & Faraone, S. V. (2000). Adoptive and biological families of children and adolescents with ADHD. *Journal of the American Academy of Child and Adolescent Psychiatry*, *39*(11), 1432–1437. doi:10.1097/00004583-200011000-00018 PMID:11068899

StokerT. B.BarkerR. A. (2020). Recent developments in the treatment of Parkinson's Disease. *F1000Research*, 862, doi:10.12688/f1000research.25634.1

Stryker, S. (1925). Encephalitis lethargica: The behavior residuals. *The Training School Bulletin*, *22*, 152–157.

Stüv, O., & Zamvil, S. S. (1999). Pathogenesis, diagnosis, and treatment of acute disseminated encephalomyelitis. *Current Opinion in Neurology*, *12*(4), 395–401. doi:10.1097/00019052-199908000-00005 PMID:10555827

Suk, H. I., Lee, S. W., & Shen, D. (2015). Latent feature representation with stacked auto-encoder for AD/MCI diagnosis. *Brain Structure & Function*, *220*(2), 841–859. doi:10.100700429-013-0687-3 PMID:24363140

Suk, H.-I., Lee, S.-W., Shen, D., & Initiative, A. D. (2014). Hierarchical feature representation and multimodal fusion with deep learning for AD/MCI diagnosis. *NeuroImage*, *101*, 569–582. doi:10.1016/j.neuroimage.2014.06.077 PMID:25042445

Suk, H.-I., & Shen, D. (2013). Deep learning-based feature representation for AD/MCI classification. *International Conference on Medical Image Computing and Computer-Assisted Intervention*, 583–590. 10.1007/978-3-642-40763-5_72

Sun, G., Tao, X., Li, N., & Xu, J. (2021). Intelligent reflecting surface and uav assisted secrecy communication in millimeter-wave networks. *IEEE Transactions on Vehicular Technology*, *70*(11), 11949–11961.

Sutton, M. A., & Carew, T. J. (2000). Parallel molecular pathways mediate expression of distinct forms of intermediate-term facilitation at tail sensory–motor synapses in Aplysia. *Neuron*, *26*(1), 219–231. doi:10.1016/S0896-6273(00)81152-6 PMID:10798406

Swaab, D. F., Chung, W. C., Kruijver, F. P., Hofman, M. A., & Hestiantoro, A. (2003). Sex differences in the hypothalamus in the different stages of human life. *Neurobiology of Aging*, *24*, S1–S16. doi:10.1016/S0197-4580(03)00059-9 PMID:12829102

Swamy, H. S., Shankar, S., Chandra, P. S., Aroor, S. R., Krishna, A. S., & Perumal, V. K. (1984). Neurological complications due to beta-propiolactone (BPL)-inactivated antirabies vaccination: Clinical, electrophysiological and therapeutic aspects. *Journal of the Neurological Sciences*, *63*(1), 111–128. doi:10.1016/0022-510X(84)90113-8 PMID:6699651

Swanson, J. M., & Castellanos, F. X. (2002). *Biological bases of ADHD--Neuroanatomy, genetics, and pathophysiology*. Academic Press.

Szegedy, C., Iofe, S., Vanhoucke, V. & Alemi, A. (2016). *Inception-v4, inception-resnet and the impact of residual connections on learning*. arXiv preprint 1602.07261

T. E. Society. (2013). *Free Epilepsy Smart-Phone App*. https://www.epilepsysociety.org.uk/free-epilepsy-smartphone-app#.WC1jamSLR8c

Tabert, M. H., Albert, S. M., Borukhova-Milov, L., Camacho, Y., Pelton, G., Liu, X., Stern, Y., & Devanand, D. P. (2002). Functional deficits in patients with mild cognitive impairment: Prediction of AD. *Neurology*, *58*(5), 758–764. doi:10.1212/WNL.58.5.758 PMID:11889240

Taffoni, F., Focaroli, V., Keller, F., & Iverson, J. M. (2014). A technological approach to studying motor planning ability in children at high risk for ASD. *2014 36th Annual International Conference of the IEEE Engineering in Medicine and Biology Society*, 3638-3641. 10.1109/EMBC.2014.6944411

Taha Ahmed, Z. A., & Jadhav, M. E. (2020). A Review of Early Detection of Autism Based on Eye-Tracking and Sensing Technology. *International Conference on Inventive Computation Technologies (ICICT)*, 160-166. 10.1109/ICICT48043.2020.9112493

Tang, H. (2017). Integration benefits and challenges on Fan-Out to enable system in package for IoT/Wearable Devices. *IEEE 19th Electronics Packaging Technology Conference (EPTC),* 1-4. doi: 10.1109/EPTC.2017.8277425

Taylor, R. (1990). Interpretation of the correlation coefficient: A basic review. *Journal of Diagnostic Medical Sonography: JDMS*, *6*(1), 35–39. doi:10.1177/875647939000600106

Tenembaum, S., Chamoles, N., & Fejerman, N. (2002). Acute disseminated encephalomyelitis: A long-term follow-up study of 84 pediatric patients. *Neurology*, *59*(8), 1224–1231. doi:10.1212/WNL.59.8.1224 PMID:12391351

Teohari, V.-M., Ungureanu, C., Bui, V., Arends, J., & Aarts, R. M. (2014). Epilepsy seizure detection app for wearable technologies. *Proceedings of the European Conference on Ambient Intelligence.*

Thiels, Aho, & Zietlow, & Jenkins. (2015). D.H. Use of unmanned aerial vehicles for medical product transport. *Air Medical Journal*, *34*, 104–108.

Thome, J., & Jacobs, K. A. (2004). Attention deficit hyperactivity disorder (ADHD) in a 19th century children's book. *European Psychiatry*, *19*(5), 303–306. doi:10.1016/j.eurpsy.2004.05.004 PMID:15276664

Thompson, N., Steck, J., & Behrman, E. (2020). A non-algorithmic approach to "programming" quantum computers via machine learning. *IEEE International Conference on Quantum Computing and Engineering (QCE)*, 63-71. doi: 10.1109/QCE49297.2020.00019

Thorndike, E. L. (1927). The refractory period in associative processes. *Psychological Review*, *34*(3), 234–236. doi:10.1037/h0072072

Tripathi, V., & Shakeel, F. (2017). Monitoring Health Care System Using Internet of Things - An Immaculate Pairing. *2017 International Conference on Next Generation Computing and Information Systems (ICNGCIS)*, 153-158, 10.1109/ICNGCIS.2017.26

Uppal, N., Wicinski, B., Buxbaum, J. D., Heinsen, H., Schmitz, C., & Hof, P. R. (2014). Neuropathology of the anterior midcingulate cortex in young children with autism. *Journal of Neuropathology and Experimental Neurology*, *73*(9), 891–902. doi:10.1097/NEN.0000000000000108 PMID:25101703

Ustun, G. (2021). Determining depression and related factors in a society affected by COVID-19 pandemic. *The International Journal of Social Psychiatry*, *67*(1), 54–63. doi:10.1177/0020764020938807 PMID:32605422

Venkatesh, C., & Bojja, P. (2020). Lung cancer detection using bio-inspired algorithm in CT scans and secure data transmission through IoT cloud. *International Journal of Advanced Computer Science and Applications*, *11*(11), 2020. doi:10.14569/IJACSA.2020.0111148

Vernon, D. J. (2005). Can neurofeedback training enhance performance? An evaluation of the evidence with implications for future research. *Applied Psychophysiology and Biofeedback, 30*(4), 347–364. doi:10.100710484-005-8421-4 PMID:16385423

Vernon, P. A., & Mori, M. (1992). Intelligence, reaction times, and peripheral nerve conduction velocity. *Intelligence, 16*(3-4), 273–288. doi:10.1016/0160-2896(92)90010-O

Villar, Vergara, LaCal, Menendez, & Sedano. (2016). Pre-clinical study on the detection of simulated epileptic seizures. *International Journal of Uncertainty, Fuzziness and Knowledge-Based Systems, 24*(2), 33–46.

Vittorias, J., Petrantonakis, P., Bolis, D., Tsiligkyri, A., Kosmidou, V., & Hadjileontiadis, L. J. (2008). NOESIS: An Enhanced Educational Environment for Kids with Autism Spectrum Disorders. *2008 Eighth IEEE International Conference on Advanced Learning Technologies*, 1019-1020. 10.1109/ICALT.2008.44

Wang, J., Wang, Q., Zhang, H., Chen, J., Wang, S., & Shen, D. (2018). Sparse Multiview Task-Centralized Ensemble Learning for ASD Diagnosis Based on Age- and Sex-Related Functional Connectivity Patterns. IEEE Transactions on Cybernetics, 49(8), 3141-3154. doi:10.1109/TCYB.2018.2839693

Wang, M.-M., & Wu, Z.-N. (2021). Transition study for asymmetric reflection between moving incident shock waves. *Journal of Fluid Mechanics, 929*, A26. doi:10.1017/jfm.2021.856

Wang, W., Lee, J., Harrou, F., & Sun, Y. (2020). Early detection of Parkinson's disease using deep learning and machine learning. *IEEE Access: Practical Innovations, Open Solutions, 8*, 147635–147646. doi:10.1109/ACCESS.2020.3016062

Wedyan, M., & Al-Jumaily, A. (2016). Early diagnosis autism based on upper limb motor coordination in high risk subjects for autism. *IEEE International Symposium on Robotics and Intelligent Sensors (IRIS)*, 13-18. 10.1109/IRIS.2016.8066059

Wegiel, J., Flory, M., Kuchna, I., Nowicki, K., Ma, S. Y., Imaki, H., ... Wierzba-Bobrowicz, T. (2015). Neuronal nucleus and cytoplasm volume deficit in children with autism and volume increase in adolescents and adults. *Acta Neuropathologica Communications, 3*(1), 1–17. doi:10.118640478-015-0183-5 PMID:25595448

Wegiel, J., Kuchna, I., Nowicki, K., Imaki, H., Wegiel, J., Ma, S. Y., ... Cohen, I. L. (2013). Contribution of olivofloccular circuitry developmental defects to atypical gaze in autism. *Brain Research, 1512*, 106–122. doi:10.1016/j.brainres.2013.03.037 PMID:23558308

Wegiel, J., Schanen, N. C., Cook, E. H., Sigman, M., Brown, W. T., Kuchna, I., ... Ma, S. Y. (2012). Differences between the pattern of developmental abnormalities in autism associated with duplications 15q11. 2-q13 and idiopathic autism. *Journal of Neuropathology and Experimental Neurology, 71*(5), 382–397. doi:10.1097/NEN.0b013e318251f537 PMID:22487857

Wells, A. (2000). *Emotional disorders and metacognition: Innovative cognitive therapy*. John Wiley & Sons Ltd.

Wells, A., & Matthews, G. (1996). Modelling cognition in emotional disorders: The S-REF model. *Behaviour Research and Therapy, 34*(11-12), 881–888. doi:10.1016/S0005-7967(96)00050-2 PMID:8990539

Wells, A., & Papageorgiou, C. (1995). Worry and the incubation of intrusive images following stress. *Behaviour Research and Therapy, 33*(5), 579–583. doi:10.1016/0005-7967(94)00087-Z PMID:7598681

Westen, D., Blagov, P. S., Harenski, K., Kilts, C., & Hamann, S. (2006). Neural bases of motivated reasoning: An fMRI study of emotional constraints on partisan political judgment in the 2004 US presidential election. *Journal of Cognitive Neuroscience, 18*(11), 1947–1958. doi:10.1162/jocn.2006.18.11.1947 PMID:17069484

White, L., Small, B. J., Petrovitch, H., Ross, G. W., Masaki, K., Abbott, R. D., Hardman, J., Davis, D., Nelson, J., & Markesbery, W. (2005). Recent clinical-pathologic research on the causes of dementia in late life: Update from the Honolulu-Asia Aging Study. *Journal of Geriatric Psychiatry and Neurology*, *18*(4), 224–227. doi:10.1177/0891988705281872 PMID:16306244

Wilder-Willis, K. E., Shear, P. K., Steffen, J. J., & Borkin, J. (2002). The relationship between cognitive dysfunction and coping abilities in schizophrenia. *Schizophrenia Research*, *55*(3), 259–267. doi:10.1016/S0920-9964(01)00211-0 PMID:12048149

Williams, D. R., & Litvan, I. (2013). Parkinsonian syndromes. *Continuum: Lifelong Learning in Neurology, 19*, 1189.

Williams-Gray, C. H., & Worth, P. F. (2016). Parkinson's disease. *Medicine*, *44*(9), 542–546. doi:10.1016/j.mpmed.2016.06.001

Williams, N. R., & Okun, M. S. (2013). Deep Brain Stimulation (DBS) at the Interface of Neurology and Psychiatry. *The Journal of Clinical Investigation*, *123*(11), 4546–456. doi:10.1172/JCI68341 PMID:24177464

Wilson, G. T. (1996). Acceptance and change in the treatment of eating disorders and obesity. *Behavior Therapy*, *27*(3), 417–439. doi:10.1016/S0005-7894(96)80025-6

Winblad, B., Palmer, K., Kivipelto, M., Jelic, V., Fratiglioni, L., Wahlund, L. O., Nordberg, A., Backman, L., Albert, M., Almkvist, O., Arai, H., Basun, H., Blennow, K., de Leon, M., DeCarli, C., Erkinjuntti, T., Giacobini, E., Graff, C., Hardy, J., ... Petersen, R. C. (2004). Mild cognitive impairment–beyond controversies, towards a consensus: Report of the International Working Group on Mild Cognitive Impairment. *Journal of Internal Medicine*, *256*(3), 240–246. doi:10.1111/j.1365-2796.2004.01380.x PMID:15324367

Wongkoblap, A., Vadillo, M., & Curcin, V. (2017). Researching Mental Health Disorders in the Era of Social Media: Systematic Review. *Journal of Medical Internet Research*, *19*(6), e228. doi:10.2196/jmir.7215 PMID:28663166

Worgan, P., Pappas, O., Omirou, T., & Collett, M. (2015). Flexible on-body coils for inductive power transfer to IoT garments and wearables. *IEEE 2nd World Forum on Internet of Things (WF-IoT),* 297-298, doi: 10.1109/WF-IoT.2015.7389069

World Health Organization. (2013). *Comprehensive mental health action plan 2013-2020.* https://www.who.int/ mental_health/action_plan_2013/en/

Wright, A. (2010). Brain scanning techniques (ct, mri, fmri, pet, spect, dti, dot). *Cerebra: Positively Different*, 1–14.

Wu, F., Rüdiger, C., Redouté, J., & Yuce, M. R. (2018). WE-Safe: A wearable IoT sensor node for safety applications via LoRa. *IEEE 4th World Forum on Internet of Things (WF-IoT),* 144-148. doi: 10.1109/WF-IoT.2018.8355234

Wu, C., Liaqat, S., Cheung, S.-c., Chuah, C.-N., & Ozonoff, S. (2019). Predicting Autism Diagnosis using Image with Fixations and Synthetic Saccade Patterns. *2019 IEEE International Conference on Multimedia & Expo Workshops (ICMEW)*, 647-650. 10.1109/ICMEW.2019.00125

Xie, S., & Krishnan, S. (2013). Wavelet-based sparse functional linear model with applications to EEGs seizure detection and epilepsy diagnosis. *Medical & Biological Engineering & Computing*, *51*(1-2), 49–60. doi:10.100711517-012-0967-8 PMID:23054383

Xiong, L., Liu, Y., Yuan, W., Lin, F., & Pan, Y. (2021). Study of the fracturing behaviour of an electrohydraulic shock wave in sandstone under static pressure. *Journal of Physics. D, Applied Physics*, *54*(49), 495503. doi:10.1088/1361-6463/ac1cb4

Yang, X.-S., Gandomi, A. H., Talatahari, S., & Alavi, A. H. (2012). *Metaheuristics in water, geotechnical and transport engineering*. Newnes.

Yang, X.-S., Karamanoglu, M., & He, X. (2014). Flower pollination algorithm: A novel approach for multiobjective optimization. *Engineering Optimization*, *46*(9), 1222–1237. doi:10.1080/0305215X.2013.832237

Yang, Y., Cao, S., Shields, G. S., Teng, Z., & Liu, Y. (2017). The relationships between rumination and core executive functions: A meta-analysis. *Depression and Anxiety*, *34*(1), 37–50. doi:10.1002/da.22539 PMID:27378739

Yen, C. T., Conley, M., & Jones, E. G. (1985). Morphological and functional types of neurons in cat ventral posterior thalamic nucleus. *The Journal of Neuroscience: The Official Journal of the Society for Neuroscience*, *5*(5), 1316–1338. doi:10.1523/JNEUROSCI.05-05-01316.1985 PMID:2987437

Youden, W. J. (1950). Index for rating diagnostic tests. *Cancer*, *3*(1), 32–35. doi:10.1002/1097-0142(1950)3:1<32::AID-CNCR2820030106>3.0.CO;2-3 PMID:15405679

Young, H., Baum, R., Cremerius, U., Herholz, K., Hoekstra, O., Lammertsma, A. A., Pruim, J., & Price, P. (1999). Measurement of clinical and subclinical tumour response using [18F]-fluorodeoxyglucose and positron emission tomography: Review and 1999 EORTC recommendations. *European Journal of Cancer*, *35*(13), 1773–1782. doi:10.1016/S0959-8049(99)00229-4 PMID:10673991

Yu, W., Liang, F., He, X., Hatcher, W. G., Lu, C., Lin, J., & Yang, X. (2018). A Survey on the Edge Computing for the Internet of Things. *IEEE Access: Practical Innovations, Open Solutions*, *6*, 6900–6919. doi:10.1109/ACCESS.2017.2778504

Zahodne, L. B., & Fernandez, H. H. (2010). Parkinson's psychosis. *Current Treatment Options in Neurology*, *12*(3), 200–211. doi:10.100711940-010-0072-y PMID:20842582

Zang, H., Zhang, S., & Hapeshi, K. (2010). A review of nature-inspired algorithms. *Journal of Bionics Engineering*, *7*(S4), S232–S237. doi:10.1016/S1672-6529(09)60240-7

Zaveri, H. P., Williams, W. J., Iasemidis, L. D., & Sackellares, J. C. (1992). Time-frequency Representation of Electrocorticograms in Temporal Lobe Epilepsy. IEEE Transactions on Biomedical Engineering, 39(5), 502–509. doi:10.1109/10.135544

Zetterberg, H., Skillbäck, T., Mattsson, N., Trojanowski, J. Q., Portelius, E., Shaw, L. M., Weiner, M. W., & Blennow, K. (2016). Association of cerebrospinal fluid neurofilament light concentration with Alzheimer disease progression. *JAMA Neurology*, *73*(1), 60–67. doi:10.1001/jamaneurol.2015.3037 PMID:26524180

Zhang, M., Ma, Y., Zheng, L., Wang, Y., Liu, Z., & Ma, J. (2019). Comparison of Neural Networks' Performance in Early Screening of Autism Spectrum Disorders Under Two MRI Principles. *2019 International Conference on Networking and Network Applications (NaNA)*, 338-343. 10.1109/NaNA.2019.00065

Zhang, Y., Dong, Z., Phillips, P., Wang, S., Ji, G., Yang, J., & Yuan, T.-F. (2015). Detection of subjects and brain regions related to Alzheimer's disease using 3D MRI scans based on eigenbrain and machine learning. *Frontiers in Computational Neuroscience*, *9*, 66. doi:10.3389/fncom.2015.00066 PMID:26082713

Zhou, W., & Piramuthu, S. (2014). Security/privacy of wearable fitness tracking IoT devices. *9th Iberian Conference on Information Systems and Technologies (CISTI)*, 1-5. doi:10.1109/CISTI.2014.6877073

Zhou, Z., Yu, H., & Shi, H. (2015). Human Activity Recognition Based on Improved Bayesian Convolution Network to Analyze Health Care Data Using Wearable IoT Device. *IEEE Access: Practical Innovations, Open Solutions*, *8*, 86411–86418. doi:10.1109/ACCESS.2020.2992584

Zuckerman, H., Pan, Z., Park, C., Brietzke, E., Musial, N., Shariq, A. S., Iacobucci, M., Yim, S. J., Lui, L. M. W., Rong, C., & McIntyre, R. S. (2018). Recognition and Treatment of Cognitive Dysfunction in Major Depressive Disorder. *Frontiers in Psychiatry*, *9*(December), 1–11. doi:10.3389/fpsyt.2018.00655 PMID:30564155

About the Contributors

Shweta Gupta has worked in Multinational Companies Like Patni Computers, Techmahindra, Reliance Infocomm and is presently an Associate Professor in Jain University, Bengaluru with academic experience of 13 years. She has expertise in Artificial Intelligence and Machine Learning with application in Cognitive Diseases.

***

Mishab A. K. is a Licensed Clinical Psychologist by profession, currently working as a Joint Director of Community Disability Management and Rehabilitation Programme (CDMRP) at the University of Calicut, Kerala, India. He did his MPhil in clinical psychology from LGBRIMH, Assam, India. He has a total of 5 years of working experience in the National Institute of Mental Health and Neurosciences (NIMHANS), and the Community Disability Management and Rehabilitation Program at the University of Calicut, India. Mishab has facilitated many workshops in national and international conferences since 2017. His key research interests are in brief psychotherapy, affective neuroscience, neuropsychology, child psychology, psychotherapy process research, and psychometric test development. He is also a trained accredited member of Solution Focused Brief Therapy. He has facilitated several introductory and advanced-level workshops on the neurodevelopmental disorder, learning disabilities, behavior therapy, and rehabilitation. He has been an organizer for many International and National conferences in India. He has published book chapters and scientific articles in national and international journals.

Sangmesh B. has completed his Ph.D. in Mechanical Engineering from VTU, Belagavi. His area of doctoral research is development of a novel cooling system used for electronic cooling application. As visionary professional, served in academics, Incubation linked intellectual property (IP) management overall 08 years of professional experience dealing with techno-commercial activities of different organizations like academic, corporate groups and central government. He was instrumental in establishment of Incubation Centre supported by Atal Innovation Mission, NITI Aayog, Govt. of India. Established numerous industry academic partnership and collaboration with foreign universities. He is also Member of IPR Think Tank constituted by DIPP, GoI. Dr. Sangmesh is a passionate social reformer also a Founder Trustee, Samanvita Trust and State Joint Secretary ISTE, Karnataka Chapter. He has many international publications to his credit in journals of high repute. He has delivered several invited talks on various scientific topics & skill development, Entrepreneurship Awareness Camp. He also has the experience of executing projects being funded by various agencies such as NITI AAYOG, GoI, DST, MSME and VGST and is currently engaged in planning, implementation and monitoring of Incubation activities at BMSIT.

Alka Bali is Professor of Pharmaceutical Chemistry at University Institute of Pharmaceutical Sciences (UIPS), Panjab University, Chandigarh. She did her B. Pharm., M. Pharm. (Pharmaceutical Chemistry) and Ph. D. from the same institute. She has an academic and research experience spanning 25 years of undergraduate and postgraduate teaching. She has expertise in the fields of pharmaceutical analysis and medicinal chemistry. Her research areas of interest include pharmaceutical analysis with focus on method development and validation, spectroscopic characterization of impurities in drugs and drug products, synthetic medicinal chemistry encompassing computer-aided drug designing (CADD), QSAR, synthesis and pharmacological evaluation of new chemical entities in the area of antipsychotics, anti-inflammatory agents and angiotensin II antagonists. She has three books, five book chapters, 40 research articles in reputed international and national journals and 60 conference papers to her credit. She is on reviewer panel of several reputed international journals including European Journal of Medicinal Chemistry, Bioorganic and Medicinal Chemistry Letters, Medicinal Chemistry Research and several others.

Nishu Bali is Associate Professor at Department of Computer Sciences, Chitkara University Campus, Punjab Campus, Rajpura, Distt Patiala, India. She has got a teaching experience of more than 15 years in various programming languages like JAVA, Python and she has taught subjects like data structures and computer graphics. Her expert area is Machine learning and Deep learning. She has to her credit publications in journals of high repute. She has been an active participant at international and national conferences.

Meenakshi Banerjee trained as a Clinical Psychologist at NIMHANS. She is currently an Assistant Professor at the Jindal School of Psychology and Counselling at the O. P. Jindal Global university. Previously she completed her two-year clinical training in 2015. Her dissertation for the MPhil was on adapting and implementing group narrative therapy for adolescents in school setting. For her PhD, she chose to study Affective Neuropsychology at the Cognitive Neuroscience Centre, NIMHANS. She studied and developed a cognitive control training program for neurocognitive deficits in depression. The thesis was a Randomised Controlled Study to analyse the effectiveness of the remediation program. As Junior Consultant at the Clinical Psychology Department, she taught and supervised MPhil Trainee Psychologists for assessment and management of clinical cases from psychiatry, neurology and neurosurgery departments. She also managed neuropsychology assessment and rehabilitation for the Geriatric Clinic at NIMHANS. Post PhD, she has been involved in research projects, with the Positive Psychology Unit at NIMHANS. She has also worked with nonprofit organisations like Sanjivani Society for Mental Health and Aarohi and for private clinics like Cadabam's Mindtalk and Reach Clinic.

Srividya Bharadwaja (PhD) finished her Bachelor of Engineering in Electronics and Communication in the year 2000. She completed her Masters degree in VLSI Design and Embedded Systems in the year 2009. She was awarded doctorate degree due to her research in designing Cryptosystems for Wireless Sensor Networks from Visvesvaraya Technological University in the year 2019. Her research interest includes Error Control Coding, Artificial Neural Networks, Artificial Intelligence, Cloud computing, Cryptography, Bio medical Image processing to name a few.

Priya Dev is working as a PhD scholar (SRF position) in clinical Neurology at the Institute of Medical Sciences, Banaras Hindu University. She has done various wet-lab studies on platelet dysfunction in cerebral stroke subtype and vascular dementia; Next-generation sequencing in stroke patients; Triple

Blinded Randomized Control Trial in patients; clinic-epidemiological study; and radiological study (CT and MRI of Bain). She has worked and assessed the post-stroke complications (such as cognitive dysfunction, insomnia, and so on) in patients. She is certified in various clinical assessment tools (such as mRS, NIHSS, MOCA, GCS, etc) and the management of stroke patients. Simultaneously, she has been looking at various multi-national projects (such as OSCAIL, INTERACT, INSTRUCT) and national projects (DST project) of her PI. All these projects were on stroke, stroke rehabilitation, care of stroke patients, Amyotrophic Lateral sclerosis patients, and so on. She did her B.Sc and M.Sc in Zoology from BHU. She has done her dissertation work on tumour genes and non-coding long RNA. She is actively involved in research and is a member of various research societies like the Indian Academy of Neurology, and Society for Neurochemistry India.

Prasad G., Assistant Professor (Sr.Gr.), Aerospace Engineering, Dayananda Sagar University, Bangalore, India. Prof. Prasad G. received his Masters degree and Bachelors degree PhD in Aeronautical Engineering from Anna University. He has 7 years of teaching experience. Prior to joining Dayananda Sagar University, he worked at Anna University. He has published 40 articles in reputed Scopus Indexed International Journals with good Impact Factor. 25 Journals related to Unmanned Aerial Vehicle and Industry 5.0. He has completed two funded project sponsored by The Institution of Engineers (India) and Tamilnadu State Council for Science and Technology. Awarded Indian National Science Academy (INSA) Visiting Scientist Programme 2019 and Awarded Science Academies' Summer Research Fellowship Programme (SRPF) 2019. He is a Professional Membership of American Institute of Aeronautics and Astronautics, Institution of Engineers, Life Member in Indian Cryogenic Council and Life Member in Shock Wave Society. Reviewer in Aircraft Engineering and Aerospace Technology, International Journal of Engine Research and Journal of The Institution of Engineers (India): Series C.

Mohammad Gouse Galety received his PhD in Computer Science in 2012 from the AU (Allahabad University, Allahabad, India). His research interests span both computer science and information science. Dr Mohammad Gouse Galety (co)author of more than a dozen journal papers and international conference proceedings indexed by the springer, Scopus, four patents, and five books. Since 1999, he served in different national and international organizations like Sree Vidyanikethan Degree College, Tirupati, India, Emeralds Degree College, Tirupati, India, Brindavan College of Engineering, Bangalore, India, Kuwait Educational Center, Kuwait, Ambo University, Ambo, Ethiopia, Debre Berhan University, Debre Berhan, Ethiopia, Lebanese French University, Erbil, Iraq. He currently serves as Assistant Professor of the Information Technology Department, Catholic University in Erbil, Erbil, Iraq. Dr Mohammad Gouse Galety teaches several courses on computer science and information technology/science engineering undergraduate and postgraduate students. His research interests cover several aspects across computer science, mainly web mining, IoT, and Networks. He is a Fellow of the IEEE. As of 2021, Google Scholar reports over 40 citations to his work.

Kavya J. is presently working in ICAR-Sugarcane Breeding Institute, Coimbatore, India. She completed MSc and BSc in Biotechnology from Avinashilingam Institute for Home Science & Higher Education for Women is a women's Deemed University in Coimbatore, Tamil Nadu, India. She is Gold Medalist in UG and PG. She cleared GATE 2019. Her research area are interdisciplinary project works.

I. Jeena Jacob is actively involved in guiding the PhD scholar, and conference chair member of the few leading conference and journal, Associate Professor, Department of CSE, GITAM University, Bangalore Campus, India.

Dinamani M. is working as an Associate Professor at Dayanandasagar College of Engineering, an Autonomous Institution affiliated to VTU. She obtained her PhD from Bangalore University in Chemistry discipline. For her PhD, she chose to study the electrochemical synthesis of inorganic solids – metal hydroxides, metal phosphates, metal carbonates and metal sulphates which are of biomaterials importance. She has got 18 years of teaching and research experience. She has published more than 20 publications in peer reviewed Journals of international recognition. Her current research interests include materials science and electrochemistry. Currently she is working on remediation of water by layered double hydroxides and nanomaterial adsorbents.

Jyothi M. S. is an Assistant Professor at Department of Chemistry, AMC Engineering College. Formerly worked as Assistant Professor in Dayananda Sagar College of Engineering, Bengaluru. She served at Center for Nano and Material Sciences, Jain University as Scientist C. She has obtained her PhD in Chemistry in 2016 from Jain University and Post-doctoral education from Chulalongkorn University, Thailand. She is a CEO of MSME registered research consultancy start-up Jorium Endeavors, which is continuously stretching out the research essentials for the needs in chemistry and pharma domain. As an academician best teaching practices, organized documentation skills and students' motivational skills are her key expertise. As a researcher, she owned several publications with accountable impact factors, several book chapters, a granted patent. She was also a part of technology transfer program at Chulalongkorn University, and the group was successful in separating a nitrogen gas from mixture of nitrogen, n-hexane and butane, which was an industrial project from PPT public company, Thailand. Her thrive for technology transformation from research and development to start-up is demonstrated and motivating.

Pavan Manjunath, PhD from Jain University Bangalore, Project and Vendor management with an extensive track record of directing major Data Science, Cloud Solution Expert and Data Analytics and other data related programs for global clients and Research scientist with industrial and academic research experience In various treading technologies (Azure Cloud, IoT, ML/AI, Block Chain, and Quantum Computing).

Bharanidharan N. received his B.E. degree in Electronics and Communication Engineering from Alagappa Chettiar College of Engineering, Karaikudi, India, in 2013; M.E. degree in Communication Systems from Thiagarajar College of Engineering, India, in 2015, and PhD degree in Information and Communication Engineering from Anna University, India, in 2020. Presently, he is working as Assistant Professor in the Department of Computer Science and Engineering at Dayananda Sagar University, Bangalore, India. His research interests include machine learning algorithms and medical image processing.

Soumya Jacob P. is a PhD scholar in Psychology from Jain Deemed-to-be University, Bangalore. Presently she is working as a Project Manager of Kerala Einstein Study affiliated to Albert Einstein College of Medicine. She has more than 10 years of experience in teaching and research. Ms. Soumya acquired her Post graduation in Neuroscience Nursing from JSS medical college, Mysore and post graduation in Applied Psychology from Annamalai University, Chidambaram. Her specializations in PhD are cognitive Psychology and Creativity. She has publications in various national and international journals.

Smitha Sasi (PhD) finished her Bachelor of Engineering in Information Technology in the year 2005. She completed her Masters degree in Digital Communication and Networking in the year 2010. She was awarded doctorate degree due to her research in space communication from Visvesvaraya Technological University in the year 2019. Her research interest includes bioinformatics, Artificial Intelligence, Cloud computing, Cryptography, Bio medical Image processing to name a few.

Harish Sudarsanan, cloud solution expert, is currently working as Program Manager at Mercedes-Benz Research and Development India, Completed my BE from Mahatma Gandhi University.

Index

www.ingramcontent.com/pod-product-compliance
Lightning Source LLC
LaVergne TN
LVHW080536300926
849162LV00007B/1620
* 9 7 8 1 7 9 9 8 9 5 3 4 3 *